Diabetes Mellitus
A Guide to Patient Care

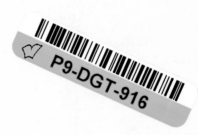

Diabetes Mellitus

A Guide to Patient Care

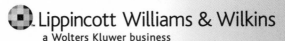

Lippincott Williams & Wilkins
a Wolters Kluwer business

Philadelphia · Baltimore · New York · London
Buenos Aires · Hong Kong · Sydney · Tokyo

Staff

Executive Publisher
Judith A. Schilling McCann, RN, MSN

Editorial Director
H. Nancy Holmes

Clinical Director
Joan M. Robinson, RN, MSN

Senior Art Director
Arlene Putterman

Art Director
Elaine Kasmer

Editorial Project Manager
Jennifer Kowalak

Clinical Project Manager
Beverly Ann Tscheschlog, RN, BS

Editor
Julie Munden

Clinical Editor
Maryann Foley, RN, BSN

Copy Editors
Kimberly Bilotta (supervisor), Scotti Cohn,
Amy Furman, Shana Harrington, Lisa Stockslager,
Dorothy P. Terry, Pamela Wingrod

Designers
Debra Moloshok (book design), BJ Crim (cover
design), Joseph John Clark

Digital Composition Services
Diane Paluba (manager), Joyce Rossi Biletz,
Donald G. Knauss

Manufacturing
Beth J. Welsh

Editorial Assistants
Megan L. Aldinger, Karen J. Kirk, Linda K. Ruhf

Design Assistant
Georg W. Purvis IV

Indexer
Barbara Hodgson

The clinical treatments described and recommended in this publication are based on research and consultation with nursing, medical, and legal authorities. To the best of our knowledge, these procedures reflect currently accepted practice. Nevertheless, they can't be considered absolute and universal recommendations. For individual applications, all recommendations must be considered in light of the patient's clinical condition and, before administration of new or infrequently used drugs, in light of the latest package-insert information. The authors and publisher disclaim any responsibility for any adverse effects resulting from the suggested procedures, from any undetected errors, or from the reader's misunderstanding of the text.

DM010806

Library of Congress Cataloging-in-Publication Data

Diabetes mellitus : a guide to patient care.
    p. ; cm.
  Includes index.
  1. Diabetes—Patients—Care. 2. Diabetes—Treatment.
I. Lippincott Williams & Wilkins.
  [DNLM: 1. Diabetes Mellitus—therapy. WK 815
D535681 2007]
  RC660.D53 2007
  616.4′62—dc22
  ISBN 1-58255-732-2 (alk. paper)   2006015256

Contents

Contributors
and consultants

●

Patricia Addie-Gentle, RN, BSN, CDE
Coordinator of Diabetes Education Program
DeKalb Medical Center
Decatur, Ga.

Judith Azok, ARNP-BC, MSN, GNP
Assistant Professor of Nursing
University of South Alabama College of Nursing
Mobile

Jo Azzarello, RN, PhD
Assistant Professor
University of Oklahoma College of Nursing
Oklahoma City

MaryAnn Edelman, RN, MS, CNS
Assistant Professor — Department of Nursing
Kingsborough Community College
Brooklyn, N.Y.

M. Susan Emerson, RN, PhD, ACNP, ANP, CDE, CNS-Med/Surg
Nurse Practitioner
Truman Medical Center — Hospital Hill
Assistant Clinical Professor
University of Missouri
Kansas City

Carmel T. Ficorelli, RN, MS, FNP
Assistant Professor, Department of Nursing
Kingsborough Community College
Brooklyn, N.Y.

Rose M. Flinchum, RN, MSEd, MS, CDE, CPT
Diabetes Educator
Methodist Hospital Diabetes Center
Gary, Ind.

Cynthia L. Frozena, RN, MSN, OCN, CHPN
Consultant/Medical Writer
Hospice Consultants of the Great Lakes
Manitowoc, Wis.

Denise Giachetta-Ryan, RN, MPA, CNOR
Associate Professor
Kingsborough Community College
Brooklyn, N.Y.

Darlene M. Gilcreast, RN, MSN, PhD, CDE
Associate Professor
University of Texas Health Science Center
San Antonio

Sandra K. Green, RN, MSN, CDE
Diabetes Educator Program Coordinator
University of Texas Medical Branch
Galveston

Linda B. Haas, RN, PhC, CDE
Endocrinology Clinical Nurse Specialist
Veterans' Administration Puget Sound Health Care System
Seattle

Sherri L. Horvat, RN,C, BSN, CDE, CPT
Diabetes Educator, Program Coordinator
The Methodist Hospitals, Inc.
Gary, Ind.

Carolyn M. Jenkins, RN, DrPH, RD, APRN-BC-ADM, CDE, FAAN
Professor
Medical University of South Carolina College of Nursing
Charleston

Karla Jones, RN, MSN
Nursing Faculty
Treasure Valley Community College
Ontario, Ore.

Coleen Kumar, RN, MS, CNS
Assistant Professor
Kingsborough Community College
Brooklyn, N.Y.

Patricia Lange-Otsuka, APRN,BC, MSN, EdD
Associate Dean of Nursing
Associate Professor of Nursing
Hawaii Pacific University
Kaneohe

Virginia Lester, RN, MSN, CNS (INACTIVE)
Assistant Professor in Nursing
Angelo State University
San Angelo, Tex.

Donna Scemons, RN, MSN, CNS, FNP-C, CWOCN
President
Healthcare Systems
Castaic, Calif.

Foreword

Caring for a patient with diabetes mellitus presents numerous challenges for the health care provider. Couple these challenges with a rising incidence, and rapidly changing treatment options and the clinician is faced with the need for an up-to-date clinical reference.

Consider some of the challenges presented by the diagnosis:
- Diabetes is a chronic illness with no cure. Health care is required over a long period.
- Many people are being diagnosed with this complex disease; incidence and prevalence seem to be rising daily.
- A wide age-range, from the very young to the elderly, can be affected. Rising incidence of type 2 diabetes, particularly in children, presents a unique set of circumstances. This diagnosis has a long-term impact on the individual as well as society at large.
- Diabetes has numerous subgroups each with its own idiosyncrasies.
- There's a broad and growing range of treatment options.
- A high potential for co-morbidities exists.

Health care providers are significantly impacted as well. Care for the patient and family with diabetes requires:
- a team approach for effective health care management (Physicians, including specialists, nurses, dietitians, physical therapists, podiatrists, and social workers, each with its own body of knowledge unique to the discipline, partner with the patient and family to maximize healthy outcomes.)
- an understanding of the unique way the diagnosis impacts the patient, family, and their quality of life
- education for health care providers to stay abreast of the rapid changes related to evidence-based standards of care
- education for the patient so that self-management of this complex disease can maximize his state of well-being
- preventive education as a component of health care management
- addressing diverse sociocultural considerations
- increasing use of technology
- acknowledgment of rising health care costs
- research dissemination.

The authors of *Diabetes Mellitus: A Guide to Patient Care* present an excellent, comprehensive resource for clinicians who must manage the care of patients with complex needs. Its use will enhance your understanding of diabetes mellitus and provide readily usable information based on the most current scientific data.

Karen A. Dadich, RN, MN, CNS
Associate Professor and Coordinator of Faculty Development
Texas Tech University Health Sciences Center, School of Nursing
Lubbock

Part 1

UNDERSTANDING DIABETES MELLITUS

Incidence and prevalence

Diabetes mellitus is a metabolic disorder characterized by hyperglycemia (elevated blood glucose level) — a direct result from a lack of insulin or insulin effect, or both. The term *diabetes mellitus* comes from the ancient Roman and Greek term meaning "the running through of sugar." The disorder can be traced back to as early as the first century A.D. Greek and Roman physicians used the term *diabetes* to describe the condition that presented with such cardinal findings of large volumes of sweet smelling urine (polyuria), intense thirst (polydipsia), and weight loss despite an increase in appetite (polyphagia).

Four general classifications of diabetes are recognized and are based on the underlying mechanism that results in hyperglycemia. (See *Classifications of diabetes mellitus*). The American Diabetes Association (ADA) also recognizes a separate classification of diabetes called *prediabetes*.

Epidemic, complex, chronic, common, modifiable, and costly are all terms used to describe diabetes. Medical advances in treatment have led to increased longevity and improved quality of life in patients with diabetes based on careful self-monitoring of blood glucose levels, use of the data to make pharmacologic and lifestyle changes, and adherence to the treatment plan. In addition, newer medications for diabetes, such as amylin hormones (pramlintide [Symlin]) and incretin mimetics (exenatide [Byetta]), work to improve the body's own glucose metabolism and insulin sensitivity, thus optimizing glycemic control and preventing long-term complications.

INCIDENCE OF DIABETES

According to the World Health Organization, approximately 150 million people worldwide have diabetes mellitus — 20.8 million of those are Americans. It's estimated that this number will most likely increase to 333 million by 2050. In addition, the Centers for Disease Control and Prevention (CDC) reported in 2005 that 1.5 million people age 20 and older were newly diagnosed with diabetes mellitus. Of these diagnosed patients, incidence was highest in the 40 to 59 age-group. (See *New cases of diabetes*, page 4.)

PREVALENCE

Overall, diabetes mellitus is considered epidemic. From 1997 through 2003, the number of new cases of diabetes increased by more than 50%. According to the CDC, diabetes affects approximately 20.8 million people of all ages in the United States, a figure that represents 7% of the population. Of those 20.8 million people, 14.6 million are diagnosed with diabetes, whereas 6.2 million people remain undiagnosed. Of those 6.2 million, between 5% and 10% have type 1 diabetes; 90% to 95% have type 2.

CLASSIFICATIONS OF DIABETES MELLITUS

Diabetes mellitus is classified according to the pathophysiologic mechanism leading to hyperglycemia. These classifications include:

■ type 1 (previously termed *insulin-dependent diabetes mellitus* [IDDM], or *juvenile-onset diabetes*)—absolute insulin insufficiency

■ type 2 (previously termed *non-insulin-diabetes mellitus* [NIDDM] or *adult-onset diabetes*)—insulin resistance with varying degrees of insulin secretory defects

■ gestational diabetes—form of glucose intolerance during pregnancy

■ other types—resulting from specific conditions, such as genetic defects of pancreatic beta cells (also known as *maturity-onset diabetes of the young,* or MODY) or insulin action; disorders involving the exocrine function of the pancreas; endocrine disorders; drugs; surgery; malnutrition; infections; and other illnesses.

Type 1 diabetes can occur at any age but it typically begins in childhood or young adulthood. Due to the absolute insulin insufficiency, exogenous insulin is necessary to achieve blood glucose control.

Type 2 diabetes is usually associated with older age, typically after age 40, but children and adolescents may be diagnosed with this type of diabetes. Obesity, family history of diabetes or gestational diabetes, impaired glucose metabolism, and physical inactivity are also associated with this type of diabetes. Type 2 diabetes is treated with diet and exercise in combination with various oral antidiabetic drugs. Treatment may also include insulin therapy.

Another growing concern is the development of prediabetes, which is believed to increase an individual's risk for developing type 2 diabetes. In prediabetes, the individual has impaired fasting glucose (IFG) levels or impaired glucose tolerance (IGT), or both. Basically, this individual has higher than normal blood glucose levels, but not high enough to be classified as diabetes. The person with IFG has a fasting blood glucose level between 100 and 125 mg/dl. The person with IGT has a blood glucose level between 140 and 199 mg/dl after a 2-hour glucose tolerance test.

Using information obtained from diabetes studies conducted between 1988 and 1994 and applying the results to the U.S. population in 2000, the CDC estimates that approximately 41 million people ages 40 to 74 would have prediabetes; 35 million would have IFG; and 16 million would have IGT. Today, it's estimated that more than 350 million people worldwide have IGT or IFG.

The International Diabetes Federation estimates that approximately 40% to 50% of people with IGT will develop type 2 diabetes. By 2025, the number of people with IGT is projected to be 472 million (9% of the adult population). However, the progression from prediabetes to type 2 diabetes isn't absolute. Studies show that such lifestyle changes as losing weight and increasing physical activity can aid in preventing or delaying diabetes and, in some cases, returning blood glucose levels to normal.

Age-related prevalence
In 2005, the CDC estimated that diabetes affects approximately 20.6 million people age 20 and older, which accounts for 9.6% of this age-group. For those older than age 60, diabetes affects 10.3 million, or approximately 20.9% of this age-group. (See *Estimated prevalence of diabetes,* page 5.)

However, people younger than age 20 aren't immune to diabetes. Approximately 176,500 people younger than

NEW CASES OF DIABETES

This graph highlights the number of new cases of diabetes diagnosed in the United States in 2005.

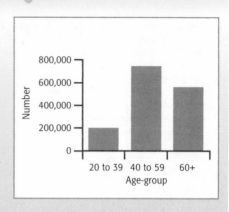

Source: National Diabetes Information Clearinghouse. National Diabetes Statistics. NIH publication. 02-3892. Fact sheet. Available at: *www.diabetes.niddk.nih.gov.*

age 20 have diabetes; thus, diabetes mellitus affects 0.22% of people in this age-group. Approximately 1 of every 400 to 600 children and adolescents has type 1 diabetes.

One of the most alarming aspects of the diabetes epidemic is the prevalence of type 2 diabetes in children and adolescents. As the rate of childhood obesity rises, type 2 diabetes — a disease that used to be seen only in adults older than age 45 — is becoming more common in younger people.

Cases of type 2 diabetes have been documented in children as young as age 4, although the data are limited regarding trends of type 2 among adolescents. Statistics from the ADA report that of the 18,000 children diagnosed with diabetes each year, 8% to 45% develop type 2. In addition, children of Native American, Black, and Latino descent are more likely to develop type 2 diabetes.

Gender-related prevalence
Historically, more women have been affected by diabetes than men. However, these statistics are changing. According to CDC estimates for 2005, approximately 10.9 million men, or 10.5% of all men age 20 and older, have diabetes. In comparison, 9.7 million women, or 8.8% of all women age 20 and older, have diabetes.

Ethnicity-related prevalence
Based on estimates for diabetes in various ethnic groups (age 20 and older), the CDC has identified that:
● approximately 8.7% (13.1 million) of Whites have diabetes
● an estimated 13.3% of Blacks have diabetes, with Blacks being almost 2 times more likely to develop diabetes than Whites
● the prevalence of diabetes in Black women is approximately 1½ times greater than in Black men; approximately one-third of Black women between ages 65 and 74 have diabetes
● Latinos are about 2 times more likely to have diabetes than Whites
● of the Latino group, Mexican Americans and Puerto Ricans have the highest prevalence of diabetes, followed by Cuban Americans; all three groups have a higher prevalence of diabetes than Whites
● approximately 12.8% of Native Americans and Inuits have diabetes, with the highest totals among Native

ESTIMATED PREVALENCE OF DIABETES

This graph shows the estimated total prevalence of diabetes for people in various age-groups older than age 20. This graph is based on estimates compiled by the Centers for Disease Control and Prevention.

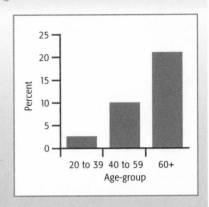

Source: National Diabetes Information Clearinghouse. National Diabetes Statistics. NIH publication. 02-3892. Fact sheet. Available at: www.diabetes.niddk.nih.gov.

Americans in the southern United States, especially southern Arizona (Pima Indians); approximately 50% of Pima Indians between ages 30 and 64 have diabetes
● Native Americans and Inuits are about 2 times more likely to have diabetes than Whites.

Although information about Asian Americans and Pacific Islanders is lacking, some studies of these groups in Hawaii show that they are twice as likely to be diagnosed with diabetes as Whites. Additional studies in California show that Asians are about 1½ times more likely to have diabetes than Whites.

CONSEQUENCES OF DIABETES

Diabetes is associated with many serious complications, including death. Based on death certificates in 2002, diabetes ranked as the 6th leading cause of death in the United States. However, this number may be erroneous because diabetes was listed on the death certificate for less than one-half of the individuals diagnosed with diabetes. Only 10% to 15% had diabetes listed as an underlying cause. Based on these numbers, the risk of death in people with diabetes

appears twice that for those who don't have the disease.

Increased risk of complications

Diabetes can affect many organs and body systems, leading to serious and, possibly, life-threatening, complications. High blood glucose levels may damage blood vessels and nerves, leading to vascular disease and neuropathies. Diabetes may also lower the body's ability to fight infection and various illnesses, leading to more complications. Additionally, people with diabetes experience acute complications directly related to blood glucose control. Moreover, gender appears to influence which complications develop. (See *How gender affects complications in diabetes*, page 6.)

Cardiovascular complications

According to the ADA, the leading cause of diabetes-related death is cardiovascular disease with four out of five deaths occurring because of this complication. It's also a major factor for morbidity associated with the disorder, which contributes to the overall cost of diabetes care.

HOW GENDER AFFECTS
COMPLICATIONS IN DIABETES

The risk of diabetes-related complications differs between women and men. Consider these findings.

Women

- Women with diabetes are at greater risk for blindness as compared to men.
- Decreased or absent sexual function occurs in about 35% of women with diabetes.
- Women with diabetes have more diabetes-related comas, nerve damage, urinary tract infections, and hypertension.

Men

- Men experience such diabetes-related complications as heart attack, stroke, kidney failure, amputation, nerve damage, impotence, and blindness.
- For the past three decades, deaths from heart disease in men with diabetes have decreased by 13%, compared to a 36% decrease in nondiabetic men.
- Symptoms of peripheral vascular disease are associated with a two to threefold risk of coronary heart disease, stroke, and cardiac failure in men with diabetes.
- Diabetic retinopathy progresses more rapidly in men before age 30.
- Amputation from a diabetes-related complication is 1.4 to 2.7 times higher in men than in women.
- An estimated 50% to 60% of men with diabetes older than age 50 have erectile dysfunction, as compared to 10% of nondiabetic men.

A person with diabetes has the same risk for developing myocardial infarction (MI) as a nondiabetic person who has a history of MI. However, adults with diabetes are 2 to 4 times more likely to die from a heart ailment than nondiabetic adults with a history of MI. Annually, these 77,000 deaths related to cardiovascular disease may be in the form of heart failure, stroke, or peripheral vascular disease. Heart disease and stroke account for 65% of deaths among people with diabetes.

Additionally, women with diabetes are at higher risk for developing cardiovascular disease than men. Data from the National Health and Nutrition Examination Survey revealed that the mortality of heart disease has decreased by 36% in nondiabetic men and 27% in nondiabetic women. The same data, however, indicated that mortality increased by 23% in women with diabetes and decreased by only 13% in men with diabetes. Yearly there are 50,000 more cardiac-related deaths among women and men with diabetes. Data also suggest that women with diabetes are less likely to survive a first MI than men with diabetes and, if women do survive, they're at higher risk for recurrence followed by heart failure. In fact, diabetes erases any protective female advantage with regard to coronary artery disease, the number one cause of death for men and women with diabetes.

The co-morbidity of hypertension affects 20% to 60% of people with diabetes. It's associated with microvascular complications related to the eyes, kidneys, and nerves. Hypertension is twice as common in diabetics as in nondiabetics. About 73% of adults with diabetes have blood pressures greater than or equal to 130/80 mm Hg.

The prevalence of hypertension in patients with diabetes is 1½ to 3 times higher than in nondiabetic patients in the same age-group. A study performed in the United Kingdom (the United Kingdom Prospective Diabetes Study) found that each 10-mm Hg decrease in mean systolic blood pressure was associated with a 12% reduction in risk for complications related to diabetes.

Ocular complications

Diabetes is the number one cause of new cases of blindness in people with diabetes between ages 20 and 74; an estimated 12,000 to 24,000 new cases of blindness occur each year more often in women than in men. Microvascular complications can lead to diabetic retinopathy and, if left untreated, to blindness. Twenty years after diagnosis, all people with type 1 and type 2 diabetes will likely have some degree of diabetic retinopathy. Data from the Diabetes Prevention Program Outcome Study presented at the ADA scientific session in June 2005 revealed that diabetic retinopathy may start to develop before the diagnosis of diabetes.

Renal complications

Diabetes is the leading cause of renal failure affecting, annually, approximately 42,000 people. Diabetic nephropathy also occurs as a result of diabetes, affecting 5% of the U.S. population. Diabetes is the leading cause of treated end-stage renal disease (ESRD) and accounts for 43% of new ESRD cases. Native Americans, Blacks, and Mexican Americans are the ethnic groups at highest risk for developing ESRD. The incidence rates of ESRD in people with diabetes in the United States have maintained an upward trend. Early intervention and treatment of kidney disease can reduce the decline in kidney function by 30% to 70%. These same interventions also help in protecting against heart, blood vessel, eye, and nerve complications.

Nervous system complications

Diabetes is responsible for 60% to 70% of mild to severe damage to the nervous system. Symptoms may present as numbness and tingling, impaired sensation or pain in the feet or hands, delayed digestion of food (gastroparesis), carpal tunnel syndrome, and other nerve problems. Approximately one-third of people with diabetes older than age 40 experience some impaired sensation in the lower extremities, primarily the feet. Sexual dysfunction may also occur as a result of nerve and blood vessel damage.

Diabetic peripheral neuropathy is a debilitating complication of diabetes and accounts for significant morbidity, predisposing the foot to ulceration and lower extremity amputation.

Amputation

Sixty percent of nontraumatic lower limb amputations result from diabetes. Annually, 82,000 amputations are performed on people with diabetes. The risk of leg amputation is 15 to 40 times greater among this population. Additionally, the risk of amputation is increased for men, with rates ranging from 1.4 to 2.7 times higher for men than for women.

Periodontal disease

Periodontal disease is more common in people with diabetes (both type 1 and type 2) than in nondiabetic patients, occurring in about one-third of this population. Additionally, periodontal disease tends to be more severe in people with diabetes. Adults and children with diabetes who have poor metabolic control are more susceptible to periodontal bacteria and dental caries. Additionally, life-threatening deep neck infections, resulting from root cavities, can lead to morbidity and mortality.

Complications of pregnancy

Complications related to pregnancy and diabetes may affect the unborn fetus as well as the mother. Approximately 2% to 5% of all nondiabetic pregnant women develop gestational diabetes, which occurs more commonly among Black, Latino, and Native American women. After the pregnancy, approximately 5% to 10% of these women are found to have type 2 diabetes, and the rest are at an increased risk (20% to 50%) of developing diabetes within the next 5 to 10 years.

Major birth defects can occur in 5% to 10% of pregnancies in which blood glucose control is poor prior to conception and during the first trimester. The risk for spontaneous abortion in these cases ranges from 15% to 20%. During the second and third trimesters, inadequate blood glucose control may lead to large birth weight infants (fetal macrosomia), which happens 2 to 3 times more often in pregnant women with diabetes than in the general population. Women with fetal macrosomia are 3 to 4 times more likely to require a cesarean delivery.

Congenital malformations in neonates born to women with diabetes are variable. For example, the rate of malformations ranges from 0% to 5% for women with diabetes who receive prenatal care, compared to 10% for those who don't receive prenatal care.

Risk of other problems
Patients with diabetes may be at increased risk for other illnesses, which can lead to more severe complications. For example, patients with diabetes who also have cardiovascular disease may be at risk for pneumococcal infection. Annually, 10,000 to 300,000 people with diabetes fall prey to complications of influenza and pneumonia — these individuals are at greater risk of dying from these respiratory complications. As a result, the CDC has developed immunization guidelines for people with diabetes.

Additional life-threatening acute complications of diabetes typically involve biochemical alterations related to glucose imbalance. These include ke-toacidosis and hyperosmolar (nonketotic) coma.

Increased costs
Due to its chronic and complex nature, diabetes is a costly disease. In 2002, $132 billion were spent on diabetes care. Of this cost, $91.9 billion were attributed to direct care expenses alone, which includes the cost of medical care and services. Of this expenditure, $23.2 billion were spent for diabetes care, $24.6 billion for chronic complications attributable to diabetes, and $44.1 billion for excess prevalence of general medical conditions. The remaining $40.1 billion were related to indirect costs, including costs for short-term, long-term, and permanent disability as well as premature death of an adult.

Obviously, the economic burden of diabetes is significant; this chronic disease requires constant intervention. However, by having a sound knowledge base about culture, disease incidence, coping strategies, and lifestyle behaviors to impact modifiable risks, health care providers can play an important role in helping to reduce costs. In addition, a focus on prevention, education, early detection through screening, and prompt treatment can help to reduce the risk of complications and overall morbidity and mortality associated with this disease.

*Selected references*_____

American Diabetes Association. "Economic Costs of Diabetes in the U.S. in 2002," *Diabetes Care* 26(3):917-32, March 2003.

American Diabetes Association. "National Diabetes Fact Sheet" [Online]. Available at: *www.diabetes.org.*

Barnett, D.M., and Krall, L.P. "History of Diabetes," in Kahn, C.R., et al. *Joslin's Diabetes Mellitus,* 14th ed. Philadelphia: Lippincott Williams & Wilkins, 2005.

Caballero, A.E. "Diabetes in Minorities in the United States," in Kahn, C.R., et al. *Joslin's Diabetes Mellitus,* 14th ed.

Philadelphia: Lippincott Williams & Wilkins, 2005.

Centers for Disease Control and Prevention. "National Diabetes Fact Sheet: General Information and National Estimates on Diabetes in the United States" [Online]. Atlanta, Ga.: U.S. Department of Health and Human Services, Centers for Disease Control and Prevention, 2005. Available at: *www.cdc.gov/diabetes/pubs/estimates05.htm.*

Centers for Disease Control and Prevention. "National Diabetes Fact Sheet: United States" [Online]. November 2003. Available at: *www.cdc.gov/diabetes/pubs/factsheet.htm.*

Diabetes and African American Women. The National Women's Health Information Center. Available at: *www.4women.gov/faq/diabetes.fre.htm.*

International Diabetes Federation. *Fight Obesity Prevent Diabetes.* Available at: *www.idf.org/home.*

"National Diabetes Education Program." National Institutes of Health and Centers for Disease Control and Prevention. Available at: *www.ndep.nih.gov/.*

National Diabetes Information Clearinghouse. "National Diabetes Statistics." NIH publication. 02-3892. Fact sheet. Available at: *www.diabetes.niddk.nih.gov.*

"Report of the Expert Committee on the Diagnosis and Classification of Diabetes Mellitus," *Diabetes Care* 25(Suppl 1):S5-S20, January 2003.

Sicree, R., et al. "The Global Burden of Diabetes," in *Diabetes Atlas*, 2nd ed. Gan, D., ed. Brussels International Diabetes Federation, pages 15-71, 2003.

Unwin, N., et al. "Impaired Glucose Tolerance and Impaired Fasting Glycaemia: The Current Status on Definition and Intervention," *Diabetic Medicine* 9(19):708-23, September 2002.

UK Prospective Diabetes Study Group. "Tight Blood Pressure Control and Risk of Macrovascular and Microvascular Complications in Type 2 Diabetes," *British Medical Journal* 317(7160):703-13, September 1998.

Causes and pathophysiology

Diabetes is a group of diseases characterized by high levels of blood glucose that results from defects in insulin production or insulin action. It's the sixth leading cause of death in the United States. Key causes include aging, unhealthy diet, obesity, and lack of exercise.

ETIOLOGY OF DIABETES

People with untreated diabetes have high blood glucose, which occurs because a person's pancreas doesn't make enough insulin or the muscle, fat, and liver cells don't respond normally to insulin, or both. Diabetes is classified primarily as type 1 or type 2. Both types are complex diseases associated with genetic mutations as well as being related to environmental factors.

Although the exact cause of diabetes is unknown, there are several factors that, when present, place a person at greater risk for the development of diabetes. These include:

- a parent or sibling with diabetes
- obesity
- age older than 45
- certain ethnic groups (particularly Native American, Black, and Latino)
- history of diabetes during pregnancy (gestational diabetes) or delivering a neonate weighing more than 9 lb (4.1 kg)
- high blood pressure

- high triglyceride levels
- high cholesterol levels.

Prediabetes

Prediabetes is metabolic state that falls somewhere between glucose homeostasis and diabetes. Individuals with prediabetes have impaired glucose tolerance (IGT) or impaired fasting blood glucose (IFG) levels, or both, and are at increased risk for developing diabetes, heart disease, and stroke.

IFG is a condition in which the fasting blood glucose level is greater than 100 mg/dl (5.6 mmol/L), but less than 126 mg/dl (7 mmol/L) after an overnight fast. The level is higher than normal but not high enough to be classified as diabetes. IGT is a condition in which the blood glucose level ranges between 140 to 199 mg/dl (7.8 to 11.1 mmol/L) after a 2-hour oral glucose tolerance test. Again, this level is higher than normal but not high enough to be classified as diabetes.

The individual with prediabetes is commonly asymptomatic. At least one of the following criteria are used to help confirm the diagnosis of prediabetes in an individual older than age 45:

- the individual identifies with one of the high-risk ethnic groups, is hypertensive, or has a serum high-density-lipoprotein (HDL) level less than 35 mg/dl

● the individual reports or exhibits: sedentary lifestyle, obesity, history of vascular disease, or a first-degree relative diagnosed with diabetes. In a cross-section sample of American adults ages 40 to 74, 40.1% were found to have prediabetes with 33.8% demonstrating IFG and 15.4% presenting with IGT. Other studies showed that lifestyle and obesity were directly linked to the development of type 2 diabetes.

Type 1 diabetes

Type 1 diabetes was previously termed *insulin-dependent diabetes mellitus* or *juvenile diabetes*. Although the disease may develop any time before age 30, it's commonly diagnosed in childhood.

In type 1 diabetes, the pancreas produces little or no insulin. Of all the people diagnosed with diabetes, only 10% have type 1. Its peak onset occurs in the second decade of life, usually between ages 10 and 14. Whites have the highest rate of developing type 1 diabetes. It's less prevalent in Latinos and has the lowest rate of occurrence in Blacks and Asians.

Factors associated with the development of type 1 diabetes may be environmental, genetic, or autoimmune.

One theory on the etiology of type 1 diabetes is that it results from damage to pancreatic beta cells from an infectious or environmental agent. Environmental agents known to induce an attack on beta cell functioning include viruses (mumps, rubella, Coxsackie B4), toxic chemicals, and cytotoxins. Exposure to cow's milk in infancy may also contribute to the development of type 1 diabetes. Bovine serum albumin (BSA), a component of cow's milk, is thought to be an environmental trigger that causes the development of antibodies for BSA. These BSA antibodies are found in children newly diagnosed with diabetes. Researchers believe that environmental factors cause the immune system to destroy the insulin-producing cells of the pancreas. A genetic predisposition makes some people more susceptible to environmental factors. Certain genetic markers have been shown to increase the risk of developing type 1 diabetes. Genes within the major histocompatibility complex located on gene 6p21 have been implicated.

Additional factors include sex hormones related to both puberty and pregnancy. If there's no family history of diabetes, the risk of developing the disease is less than 1%. If an individual is an identical twin whose twin has type 1 diabetes, the risk of developing the disease increases to 25% to 50%. If either parent has diabetes, the risk of developing type 1 diabetes increases. The risk is greater if the individual's father has type 1 diabetes. If an individual's mother has type 1 diabetes, the risk of developing the illness depends on the mother's age at the time of the individual's birth. The exact reason for this is still unknown.

Type 1 diabetes is considered an autoimmune disease when the pancreas shows lymphocytic infiltration and destruction of insulin-secreting cells of the islets of Langerhans, ultimately causing insulin depletion. It develops when the body's immune system destroys pancreatic beta cells. Of the patients with type 1 diabetes, 85% have circulating islet cell antibodies, especially human leukocyte antigens (HLAs), such as HLA-DR3 and HLA-DR4. In addition, the majority of these individuals also have detectable anti-insulin antibodies. Most islet cell antibodies are directed against glutamic acid decarboxylase within pancreatic beta cells.

Measurement of a substance called C-peptide, which is a component of *proinsulin* (the precursor to insulin), can be used to determine if the patient is capable of secreting endogenous insulin. If C-peptide isn't present, total beta cell failure has occurred. This is the basis for a diagnosis of type 1 diabetes.

In type 1 diabetes, more than 90% of the insulin-producing cells of the pancreas are permanently destroyed. However, the rate of beta cell destruction varies. In infants and children, destruction is usually rapid; whereas in adults, the destruction is slow.

Type 2 diabetes

Type 2 diabetes is more common than type 1, accounting for up to 90% or more of all cases of diabetes. It usually occurs in adulthood, and it occurs in 3% to 5% of Americans younger than age 50. This rate increases to 10% to 15% in Americans older than age 50. Although the exact cause is unknown, it's believed that, unlike type 1 diabetes, pancreatic beta cell destruction doesn't occur.

Type 2 diabetes is more common in people of Native American, Latino, and African descent. Compared with Whites, diabetes rates are about 60% higher in Blacks and 110% to 120% higher in Mexicans and Puerto Ricans. However, Native Americans have the highest rates of diabetes in the United States. For example, among adult Pima Indians, 50% have type 2 diabetes. The prevalence of type 2 diabetes is likely to increase because the population is aging and Latinos and other minority groups are becoming a major portion of the United States' population. People who have migrated to Western cultures from East India, Japan, and Australian Aboriginal cultures are also more likely to develop type 2 diabetes than those who remain in their native countries due to the American diet and sedentary lifestyle.

Type 2 diabetes is strongly familial. However, only recently have some genes been consistently associated with increased risk for type 2 diabetes in certain populations.

Genetic, functional genomic, and transgenic research have identified coactivators (PGC-1 alpha and PGC-1 beta) as regulators of mitochondrial number and function. They regulate glucose and fat oxidation in muscle and fat tissue, gluconeogenesis in the liver, and even glucose-regulated insulated secretion in beta cells. PGC-1 alpha and PGC-1 beta messenger ribonucleic acid levels and the mitochondrial genes they regulate are decreased in the muscles of patients with type 2 diabetes.

Type 2 diabetes results from insulin resistance in muscle (leads to decreased glucose uptake) and in the liver (results in increased gluconeogenesis) in conjunction with declining beta cell function. The pancreas doesn't make enough insulin to keep blood glucose levels normal.

Type 2 diabetes is becoming more common due to the growing number of older Americans, increasing obesity, and lack of exercise. Approximately 80% to 90% of people with type 2 diabetes are obese. Because obesity causes insulin resistance, obese people need greater amounts of insulin to maintain normal blood glucose levels. Obesity is determined by calculating the individual's body mass index or the waist-to-hip ratio. Studies have shown that a waist-to-hip ratio greater than 0.76 increases the person's risk. (See *Determining body mass index*.)

Because of its slow onset (sometimes developing over the course of several years), type 2 diabetes may be considered by some to be a milder form of diabetes, commonly controlled with diet, weight loss, and oral medication. However, patients with type 2 diabetes are at risk for complications, just as those with type 1 diabetes.

In type 2 diabetes, the pancreas may produce adequate insulin. However, cells have become resistant to the insulin produced. Subsequently, the insulin isn't able to work as efficiently as it should. Symptoms of type 2 diabetes can begin so gradually that a person may not know that he has this type of diabetes. Early signs are lethargy, extreme thirst, and frequent urination.

DETERMINING BODY MASS INDEX

Body mass index (BMI) is a mathematical calculation that's based on the person's weight in kilograms and his height in meters squared. To calculate BMI, divide the weight in kilograms by the height in meters squared: BMI = weight (kg)/height (m^2).

For example, if a patient weighs 165 lbs and is 5′ 6″ tall, first convert his weight to kilograms by dividing 165 by 2.2 (2.2 lb = 1 kg). The patient weighs 75 kg.

Next, convert the patient's height to meters by dividing his height in inches (66) by 39.4 (39.4 in = 1 m). The patient's height is 1.68 meters.

Then calculate the BMI: 75 kg /(1.68 m)^2 = 75/2.82

Other symptoms may include sudden weight loss, slow wound healing, urinary tract infections, gum disease, or blurred vision. It isn't unusual for type 2 diabetes to be detected while a patient is seeing a physician about another health concern that's actually being caused by the undiagnosed diabetes.

Individuals at high risk for developing type 2 diabetes mellitus include those who:
● are obese (more than 20% above their ideal body weight)
● have a relative with diabetes mellitus
● belong to a high-risk ethnic population (Black, Native American, Latino, or Native Hawaiian)
● have been diagnosed with gestational diabetes or have delivered a neonate weighing more than 9 lb (4.1 kg)
● have high blood pressure (140/90 mm Hg or above)
● have an HDL; (sometimes called the "good" cholesterol) level less than or equal to 35 mg/dl
● have a triglyceride level greater than or equal to 250 mg/dl
● have had IGT or IFG levels on previous testing
● ingest alcohol in large amounts
● lead a sedentary lifestyle
● consume a high-fat diet
● are older.

The incidence of type 2 diabetes increases with age. In the United States,

more than 40% of patients with diabetes are age 65 and older, with several contributing factors. As the population ages, activity levels decrease, lean body mass decreases, and adipose tissue increases contributing to insulin resistance. Also with aging, the production of insulin decreases. The use of medications, such as diuretics and corticosteroids, as well as surgical procedures may also raise the risk of developing type 2 diabetes.

The consequences of uncontrolled and untreated type 2 diabetes, however, are just as serious as those for type 1 diabetes.

Other types of diabetes

Other types of diabetes have a specific etiology and include diabetes related to:
● genetic defects in beta cell function (frequently associated with hyperglycemia before age 25; commonly referred to as *maturity-onset diabetes of the young*; insulin secretion is impaired but there are minimal to no defects in insulin action)
● genetic defects in insulin action (commonly involving mutation of the insulin receptor)
● diseases of the exocrine pancreas (such as pancreatitis, trauma, infection, and pancreatic carcinoma)
● endocrinopathies (such as excess hormone secretion associated with acro-

CLASSIFICATION OF DIABETES BASED ON ETIOLOGY

Although the exact cause of diabetes mellitus is unknown, there are many identified risk factors for the development of both type 1 and type 2 diabetes. Type 1 is linked to genetics, ethnicity, and environmental triggers. Type 2 is linked to genetics, lifestyle, family history, weight, body mass index, ethnicity, and co-morbidity. In addition, researchers have also identified a prediabetic condition involving impaired glucose tolerance or impaired fasting blood glucose levels, which increases the risk of developing diabetes. Additionally, there are other types of diabetes with a known etiology.

1. Type 1 diabetes (beta cell destruction)
   a. Immune mediated
   b. Idiopathic
2. Type 2 diabetes (range from predominant insulin resistance with relative insulin deficiency to predominant secretory defect with insulin resistance)
3. Prediabetes
4. Other causes of diabetes
   a. Genetic defects of beta cell function
      i. Chromosome 12m hepatocyte nuclear factor (HNF)-1alpha (maturity-onset diabetes of the young [MODY]3)
      ii. Chromosome 7, glucokinase (MODY2)
      iii. Chromosome 20, HNF-4alpha (MODY1)
      iv. Mitochondrial deoxyribonucleic acid
   b. Genetic defects in insulin action
      i. Type A insulin resistance
      ii. Leprechaunism
      ii. Rabson-Mendenall syndrome
      iv. Lipoatrophic diabetes
   c. Diseases of the exocrine pancreas
      i. Pancreatitis
      ii. Trauma, pancreatectomy
      iii. Neoplasia
      iv. Cystic fibrosis
      v. Hemochromatosis
      vi. Fibrocalculous pancreatopathy
   d. Endocrinopathies
      i. Acromegaly
      ii. Cushing's syndrome
      iii. Glucagonoma
      iv. Pheochromocytoma
      v. Hyperthyroidism
      vi. Somatostatinoma
      vii. Aldosteronoma
   e. Drug- or chemical-induced
      i. Vacor
      ii. Pentamidie
      iii. Nicotinic acid
      iv. Glucocorticoids
      v. Thyroid hormone
      vi. Diazoxide
      vii. Beta-adrenergic agonists
      viii. Thiazides
      ix. Dilantin
      x. Alpha-interferon
   f. Infections
      i. Congenital rubella
      ii. Cytomegalovirus
   g. Uncommon forms of immune-mediated diabetes
      i. "Stiff-man" syndrome
      ii. Anti-insulin receptor antibodies
   h. Other genetic syndromes associated with diabetes
      i. Down syndrome
      ii. Klinefelter's syndrome
      iii. Turner's syndrome
      iv. Wolfram's syndrome
      v. Friedreich's ataxia
      vi. Huntington's chorea
      vii. Laurence-Moon-Biedle syndrome
      viii. Myotonic dystrophy
      ix. Porphyria
      x. Prader-Willi syndrome
5. Gestational diabetes

Adapted from Report of the Expert Committee on the Diagnosis and Classification of Diabetes Mellitus. *Diabetes Care* 26(Suppl 1):S5-S20, January 2003, with permission of the publisher.

megaly, Cushing's syndrome, pheochromocytoma)
● drugs or chemicals, such as nicotinic acid, glucocorticoids, alpha-interferon, and toxins
● immune mediation and other genetic syndromes, such as Down syndrome, Klinefelter's syndrome, and Turner's syndrome.

In addition, pregnancy may be responsible for causing glucose intolerance — also known as *gestational diabetes*. (See *Classification of diabetes based on etiology*.)

PATHOPHYSIOLOGY
The development of diabetes mellitus is a result of three major factors: the pancreas doesn't make enough (or any) insulin, which is the primary cause of type 1 diabetes; the body is unable to recognize its own insulin and use it properly in the cells of the muscles, liver, and fat; or a combination of these two factors.

Understanding what happens in diabetes first requires understanding the normal process of food metabolism.

Overview of food metabolism
Every cell in the human body needs energy to function. Although the body can derive energy from fats and proteins, the body's primary energy source is glucose. Glucose is a simple sugar that's obtained from the digestion and metabolism of carbohydrates.

Several steps occur when food is digested:
● Glucose enters the bloodstream.
● The pancreas, via the beta cells of the islets of Langerhans, secretes insulin that moves glucose from the bloodstream into muscle, fat, and liver cells, where it can be used as fuel.

Carbohydrates are broken down in the small intestine and the glucose in digested food is then absorbed by the intestinal cells into the bloodstream. This glucose circulates in the blood as an available energy source for any cells that need it. However, glucose can't enter the cells alone, it needs insulin to aid its transport.

Glucoregulatory hormones
The glucoregulatory hormones, secreted by the pancreas, are designed to maintain circulating glucose concentrations within a relatively narrow range. These hormones include insulin, glucagon, and amylin among others. Insulin is a hormone produced by the beta cells of the islets of Langerhans in the pancreas. Glucagon is a hormone produced by the alpha cells of the pancreas. Together, these hormones are the prime regulators of glucose metabolism. Amylin (identified in the late 1980s) is produced by the pancreatic beta cells. Insulin and amylin both have similar low fasting glucose concentrations and increases in glucose levels with nutrient intake. Amylin works in conjunction with insulin to regulate the glucose levels.

Two other hormones have been identified as playing a role in glucose metabolism and insulin secretion. These hormones, called *incretins*, are produced by the GI tract in response to food intake. In turn, these hormones stimulate insulin secretion. The two major incretin hormones are gastric inhibitory polypeptide (GIP), also known as *glucose-dependent insulinotropic polypeptide*, and glucagon-like peptide-1 (GLP-1). Both hormones are secreted by specialized cells in the GI tract: GIP by the potassium cells in the duodenum and proximal jejunum; GLP-1 by specialized cells in the ileum and colon. Studies have shown that both hormones are secreted in response to food ingestion. GIP is primarily stimulated by the ingestion of carbohydrate and lipid-rich foods. With both hormones, their release ultimately leads to an increase in insulin secretion only when glucose concentrations are elevated. It has also been noted that GLP-1 has an effect on food intake. Studies have shown that GLP-1 reduces food intake over the short-term in healthy individuals and

FDA APPROVES INCRETIN MIMETIC AGENT

The U.S. Food and Drug Administration (FDA) recently approved the use of exenatide (Byetta), a synthetic form of the naturally occurring incretin, glucagon-like peptide-1, for the treatment of type 2 diabetes in combination with metformin and sulfonylureas. Studies revealed that the drug enhanced insulin secretion in response to glucose when ingested in the fasting state. The drug also helped improve postprandial glucose levels.

Results of studies indicated that close to one-half of the patients who received the drug experienced glycosylated hemoglobin levels less than 7% (the goal for glycemic control). Additionally, the drug was shown to help patients lose significant amounts of weight—a benefit for those with type 2 diabetes. Other benefits, such as a reduction in diastolic blood pressure, triglyceride levels, and high-density lipoprotein levels, also occurred.

---

those with type 2 diabetes. Although still unclear, it's thought that GLP-1's effect may be due to a reduction in the gastric emptying rate that results in a prolonged feeling of satiation. (See *FDA approves incretin mimetic agent.*)

Insulin action

Insulin bonds to a receptor site on the outside of a cell and acts like a key, unlocking the doorway into the cell through which glucose can enter. In addition to helping glucose enter the cells, insulin is also important in regulating the levels of glucose in the blood. Insulin helps control postprandial glucose in three ways:

● Initially, insulin signals the cells' insulin-secreting tissues, primarily skeletal muscle, to increase their uptake of glucose.

● Next, insulin acts on the liver to inhibit gluconeogenesis (formation of glucose molecules from noncarbohydrates including amino acids supplied from muscle tissue and glycerol supplied from fat; molecules are released into the circulation or stored in the liver as glycogen).

● Finally, insulin simultaneously inhibits glucagon secretion from pancreatic alpha cells, thus signaling the liver to stop producing glucose via glycogenolysis (the breakdown of glycogen to glucose by the liver) and gluconeogenesis.

After a meal, an individual's blood glucose level rises. In response to the increased glucose level, the pancreas normally releases insulin into the bloodstream to help glucose enter the cells, subsequently lowering blood glucose levels. When the blood glucose level is lowered, insulin released from the pancreas is reduced. Amylin suppresses postprandial glucagon release as well as decreases the rate of gastric emptying. The net effect is reduced glucose output by the liver following ingestion and a decreased rate of nutrients available for absorption in the small intestine. All of these actions reduce blood glucose. (See *Maintaining glucose balance.*)

Insulin also stimulates fat synthesis and promotes triglyceride storage in fat cells, protein synthesis in the liver and muscle, and proliferation of cell growth. Some of the glucose ingested during a meal can be converted to concentrated energy sources like glycogen or fatty acids and saved by the body for later use.

MAINTAINING GLUCOSE BALANCE

Glucose levels are maintained within narrow limits in the blood. The liver and the pancreas work together to control the body's fuel supply.

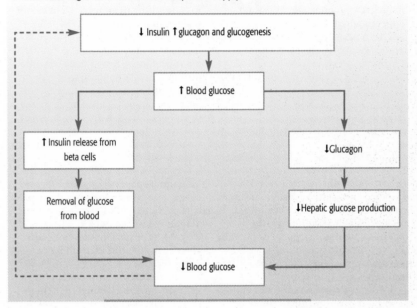

Mechanism of hyperglycemia

Hyperglycemia results when glucose remains in the bloodstream rather than being transported to the cells. This occurs when there's inadequate or no insulin produced or when the cell doorway no longer recognizes the insulin key.

With hyperglycemia, the body attempts to dilute the high level of glucose in the blood by drawing glucose-laden water out of the cells and into the bloodstream. It then excretes the glucose with water as urine. While the body is trying to rid the blood of higher concentration of glucose, the cells are starving for glucose and causing the individual to feel extreme hunger. To provide energy for the starving cells, the body converts fats and proteins to glu-

cose, releasing ketones in the blood as the end product of fat metabolism. Ketones are also excreted in the urine to maintain blood and pH and prevent ketoacidosis.

Type 1 diabetes

Type 1 diabetes mellitus is a catabolic disorder resulting in hyperglycemia. It's characterized by the autoimmune destruction of pancreatic beta cells, islet cell antibody-mediated insulitis, and complete insulinopenia. Approximately 95% of individuals with type 1 diabetes demonstrate the presence of antigen-specific markers that identify their genetic susceptibility to the disorder. Heavy lymphocytic infiltrates appear in and around islets. The number and size of islets are eventually destroyed, leading to decreased insulin production and glucose intolerance.

Type 1 diabetes is characterized by insulin deficiency, often complete deficiency. Due to this deficiency, glucose can't enter muscle and adipose tissue. In addition, the production of glucose in the liver (gluconeogenesis) is no longer opposed.

Overproduction of glucagon by pancreatic alpha cells stimulates glycogenolysis and gluconeogenesis. Gluconeogenesis occurs mainly in the liver but also occurs to a limited extent in the kidney and small intestine. As a result, blood glucose levels rise.

As glucose levels rise, the tubular absorptive capacity of the kidneys is exceeded and glucose (and water) is lost in the urine. This results in glycosuria and osmotic fluid loss that eventually leads to hypovolemia. Because insulin is unavailable, the tissues begin to starve. Neural tissue in the brain responds to this emergency by stimulating appetite. Classic symptoms, such as polydipsia, polyuria, and polyphagia, occur.

Prolonged insulin deficiency and other hormonal influences (increased levels of catecholamines, cortisol, glucagons, and growth hormone in part caused by hypovolemia, physical stress, or insulin deficiency itself) lead to the breakdown of fat in body tissues. As the catabolic process continues, metabolism of fat stored in adipose tissue leads to the production of fatty acids, which are broken down to ketoacids in the liver. In addition, hepatic gluconeogenesis, in response to tissue glucose deprivation, is responsible for the increased production of ketoacids. Normally, ketoacids can be used by neural and muscle tissue for energy metabolism. However the amount of ketoacids is too great. As a result, the normal pathway becomes saturated and the pH of the blood falls (6.8 to 7.3). Ketone bodies present in the urine ultimately increase the osmotic fluid loss. Metabolic acidosis ensues as the bicarbonate concentra-

tion decreases, resulting in diabetic ketoacidosis (often the initial symptom of the person with newly diagnosed type 1 diabetes).

In response to metabolic acidosis, extracellular hydrogen ions are exchanged for intracellular potassium ions, resulting in an increase in serum potassium levels (transient hyperkalemia). As a result, excess potassium is excreted into the urine leading to a net potassium loss. As total body water decreases, losses of sodium, magnesium, and phosphorus also occur. However, serum electrolyte levels may be normal or elevated due to hypovolemia. Hypovolemia is also responsible for an increased hematocrit, serum osmolality, white blood cell count, and hemoglobin, protein, and creatinine levels. Lactic acidosis may also be present because of hypovolemia. Prolonged lack of protein synthesis and increased degrading of protein leads to muscle wasting and weight loss. Hypovolemic shock can also occur and lead to death if not treated promptly.

Compensation for metabolic acidosis results in deep labored respirations (Kussmaul's respirations) that are "fruity" in odor. This compensation eventually results in lowered partial pressure of arterial carbon dioxide values (compensatory respiratory alkalosis). (See *Understanding the effects of insulin deficiency.*)

Type 2 diabetes

In type 2 diabetes, the pancreas actually makes enough insulin; however, because the cell doesn't recognize the insulin, body tissue cells exhibit resistance.

Glucose enters the circulation from ingested nutrients in the GI tract as well as from the hepatic processes of glycogenolysis and gluconeogenesis. Because of the resistance to insulin, circulating glucose can't be metabolized.

Despite the availability of insulin, hyperglycemia occurs leading to similar but not identical signs and symptoms of

UNDERSTANDING THE EFFECTS OF INSULIN DEFICIENCY

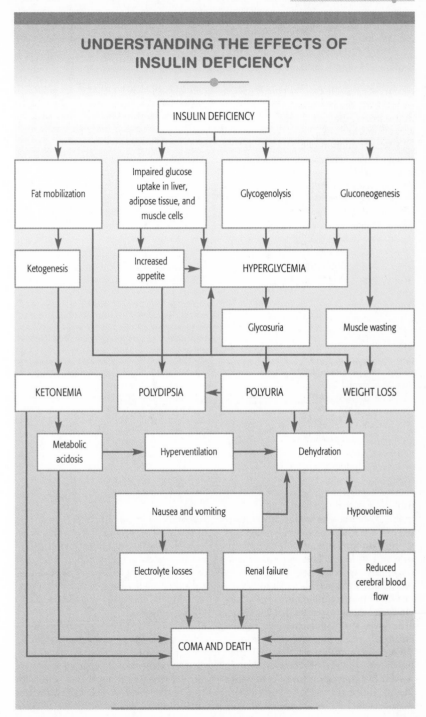

UNDERSTANDING TYPE 2 DIABETES

In type 2 diabetes, glucose enters the circulation from the ingested nutrients in the GI tract as well as from the hepatic processes of glycogenolysis and gluconeogenesis. The body tissue cells exhibit resistance to insulin and subsequently the circulating glucose cannot be metabolized. This illustration highlights the key risks factors and subsequent events associated with the development of type 2 diabetes.

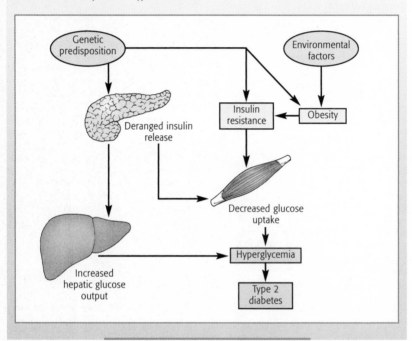

type 1 diabetes. The initial symptoms of polyuria, polydipsia, and polyphagia are present but in a more subtle form than in type 1 diabetes. The presence of endogenous insulin in type 2 diabetes suppresses the lipolysis that leads to the production of ketone bodies and subsequent ketoacidosis associated with type 1 diabetes. (See *Understanding type 2 diabetes*.)

A more common occurrence in patients with type 2 diabetes is hyperosmolar hyperglycemic nonketotic syndrome, especially in those who can't respond independently to the sensation of thirst. This condition is characterized by high plasma osmolarity, blood glucose in excess of 600 mg/dl, the absence of ketoacidosis, and sensory depression. It's a life-threatening event, resulting in 10% to 50% mortality in patients older than age 64.

Diabetes in elderly people

Latent autoimmune diabetes of aging (LADA) refers to a slow, progressive form of type 1 diabetes that accounts for 10% of cases seen in elderly people. Initially, these individuals don't require insulin to manage the condition, even though the immune markers of type 1 diabetes are present. Consequently, a number of cases progress to dependence on insulin. The evidence suggests that in LADA, the genetic predisposition is less marked than in patients diagnosed at younger ages. Both type 1 diabetes and LADA have features in common, such as insulitis and the presence of antibodies. Progression to beta cell destruction varies according to the age when hyperglycemia is diagnosed. What this means is that when the age of diagnosis is more advanced as in the LADA patients, the amount of remaining beta cell mass is higher, and the need for insulin control may be delayed.

Selected references

American Diabetes Association. "National Diabetes Fact Sheet" [Online]. Available at: *www.diabetes.org.*

American Diabetes Association. "Report of the Expert Committee on the Diagnosis and Classification of Diabetes Mellitus," *Diabetes Care* 26(Suppl. 1):S5-S20, January 2003.

Aronda, V.R. and Henry, R.R. "Incretin Hormones in Diabetes and Metabolism," Medscape Continuing Medical Education. May 18, 2004. Available at: *www.medscape.com/viewprogram/ 3075_pnt.*

Aronoff, S.L., et al. "Glucose Metabolism and Regulation: Beyond Insulin and Glucagon," *Diabetes Spectrum* 17(3):183-90, July 2004.

Centers for Disease Control and Prevention. "National Diabetes Fact Sheet: General Information and National Estimates on Diabetes in the United States" [Online]. Atlanta, Ga.: U.S. Department of Health and Human Services, Centers for Disease Control and Prevention, 2005. Available at: *www.cdc.gov/diabetes/pubs/ estimates05.htm.*

Copstead, L., and Banasik, J. *Pathophysiology,* 3rd ed. Philadelphia: W.B. Saunders Co., 2005.

Franz, M.J., ed. *Diabetes and Complications: A CORE Curriculum for Diabetes Education,* 4th ed. Chicago: American Association of Diabetes Educators, 2001.

"Gluconeogenesis: Regulation of Glycolysis and Gluconeogenesis" [Online]. Available at: *www.rpi.edu/dept/bcbp/ molbiochem/MBWeb/mb1/part2/ gluconeo.htm.*[2005 November 5].

Hussain, A.N., and Vincent, M.T. "Diabetes Mellitus, Type 1" [Online]. Available at: *www.emedicine.com/ MED/topic546.htm.*

National Diabetes Education Program National Institutes of Health and Centers for Disease Control and Prevention. Available at: *www.ndep.nih.gov.*

National Diabetes Information Clearinghouse. National Diabetes Statistics. NIH publication. 02-3892. Fact sheet. Available at: *www.diabetes.niddk.nih.gov.*

Ratner, R.E. "Expert Column: Therapeutic Role of Incretin Mimetics," *Medscape Diabetes and Endocrinology* 7(1) [Online]. Available at: *www.medscape. com/viewarticle/506475_print.* [2005 June 27].

Shuldiner, A.R., and McLenithan, J.C. "Genes and Pathophysiology of Type 2 Diabetes: More Than Just the Randle Cycle All Over Again," *The Journal of Clinical Investigation* 114(10):1414-417, November 2004.

Rorsman, P. "Insulin Secretion: Function and Therapy of Pancreatic Beta-cells in Diabetes," *British Journal of Diabetes and Vascular Disease* 5(4):187-91, 2005. Available at: *www.medscape.com/viewarticle/ 514155?src=search.*

Tuomilehto, J., et al. "Prevention of Type 2 Diabetes Mellitus by Changes in Lifestyle Among Subjects with Impaired Glucose Tolerance," *The New England Journal of Medicine* 344(18): 1343-350, May 2001.

Assessment and diagnosis

Diabetes is typically classified as type 1 or type 2 diabetes mellitus, gestational diabetes, and other specific types depending on the underlying cause. All types of diabetes mellitus involve hyperglycemia and its associated signs and symptoms. However, some differences do exist in terms of patient presentation.

TYPE 1 CLINICAL PICTURE

A diagnosis of type 1 diabetes requires a genetic predisposition in addition to an environmental trigger (see chapter 2 for a more in-depth description of causes). With type 1 diabetes, considered an autoimmune disease, the destruction of beta cells can take place over as many as 9 years. In fact, 80% to 90% of functioning beta cells are completely destroyed before the onset of hyperglycemia and associated symptoms. With glucose traveling freely and building up in the blood, hyperglycemia ensues. Subsequently, the body attempts to rid itself of excess glucose via the renal system; the renal threshold is approximately 180 mg/dl for most individuals. Therefore, excess glucose appears in the urine (*glycosuria*), which leads to excessive urination (*polyuria*) and an acute state of dehydration. This leads to excessive thirst (*polydipsia*).

Excessive appetite (*polyphagia*) is a direct result of the body's attempt to increase glucose intake for energy pro-

duction. However, due to the lack of insulin, further hyperglycemia ensues.

The severity of polyuria, polydipsia, and polyphagia are in direct proportion to the level of hyperglycemia.

The patient with type 1 diabetes usually demonstrates rapid weight loss as a result of a reduction in subcutaneous fat and muscle wasting. Because the body can't utilize insulin for glucose transport into the cell, it begins to consume stored protein and fat for energy production. Lipolysis (breakdown of fat for energy), gluconeogenesis (production of new glucose by the liver), and glycogenolysis (breakdown of liver-stored glycogen into glucose) lead to the release of increased amounts of free fatty acids (FFA) and glycerol. The release of hepatic enzymes in response to low insulin levels leads to the conversion of FFA to ketone bodies.

As ketones accumulate, a state of acidosis develops. As the body attempts to neutralize the ketosis, additional symptoms develop including chest pain secondary to Kussmaul's respirations (rapid breathing not related to activity), acute abdominal pain secondary to hepatic gluconeogenesis, and severe dehydration secondary to the hyperosmotic state. When patients arrive at the emergency department with the initial onset of type 1 diabetes, they're usually in a state of diabetic ketoacidosis (DKA). (See *Events leading to DKA*. Also see

EVENTS LEADING TO DKA

Patients with type 1 diabetes commonly demonstrate diabetic ketoacidosis (DKA). This flowchart highlights the major events that occur due to the insulin deficiency.

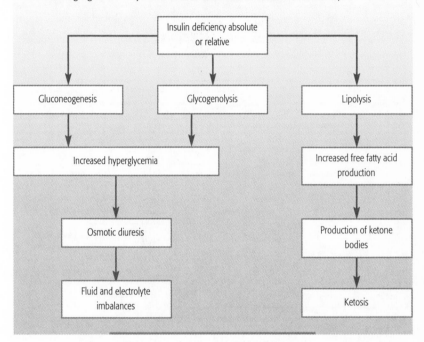

chapter 10 for a more in-depth discussion of DKA.)

Latent Autoimmune Diabetes in Adults (LADA) is a slower and more progressive destruction of the beta cells, but results in the same lack of insulin seen in type 1 diabetes. As many as 10% of people diagnosed with type 2 diabetes who require insulin regimens, may in fact have LADA. The differentiation of type 2 diabetes requiring insulin therapy from LADA can be made in 90% of the cases through testing for islet cell antibodies, anti-insulin antibodies, or autoantibodies to glutamic acid decarboxylase.

TYPE 2 CLINICAL PICTURE

With type 2 diabetes, hyperglycemia also occurs. Like type 1 diabetes, the patient experiences polyuria, polydipsia, and polyphagia. The similarities end there, however. Type 2 diabetes is commonly seen in people older than age 30 (although it may develop at any age). However, according to the American Association of Diabetes Educators (AADE), type 2 diabetes now accounts for 30% to 50% of childhood-onset diabetes. This increased incidence in children is a direct reflection of the lifestyle choices being made. As children are less physically active and making poor food choices, their weight is increasing;

DIFFERENTIATING TYPE 1 AND TYPE 2 DIABETES

Although type 1 and type 2 diabetes both involve hyperglycemia, other signs and symptoms present differently. This chart highlights these differences.

	TYPE 1 DIABETES	TYPE 2 DIABETES
Symptom onset	Rapid	Gradual
Age of onset	Younger than age 30	Older than age 30
Duration of symptoms from onset	Less than 2 days	More than 2 days
Polyuria	Yes	Yes
Polydipsia	Yes	Yes
Polyphagia	Yes	Yes
Body type	Thin, emaciated	Obese, increased abdominal girth
Weight change	Weight loss	Possible loss, but usually weight gain or weight staying the same
Vision change	Yes	Yes
Skin change	No	Dry, itchy skin
Wounds	Not usually present at time of diagnosis	Typically slow to heal
Strength	Weak and tired	Weak and tired

therefore, insulin resistance increases, resulting in type 2 diabetes.

The onset of symptoms of type 1 diabetes is rapid and requires immediate medical attention; however, symptoms of type 2 diabetes are more subtle and tend to develop over a longer period of time. (See *Differentiating type 1 and type 2 diabetes.*)

With type 2 diabetes, insulin is present, but there may be difficulty with production or with insulin resistance. Thus, ketones are rarely present in the body, and the person doesn't develop ketoacidosis.

With the continued production of insulin, although it may be less than

what's required by the body at that time or may be used inadequately by the body, glucose isn't able to be transported into the muscle and fat cells. As a result, symptoms may be dismissed by the individual as normal signs of aging. For example, polyuria is usually present, but it's typically blamed on the use of diuretics or the individual's increased thirst and increased liquid intake, which leads him to urinate more frequently. Polyphagia is another commonly misconstrued sign that the person may attribute to an increased desire to eat, with the subsequent increase in visceral fat being viewed as a natural result. Finally, vision changes are typical-

LABORATORY VALUE COMPARISONS

The degree of hyperglycemia as well as other laboratory test results typically differ in type 1 and type 2 diabetes. This chart highlights these differences.

Laboratory value	Type 1 diabetes	Type 2 diabetes
Blood glucose levels	Usually over 300 mg/dl	Usually over 600 mg/dl
Sodium level	Normal or low	Normal or high
Potassium level	High, normal, or low	High, normal, or low

Blood gas levels
    pH
    bicarbonate level
	
	Low
	Low
		
		Normal
		Normal

Serum osmolality	Less than 320 mmol/kg	More than 320 mmol/kg
Ketones	Positive	Usually negative

ly thought of as secondary to advancing years or the need for new prescription lenses.

Weight distribution associated with the onset of type 2 diabetes is usually an increased abdominal girth, with smaller, thinner extremities. Individuals are commonly referred to as having an apple-shape. In addition, they tend to have more fat deposits on the face and neck.

Symptoms present at the time of diagnosis are a reflection of the level of hyperglycemia and the extent of dehydration; many individuals with type 2 diabetes have the same hallmark symptoms as seen in type 1. Other signs and symptoms develop due to the prolonged state of hyperglycemia. The length of time a person with type 2 diabetes can go undiagnosed ranges from 6½ to 12 years. This time frame, however, doesn't include the length of time for which they have had glucose intolerance.

⚡ **ALERT** *Remember, type 1 dia-betes usually has a rapid onset, typically with polydipsia, polyuria,*

polyphagia, weakness, weight loss, dry skin, and ketoacidosis. Type 2 diabetes is typically slow and insidious in onset and usually unaccompanied by overt symptoms.

Hematologically, type 1 and type 2 diabetes also differ. The presence of ketones in type 1 diabetes leads to signs of acidosis and metabolic compensation as well as a weak respiratory alkalosis; whereas type 2 diabetes may present with ketones measuring less than 2+ in a 1:1 dilution, which isn't enough to cause a state of acidosis. For example, blood gases vary with ketoacidosis, resulting in a lowered, more acidic pH value. The bicarbonate level will be affected as the body attempts to eliminate, or blow off, the ketone bodies via the respiratory system. Because of the severe dehydration, both types result in altered electrolyte levels, but in different ways. (See *Laboratory value comparisons*.)

ASSESSMENT FINDINGS FOR TYPE 1 AND TYPE 2 DIABETES

———●———

This chart provides a comparative review of findings based on body systems that you may assess in a patient with type 1 and type 2 diabetes.

AREA OF ASSESSMENT	TYPE 1 DIABETES	TYPE 2 DIABETES
Integumentary	■ Hot, dry, flushed face ■ Cool extremities ■ Dry mucous membranes ■ Poor skin turgor ■ Temperature elevated, or decreased	■ Hot, dry, flushed face or possible normal ■ Cool extremities ■ Dry mucous membranes ■ Poor skin turgor ■ Temperature elevated ■ Taut, shiny, hairless skin in lower extremities ■ History of slow healing wounds
Oral	■ Normal	■ Evidence of periodontal disease, such as gingivitis, caries, loss of teeth, broken teeth, burning tongue, or gingival bleeding
Ocular	■ Blurry vision ■ Dry, gritty eyes ■ Usually normal vision at diagnosis ■ Sunken eyeballs ■ Soft eyeballs ■ Hypotonia	■ Blurry vision ■ Dry, gritty eyes ■ Retinopathy ■ Sunken eyeballs ■ Soft eyeballs ■ Hypotonia
Cardiovascular	■ Hypotension or orthostatic hypotension (drop of 20 mm Hg when going from sitting to standing within 1 minute's time) ■ Weak, thready pulse ■ Electrocardiogram (ECG) changes ■ Decreased jugular vein filling ■ Tachycardia or bradycardia	■ Low, normal, or high blood pressure ■ Orthostatic hypotension ■ Rapid, thready pulse ■ Signs of shock ■ ECG changes ■ Decreased jugular vein filling ■ Tachycardia
Respiratory	■ Kussmaul's respirations, or hyperpnea ■ Acetone breath (fruity odor) ■ Complaints of shortness of breath unrelated to level of exertion	■ Normal
Neurologic	■ Mentation changes including alert, stuporous, or comatose ■ Hyporeflexia	■ More likely to have mentation changes including lethargy, mild to severe confusion, coma ■ Hemiparesis, hemisensory deficits, aphasia, and seizures ■ Normal, decreased, or increased reflexes ■ Positive Babinski's sign
Gastrointestinal	■ Nausea, vomiting ■ Decreased bowel sounds ■ Abdominal bloating	■ Normal to mild nausea ■ Constipation

ASSESSMENT FINDINGS FOR
TYPE 1 AND TYPE 2 DIABETES *(continued)*

AREA OF ASSESSMENT	TYPE 1 DIABETES	TYPE 2 DIABETES
Renal	■ Dark, concentrated, sticky urine, high specific gravity ■ Polyuria ■ Nocturia ■ Bedwetting in children previously trained	■ Sticky urine ■ Polyuria
Neuromuscular	■ Muscle weakness ■ Muscle wasting ■ Decreased muscle tone	■ Muscle weakness
General	■ Polydipsia ■ Polyphagia or anorexia ■ Weight loss (up to 30% of total body weight in young children) ■ Increased irritability	■ Polydipsia ■ Normal appetite or polyphagia ■ Weight loss or gain ■ Possible increased irritability

EVALUATION OF SYSTEMIC EFFECTS

All human tissues come in contact with blood because it's responsible for oxygenating these tissues. When the blood glucose level is high, those hyperglycemic levels also affect the tissues throughout the body. Diabetes can cause signs and symptoms as well as complications in all areas of the body secondary to hyperglycemia. Often, it's the emergence of a complication of diabetes that causes a person to visit his health care provider, which in turn leads to the diagnosis of type 2 diabetes for the first time.

The negative consequences of chronic hyperglycemia are generally divided into macrovascular and microvascular complications. In addition to this, other long-term complications of diabetes center on the nervous system resulting in neuropathy. (See *Assessment findings for type 1 and type 2 diabetes.*)

Cardiovascular

Individuals with type 2 diabetes commonly present with hypertension and hyperlipidemia, secondary to the insulin resistance. The common lipid profile for a person with diabetes includes a low high-density-lipoprotein level, an elevated low-density-lipoprotein level, and an elevated triglyceride level. Due to insulin resistance, endogenous insulin production increases, leading to a state of hyperinsulinemia. As insulin levels increase, the amount of tubular reabsorption of sodium also increases, leading to increased blood volume, which in turn leads to increased blood pressure. This can occur in children with type 2 diabetes as well.

Hypertension is diagnosed when blood pressure is greater than or equal to 140/90 mm Hg. It's also one of the major risk factors for cardiovascular disease. Type 2 diabetes is also considered

TREATMENT OF
HYPERGLYCEMIC-INDUCED DEHYDRATION

If your patient exhibits dehydration as a result of hyperglycemia, follow these steps:
1. Correct fluid and electrolyte imbalances.
2. Correct hyperglycemia and maintain euglycemia, correcting acidosis in type 1 diabetes.
3. Prevent complications caused by the treatment of hyperglycemia, such as hypoglycemia or other fluid and electrolyte imbalances.
4. Treat underlying medical conditions.
5. Provide education for the ongoing self-management of diabetes in correlation with physician-directed care.

an independent risk factor for cardiovascular disease, as is hypertension. Subsequently, the American Diabetes Association (ADA) recommends keeping blood pressure at less than 130/80 mm Hg for adults and to the 90th percentile for the corresponding age-group for children.

Hyperglycemia leads to dehydration, and the person with type 1 diabetes tends to be hypotensive as a result of decreased intravascular volumes caused by severe dehydration. When blood pressure drops, typically the cardiovascular system responds with a rapid heartbeat. This may be identified as a weak, thready pulse.

A person with type 1 diabetes may also have a diagnosis of hypertension. However, because the hypertension is commonly secondary to nephropathy, the person is less likely to have hypertension at the time of diagnosis than the person with type 2 diabetes.

Fluids and electrolytes
Dehydration due to polyuria is common. Other signs of dehydration seen in both type 1 and type 2 diabetes include poor skin turgor and dry mucous membranes (despite the patient's excessive fluid intake). Older adults commonly lose the ability to sense when they're thirsty and don't respond by drinking extra fluids, thereby contribut-

ing further to the severity of the dehydration. Decreased jugular vein filling can be seen from below when the patient is in a supine position.

With profound dehydration, the patient may develop sunken eyeballs, or soft eyeballs. If fixed, dilated pupils and hypotonia (uncoordinated eye movements) are detected; these are very late signs and suggestive of a poor prognosis.

Dehydration can prove to be the most critical problem for a person with severe hyperglycemia. The patient needs I.V. fluid replacement and close, frequent monitoring. Initially, fluid replacement for an adult depends on the degree of dehydration and the patient's cardiovascular status, which may be severely compromised, especially if the patient is elderly. (See *Treatment of hyperglycemic-induced dehydration.*)

Potassium imbalances
Insulin is one of the mediators, or regulators, of potassium levels within the body, and a relative or absolute insulin deficiency also affects potassium levels. Insulin assists with the movement of potassium into liver and muscle cells, so the lack of insulin leads to an increase in serum potassium levels. As insulin is administered to correct hyperglycemia, potassium follows glucose into the cells, thereby leading to the opposite effect, a hypokalemic state.

ECG FINDINGS WITH POTASSIUM IMBALANCES

These rhythm strips highlight the electrocardiogram (ECG) changes seen with potassium imbalances in a patient with diabetes.

Hyperkalemia

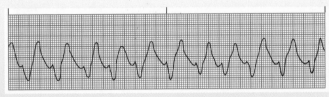

- *P wave:* Widened, flat
- *PR Interval:* Prolonged
- *QRS interval:* Widened, decreased R wave amplitude

- *T wave:* Tall, tented
- *ST segment:* Depressed
- *U wave:* Absent

Hypokalemia

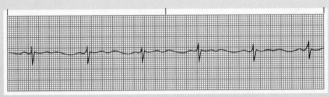

- *P wave:* Slightly peaked
- *PR Interval:* Normal
- *QRS interval:* Normal

- *T wave:* Flattened
- *ST segment:* Depressed
- *U wave:* Prominent

Changes in serum potassium levels can be noted on the patient's electrocardiogram (ECG). A flat T wave or a U wave frequently represents hypokalemia, whereas a spiked or peaked T wave indicates hyperkalemia, along with a widened QRS interval. (See *ECG findings with potassium imbalances.*)

Bradycardia rhythms can develop with hyperkalemia, which can lead to cardiac irritability and the increased potential for arrhythmias. Serial ECGs can reflect the changes in potassium levels as the patient is rehydrated and the hyperglycemia corrected.

Based on potassium levels, potassium most likely will be added to the patient's I.V. fluids at some point, because insulin will push potassium into the cells when transporting glucose from the bloodstream. In addition, the serum potassium levels decline with correction in blood osmolality. This decline is further compounded by the renal excretion of potassium secondary to increased hydration and renal perfusion.

If the patient has hypokalemia, signs and symptoms include skeletal muscle weakness, decreased or absent deep tendon reflexes, arrhythmias, shallow or gasping respirations, vomiting, paralytic ileus, and the inability to concentrate urine. Hypokalemia can develop rapidly and be fatal. Diligent, focused assessment is necessary.

If the patient has hyperkalemia, signs and symptoms include skeletal muscle weakness, numbness and tingling, and possible respiratory paralysis due to progression of the weakness. Milder manifestations include neuromuscular irritability, such as restlessness, stomach cramps, and diarrhea.

Integumentary

Changes in the skin occur with blood glucose fluctuations. With high levels, the skin is typically hot, dry, and flushed. Body temperature may be elevated due to hyperthermia, secondary to the acute onset of severe dehydration and the increase in the release of catecholamines, which also contributes to a flushed, hot face. However, if there's cardiac involvement, the person may present with cool skin, or even clammy skin that's more commonly associated with hypoglycemia. This sign can be due to the involvement of autonomic neuropathy, leading to more atypical signs and symptoms as opposed to the expected angina.

The skin on the lower extremities is typically described as taut and shiny, with hair loss. With a decrease in circulation to the lower extremities, hair is lost because circulation is focused on more important tissues and structures. Additionally, with the decrease in circulation to the lower extremities, and the sustained increase in blood glucose levels, wounds heal more slowly, particularly when they're located on the lower leg or foot.

Neurologic

For a person with diabetes who's in a hyperosmolar hyperglycemic state, the level of dehydration can be such that the viscosity of the blood tends to be markedly elevated (greater than 320 mmol/kg). This may cause focal neurologic signs, such as hemiparesis, hemisensory deficits, and aphasia. Mentation changes may also result from the serum osmolality, more so than from the dehydration itself. Only on serological review is hyperglycemia identified and noted.

Just as a person can present with cardiovascular manifestations or complications, such as an acute myocardial infarction, a patient may also present with an acute stroke. According to the AADE, studies show the rate of mortality after a stroke for a person with diabetes is 3 to 5 times higher than in a nondiabetic person, regardless of gender.

Hyperglycemia triggers changes in the metabolism of proteins, lipids, and other factors leading to the production of advanced glycosylated end products or oxidative stress. (See *Development of diabetic autonomic neuropathy*.) Oxidative stress prevents oxygen and other nutrients from reaching the cell and, without oxygen, the cells die. The result is autonomic neuropathy, the inability of the nerves of the autonomic nervous system to respond as expected. Although typically a late symptom, autonomic neuropathy can lead to gastric symptoms and erectile dysfunction.

Gastrointestinal

Compounding the difficulty in identifying the true cause of diabetes in an undiagnosed person can be the involvement of the GI system. Especially in type 1 diabetes, the presence of nausea and vomiting can be misconstrued as stomach flu. In some individuals, the acute abdominal symptoms can also be mistaken for appendicitis requiring immediate emergency surgery because the person can develop absent bowel sounds, rebound tenderness, or a rigid abdomen.

Nausea and vomiting are milder and less common in type 2 diabetes. The abdominal pain, nausea, and vomiting in type 1 diabetes are believed to be related to the ketosis or acidotic state, there-

DEVELOPMENT OF DIABETIC AUTONOMIC NEUROPATHY

The underlying cause of autonomic neuropathy is hyperglycemia, which may lead to abnormal nerve responses to stimuli, damaged or dysfunctional nerves, or actual nerve cell demise. This flowchart shows the sequence of events leading to autonomic neuropathy.

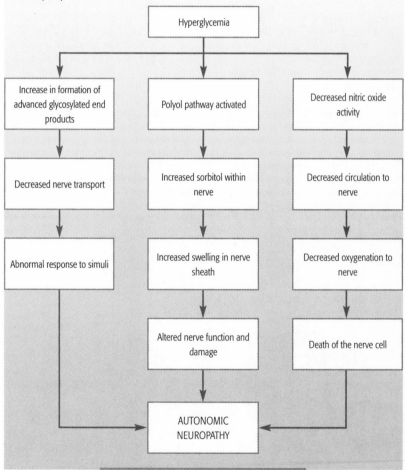

by explaining why people with type 2 diabetes experience them to a lesser degree.

Ocular

People with high glucose levels may also exhibit vision changes, which they may not mention unless questioned directly about them. Blurry vision is common when glucose levels have exceeded the renal threshold. As the kidney attempts to rid the body of excess glucose, it pulls fluids from various parts of the body. The eye is one of these areas. Transient osmotic changes in the lens occur, directly related to the fluctuating glucose levels. However, vision may not return to normal for as long as 6 to 8 weeks after blood glucose stabilization.

Ironically, if a person is experiencing hypoglycemia, vision is also affected. Dimming of vision, bright flashing lights, and double vision are commonly reported during these episodes. These changes disappear immediately when euglycemia is reached.

Retinopathy can also be detected in a person with hyperglycemia, but it tends to occur more frequently with type 2 diabetes. That's because type 1 symptoms occur more rapidly, and a long period of elevated glucose levels prior to diagnosis is lacking. However, the person with type 2 diabetes may be undiagnosed for an extended period and may have had a more prolonged hyperglycemic state.

Diabetes remains the single greatest cause of blindness in the United States, with diabetics being 25 times more likely to have eye disease than the rest of the population. At the time of diagnosis, more than 1 in 5 patients with type 2 diabetes already have retinopathy. Based on this staggering statistic, screening for retinopathy must be included as early in the process as possible. The degree of retinopathy relates directly to glycemic control as well as blood pressure control.

The retina is the structure of the eye that's responsible for focusing images and light. Those images are then relayed along the optic nerve to the brain for interpretation of the image viewed. Retinopathy occurs in various stages as a result of the length of time the retina has been exposed to adverse conditions; the more advanced the stage, the more

IDENTIFYING DIABETIC RETINOPATHY

These illustrations depict two of the possible changes that may occur with diabetic retinopathy: small retinal hemorrhages and microaneurysms.

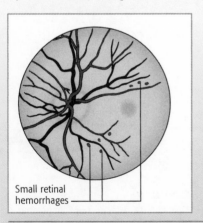

Small retinal hemorrhages

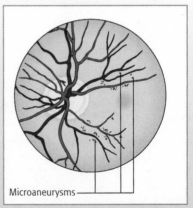

Microaneurysms

Source: Weber, J., and Kelly, J. *Health Assessment in Nursing*, 3rd ed. Philadelphia: Lippincott Williams & Wilkins, 2007.

severe the condition. Non-proliferative diabetic retinopathy (NPDR) involves the development of microaneurysms, the leaking of fluid and lipids from blood vessels, actual hemorrhages from the vasculature, and soft exudates caused by nerve fiber layers infarcting, referred to as cotton-wool spots. NPDR doesn't affect the visual field. It progresses to proliferative retinopathy (see chapter 9, Management of complications, for more information). (See *Identifying diabetic retinopathy*.)

If new blood vessels (neovascularization) begin to develop on their own in response to retinal ischemia, the retinopathy has progressed to proliferative diabetic retinopathy. The difficulty with neovascularization is that these new blood vessels are extremely fragile and are at increased risk for rupture, further compounding the problem.

According to the AADE, more than 90% of all vision loss can be prevented if retinopathy is identified early and the person receives appropriate treatment. Individuals with type 2 diabetes need to have an annual dilated eye examination starting with the year of their diagnosis. Individuals with type 1 diabetes should have annual dilated eye examinations starting within 5 years of diagnosis.

Renal

Just as the eye is comprised of microvasculature, so too is the renal system. Thus, the person with diabetes requires regular screening for renal involvement. If the individual has a history of hypertension, which is now aggravated by hyperglycemia and dehydration, blood urea nitrogen and creatinine levels may be elevated. Serum creatinine is an indirect measure of glomerular filtration rate, and slight elevations may represent a major loss of renal function. Acute renal failure can be caused by dehydration and, if unidentified and untreated, can progress to chronic renal failure.

Blacks with diabetes are 4 to 5 times more likely to develop end-stage renal disease (ESRD) than Whites with diabetes. Latinos and Native Americans have an even greater risk, with an average 6.3 times greater incidence than Whites. Due to the higher rates of insulin resistance, type 2 diabetes, and hypertension in these populations, initial urine examinations should include screening for microalbuminuria as well as specific gravity and infections.

Non-system-specific manifestations

Periodontal disease is ranked as the sixth most common complication of diabetes. Poor oral hygiene, in combination with hyperglycemia, is the most common reason. The immune system is compromised when a person is in a hyperglycemic state, which leads to increased susceptibility to infections. When good oral hygiene isn't practiced, the bacteria remain in direct contact with a compromised gum line (due to the hyperglycemia), thereby exposing the person to an increased risk of periodontal disease.

DIAGNOSIS

Criteria are highly specific for a diagnosis of diabetes mellitus. Definitive guidelines have been established for populations that should be screened.

Blood tests

The ADA publishes a Position Statement on the Clinical Practice Recommendations for caring for a person with diabetes. According to *Diagnosis and Classification of Diabetes Mellitus*, there are three ways in which diabetes can be diagnosed conclusively. They include a casual plasma glucose level with overt symptoms of diabetes, fasting plasma glucose level, and an oral glucose tolerance test.

Glucose binds to hemoglobin, particularly the glycosylated hemoglobin (HbA_{1c}) component. The average lifespan of a red blood cell is 90 to 120 days, thereby reflecting the average blood glucose level for 3 months. However, HbA_{1c}, isn't considered a reliable

LABORATORY TEST RESULTS AND THEIR IMPLICATIONS

This chart identifies the results of two blood tests used for diagnosing diabetes.

	NORMAL	PREDIABETES	DIABETES
Fasting plasma glucose	< 100 mg/dl	100 to 125 mg/dl	≥ 126 mg/dl
Casual plasma glucose	< 140 mg/dl	140 to 199 mg/dl	≥ 200 mg/dl

indicator for diagnosis of diabetes. The drawbacks of the HbA_{1c} test, as identified by Richard K. Bernstein, a recognized expert on diabetes and its complications, are that it's an average value. Additionally, he states that blood glucose may need to be elevated as long as 24 hours in order to have a long-term effect on the HbA_{1c} level. Therefore, if a person demonstrates hyperglycemia only postprandially and returns to euglycemic or even hypoglycemic levels the remainder of the time, the results of the HbA_{1c} may appear to be in the normal range. However, damage is still being done to tissues and organs from the bouts of hyperglycemia. As a result, this test should be reserved for use as a measure of glycemic control in an established patient with diabetes. After an individual is determined to have diabetes, a baseline HbA_{1c} level should be drawn for comparison in 3 months, but not as a diagnostic tool. (See *Laboratory test results and their implications*.)

Casual plasma glucose
A casual plasma glucose (CPG) level refers to a blood glucose level obtained randomly during the day, without regard to previous intake of food. The diagnosis of diabetes can be made when this level is greater than or equal to 200 mg/dl, along with signs and symptoms suggestive of diabetes. Those signs and symptoms include polyuria, poly-

dipsia, and unexplained weight loss. In the event that signs and symptoms aren't present, the test would need to be repeated on a subsequent day. In the presence of unequivocal hyperglycemia, the diagnosis may be made based on the results of the initial test.

Fasting plasma glucose
The most commonly used tool for diagnosing diabetes is the fasting plasma glucose (FPG) test. It's the preferred test in children and non-pregnant adults. An FPG greater than 125 mg/dl is definitive for diabetes.

An FPG of 100 to 125 mg/dl indicates impaired fasting glucose. A CPG of 140 to 199 mg/dl leads to the diagnosis of impaired glucose tolerance. These FPG and CPG results together are now considered signs of prediabetes; the numbers are above normal and high enough to cause structural damage, but not high enough to be diagnosed as having diabetes. Prediabetes is a risk factor for the development of diabetes in the future and for cardiovascular disease.

Oral glucose tolerance test
An oral glucose tolerance test (OGTT) isn't recommended for routine use in diagnosing diabetes. According to the ADA, the test is poorly reproducible, more time-consuming, and more expensive than the FPG. Results can also

URINALYSIS RESULTS ASSOCIATED WITH HYPERGLYCEMIA

Routine urinalysis can be an indicator of the need for further screening for diabetes. This chart identifies some typical characteristics associated with hyperglycemia.

CHARACTERISTICS	RESULTS
Odor	Strong, sweet smell (diabetic ketoacidosis [DKA])
pH	Decreased
Protein	Increased
Glucose	Increased
Specific gravity	Increased
Ketones	Present for DKA

be affected by normal aging, smoking during the test, stress, exercise during the test, and inadequate caloric intake in the days before the test. Drugs can also interfere with the test results. They include antihypertensives, anti-inflammatory drugs, aspirin, beta-adrenergic blockers, furosemide, nicotine, hormonal contraceptives, psychiatric drugs, steroids, and thiazide diuretics.

However, the OGTT can be useful if a person is recognized as having an impaired fasting glucose level that falls within the prediabetes range, or has a clinical condition such as neuropathy indicative of chronic hyperglycemia that isn't showing up on the FPG.

For an OGTT, laboratory guidelines indicate that an adequate diet must be consumed before the test for at least 3 days. The diet should contain an average of 150 g of carbohydrate per day. On the day of the test, the patient fasts for 12 hours.

An FPG is taken, and if the result is over 200 mg/dl, an OGTT isn't conducted because this level is considered

unequivocal hyperglycemia in a fasting state. If the FPG results are below 200 mg/dl, the patient is asked to drink a 75 to 100 g glucose load. A diagnosis of diabetes is made if the result of a 2-hour postload glucose result is greater than or equal to 200 mg/dl. In a child, the glucose load would be calculated at 1.75 g/kg body weight, to a maximum of 75 g. In the absence of unequivocal hyperglycemia, the test should be repeated on a subsequent day. A third testing isn't recommended for routine clinical use.

Urine tests

Routine urinalysis isn't used for the diagnosis of diabetes, but can be an indicator of the need for further screening with one of the blood tests previously mentioned. (See *Urinalysis results associated with hyperglycemia*.) At the point that glucose is detected in the urine, the renal threshold has been reached, thus causing the kidneys to excrete excess glucose in the urine. Glycosuria isn't always considered abnormal and can be present in pregnancy, after a high-carbohydrate meal, or if there has been damage to the renal tubules as in kidney disease. In addition, certain drugs, such as cephalosporins, diuretics, estrogens, lithium, nafcillin, nicotinic acid in large doses, and I.V. glucose infusions, can cause increased urine glucose levels.

Evidence of protein (albumin) in the urine indicates damage to the glomerular filtration membrane. Urinary microalbuminuria shouldn't be ignored. Microalbuminuria is an early indicator of impending kidney disease and if treated can prevent or delay progression to ESRD. Many people with type 2 diabetes have had an existing state of hyperglycemia for an indeterminate amount of time and, when in combination with hypertension, renal disease can be present at the time of diagnosis.

Proteinuria may result from other conditions, such as preeclampsia, nephritic syndrome, glomerulonephritis, amyloidosis, and multiple myeloma. False positives may arise from severe emotional stress, excessive exercise, cold baths, use of radiopaque dye within the previous 3 days, or urine contaminated by vaginal secretions. Medications causing increased protein levels include aminoglycosides, amphotericin B, cephalosporins, griseofulvin, lithium, methicillin, nafcillin, nephrotoxic drugs, oxacillin, penicillin G, phenazopyridine, polymixin B, salicylates, sulfonamides, tolbutamide, and vancomycin.

Ketonuria is generally indicative of DKA and type 1 diabetes. However, other interfering factors may be present. For example, a diet severely restricted in carbohydrates and high in protein and fat can also lead to ketonuria. Drugs, such as isoniazid, isopropanol, levodopa, phenazopyridine may also be a cause. Acute febrile illness, especially in infants and children will also result in the production of ketones.

Diabetes mellitus is a systemic condition, with multisystem involvement.

As a result, the assessment of an individual presenting with diabetes needs to be evaluated for more than the presence of elevated glucose levels.

Selected references

American Association of Diabetes Educators. *A Core Curriculum for Diabetes Education: Diabetes and Complications,* 5th ed. Chicago: American Association of Diabetes Educators, 2003.

American Association of Diabetes Educators. *A Core Curriculum for Diabetes Education: Diabetes in the Life Cycle and Research,* 5th ed. Chicago: American Association of Diabetes Educators, 2003.

American Diabetes Association. "Diagnosis and Classification of Diabetes Mellitus," *Diabetes Care* 28(Suppl 1):S37-S42, Janurary 2005.

American Diabetes Association. "Standards of Medical Care in Diabetes," *Diabetes Care* 28(Suppl 1):S4-S36, January 2005.

Bernstein, R.K. *Dr. Bernstein's Diabetes Solution.* Boston: Little, Brown & Co., 2003.

Huether, S.E., and McCance, K.L. *Understanding Pathophysiology,* 2nd ed. St. Louis: Mosby–Year Book, Inc., 2000.

Kaufman, F.R. *Diabesity: The Obesity-Diabetes Epidemic that Threatens America—and What We Must Do To Stop It.* New York: Bantam Books, 2005.

Pagana, K.D., and Pagana, T.J. *Diagnostic and Laboratory Test Reference,* 5th ed. St. Louis: Mosby–Year Book, Inc., 2001.

Thompson, J.M., et al. *Clinical Nursing,* 5th ed. St. Louis: Mosby–Year Book, Inc., 2002.

Vascular Complications of Diabetes, 2nd ed. Cambridge, Mass: Blackwell Scientific Pubs., 2005.

4

Prevention

With the prevalence of diabetes rising so rapidly, strategies directed toward prevention of this epidemic assume the utmost importance. Prevention of type 1 diabetes, while the subject of much research, is still elusive. However, evidence indicates that type 2 diabetes can be prevented.

RESEARCH INITIATIVES

Several randomized controlled clinical trials in different settings have demonstrated that type 2 diabetes can be delayed or even prevented.

Studies worldwide

In a Finnish study, 522 overweight, middle-age subjects with elevated blood glucose levels were randomized to intervention or control groups. The control group received minimal information about meal planning and exercise. The intervention group received extensive education on meal planning, including lowering fat intake to less than 30% of total calories, increasing fiber intake to 15 g per 1,000 calories consumed, and losing 5% or more of their body weight. In addition, they received education on exercising a minimum of 30 minutes per day. After 1 year, total weight loss was 9.2 lb (4.2 kg) in the intervention group and 1.8 lb (0.8 kg) in the control group. In addition, the intervention group showed decreased waist girth and blood glucose and insulin levels. Follow-up averaged 3.2 years, at which time 27 subjects in the intervention group and 59 in the control developed type 2 diabetes. This indicates that the lifestyle changes used in this study were able to decrease the incidence of type 2 diabetes in the intervention group by 58%.

In another study, conducted in China, 5,778 subjects were randomized to an intervention group, which received intensive education on meal planning and exercise targeted at reducing caloric intake and increasing activity levels, or a control group, which received general instructions for meal planning and exercise. After a 6-year follow-up, the intervention group showed a 38% decrease in the incidence of type 2 diabetes compared to the control group.

Diabetes Prevention Program

In the United States, the Diabetes Prevention Program (DPP) was a multicenter randomized controlled trial involving 3,324 adults with impaired glucose tolerance. Subjects were purposely recruited to include various ethnic groups, such as Native Americans, Asians, Blacks, and subjects older than age 60. Subjects were randomized to three groups. One group received 850 mg of metformin twice daily, one received an intensive lifestyle intervention, and the third (the control group) received a placebo and routine meal planning and exercise advice. After a

3-year follow-up, the incidence of type 2 diabetes was 28.9% in the control group, 21.7% in the metformin group, and 14.4% in the intensive lifestyle group. This translates to a 31% reduction in the development of diabetes in the metformin group and a 58% reduction in the lifestyle group.

The goals of the lifestyle intervention were a 7% weight loss, maintenance of that loss, and 150 minutes of physical activity, similar to brisk walking, per week. The lifestyle intervention, taught by specialized case managers, consisted of 16 education sessions using a standard curriculum focused on behavioral self-management strategies for weight loss and maintenance, increase in activity level, and behavior modification. Sessions were done on a one-to-one basis, followed by group sessions for reinforcement. There was frequent contact with participants, supervised activity sessions, and motivational campaigns and individualization of approaches tailored to address ethnic diversity. All interventions incorporated an extensive network for feedback and clinical support. Whereas the lifestyle intervention was effective in all subgroup studies, it was most effective in the older, leaner subjects; the metformin intervention was most effective in the younger, more obese subjects. Additional detailed information about the DPP and the curriculum and activities used are available at no cost at: *www.diabetes.niddk.nih.gov/dm/pubs/preventionprogram/index.htm*.

The interventions used in the DPP were also cost effective. In order to prevent one case of type 2 diabetes using lifestyle intervention, 6 patients needed to be treated; however, using metformin, 13 subjects needed to be treated to prevent one case of the disease.

Other studies

Several studies, in addition to the DPP, have looked at the prevention of type 2 diabetes using medications. The STOP-NIDDM (non-insulin-dependent diabetes mellitus, now called *type 2 diabetes*) study, done in several European countries, showed that acarbose, an alpha glucosidase inhibitor, prevented the progression to type 2 diabetes in subjects with impaired glucose tolerance by 25% over 3 years. In addition, treatment with acarbose increased the reversion to normal glucose tolerance, although there was a 30% drop-out rate, most likely due to the drug's adverse effects. Although the design, methodology, and results of this study have been questioned, it has provided some impetus for current research.

The Troglitazone in Prevention of Diabetes (TRIPOD) study — a placebo controlled study — showed that the insulin sensitizer, troglitazone, could delay or prevent the development of type 2 diabetes in Latino females who had gestational diabetes. After 30 months, treatment with troglitazone significantly prevented the incidence of type 2 diabetes in these high-risk women. However, troglitazone is no longer available and it isn't known if the currently available insulin sensitizers, pioglitazone and rosiglitazone, would have the same effect.

PREVENTION STRATEGIES

The DPP is considered the landmark study in the United States, demonstrating that type 2 diabetes can be prevented. However, it may not be feasible to translate the lifestyle change methodology used in the DPP to "real world settings." Therefore, identification of strategies that can be used in varied settings is important.

Risk factor identification

One of the first steps in preventing type 2 diabetes is to identify those individuals at high risk for developing this disorder. Diabetes is more common in people older than age 60, in those who are obese, and in those who have sedentary lifestyles. In addition, risk factors for type 2 diabetes include a family history of type 2 diabetes, and ethnicity, such as in Blacks, Asians, Latinos, and Pacific Islanders. (For more information about risk factors for diabetes, see chapters 2 and 3.)

If you suspect that a patient might be at risk for type 2 diabetes, you can suggest that he take the diabetes risk test at the American Diabetes Association (ADA) Web site: *www.diabetes.org/risk-test.jsp.* (See *Diabetes risk test,* pages 40 and 41.)

Because of the frequency with which impaired glucose tolerance (IGT) and fasting plasma glucose (FPG) progress to type 2 diabetes, the ADA uses the term "prediabetes" to refer to these conditions. Individuals with prediabetes have fasting blood glucose levels between 100 and 125 mg/dl.

Lifestyle changes

A major area of diabetes prevention involves lifestyle changes, which can be addressed at several levels. These levels include communities; specific settings, such as businesses, schools, and health care settings; and individual encounters with at-risk patients.

Community interventions

Because major risk factors for type 2 diabetes are related to lifestyle, community interventions to address lifestyles are appropriate. Interventions targeted at weight loss or even weight maintenance can significantly decrease the progression of prediabetes to diabetes.

Community interventions focused on increasing activity levels have also shown success. These activities can include exercise in senior centers, parks, churches, and shopping malls, which frequently encourage "group mall walks" before businesses open. Community efforts have been effective in other chronic diseases, such as cancer and atherosclerosis. Lessons from these conditions show that community interventions must be specific for a particular area, taking into consideration the cultural preferences of the people and the geography and history of the area.

Geography and history can influence the community's ability and desire to change. Keep in mind that what works in one community may not work in another.

Community efforts to prevent diabetes are most productive if they focus on healthy eating to enhance weight control and prevent the obesity that commonly leads to type 2 diabetes. The link between obesity and diabetes is so close that the term "diabesity" is commonly used.

In a Canadian indigenous population, behavior change was targeted using environmentally supportive interventions. The interventions included walking groups, cooking demonstrations, media support, and local promotion. The intervention community was compared to two other communities without the interventions. The intervention community showed significantly decreased body mass index and waist girth, increased knowledge about diabetes, and increased "sweat producing" activity.

In another study, a church-based intervention in New Zealand compared two groups of Western Samoans. The intervention involved diabetes awareness sessions, cooking classes, and exercise groups. The intervention churchgoers showed weight stability (as opposed to weight gain in the comparison group), a significant reduction in waist girth, and an increase in diabetes knowledge and regular physical activity.

One community in Sweden worked with local eating places, including fast food eateries, to list the nutritional breakdown of foods that were served so that consumers would know what they were ordering. As a result, they had the opportunity to choose more healthy foods if they wished. Along with restaurant cooperation, the value of healthy eating was presented in broadcasts and printed in the local media.

Another important community effort is to increase the activity level of its inhabitants. As a society, we're less physi-

DIABETES RISK TEST

The test below, developed by the American Diabetes Association (ADA), determines a person's risk for developing type 2 diabetes. You can print out the test and go over it with the patient or have him take the test on his own. An online version is available at the ADA web site: *www.diabetes.org/risk-test.jsp*.

Risk test
Could your patient have diabetes and not know it?
To find out if your patient is at risk, have him write in the points next to each statement that's true for him. If a statement is *not* true, instruct him to write a zero. Then have him add all the points to get his total score.

	Yes	No
1. My weight is equal to or above that listed in the chart at right.	5 pts	0 pts
2. I am under 65 years old and I get little or no exercise during a usual day.	5 pts	0 pts
3. I am between 45 and 64 years of age.	5 pts	0 pts
4. I am 65 years old or older.	9 pts	0 pts
5. I am a woman who has had a baby weighing more than nine pounds at birth.	1 pts	0 pts
6. I have a sister or brother with diabetes.	1 pts	0 pts
7. I have a parent with diabetes.	1 pts	0 pts

Total points: _____ _____

Scoring 3 to 9 points
Your patient is probably at low risk for currently having diabetes, but may be at future risk, espcially if he's Hispanic, Black, Native American, Asian, or a Pacific Islander.

Scoring 10 or more points
Your patient is at greater risk for having diabetes and should be thoroughly assessed for diabetes at his next office visit.

cally active than we were a century ago, or even a few decades ago. Our mechanized and busy lives often preclude the physical activity necessary for good health and disease prevention, particularly type 2 diabetes. Community efforts targeting this sedentary behavior have been shown to be successful. In one study, researchers showed that creating a supportive environment for increased activity, media involvement, and advertisement of planned activities increased participation in a walking campaign by 33%.

Business interventions
Businesses are another likely location for interventions to prevent type 2 dia-

betes. In New Zealand, the Polynesian workforce in hospitals was studied. The intervention consisted of an educator presenting information, a video, and a 4-month exercise program. After 4 months, the intervention group had more diabetes knowledge and did more exercise compared to baseline. The control group did less exercise than at baseline. One study showed that use of colorful signs near elevators increased the use of stairs.

Group interventions
Group interventions have also targeted youth, the population where prevention of type 2 diabetes can be most effective. A study of adolescent Zuni Pueblo Indi-

At-risk weight chart body mass index

Height without shoes	At-risk weight chart body mass index	Height without shoes	At-risk weight chart body mass index
4'0'	129	5'7"	172
4'1"	133	5'8"	177
5'0"	138	5'9"	182
5'1"	143	5'10"	188
5'2"	147	5'11"	193
5'3"	152	6'0"	199
5'4"	157	6'1"	204
5'5"	162	6'2"	210
5'6"	167	6'3"	216
		6'4"	221

If you weigh the same or more than the amount listed for your height, you may be at risk for diabetes.

Adapted from *www.diabetes.org/risk-test.jsp*. The American Diabetes Association: Alexandria, Virginia, with permission of the publisher.

ans implemented changes that modified the food supply in schools, established supportive networks, emphasized physical activity at teen wellness centers, and provided diabetes education in school. This study showed significant reductions in the consumption of sugary drinks and an increase in glucose-insulin ratios, indicating a decrease in insulin resistance.

In another study involving fifth graders on the Texas-Mexico border, teachers varied in who they presented a lifestyle intervention program to. The study showed that whereas there were no differences in outcomes based on how the intervention program was administered, the program was effective in increasing knowledge, self-efficacy, and nutrition and exercise behaviors. An additional study in Mexican fourth-grade students in San Antonio, Texas, used four social systems — parents, classroom, school cafeteria, and after-school care, to reduce dietary fat intake and nutritional behavior change. There were significant reductions in fat intake and in fat as a percentage of total calories, and increases in the consumption of fruits and vegetables.

It has been shown that an increase of sugary beverages is the leading cause of increased sugar in the diet of children and is associated with obesity as well as insulin resistance and impaired insulin secretion. However, many schools are reluctant to give up vending machines becuase they're a significant source of income. Nonetheless, interventions targeted at removing or decreasing the choices of sugary beverages from vending machines, or even removing the vending machines themselves, seems warranted. Efforts to this end will require the support of parents, teachers, policy makers, and businesses.

Weight control

When working with individuals at risk for type 2 diabetes, health care providers can use several strategies to help those individuals lose weight. These strategies include diet and exercise, behavioral changes, bariatric surgery, and medications.

Diet and exercise

The National Weight Control Registry (NWCR) contains the names of over 3,000 individuals who have lost at least 30 lb (13.6 kg) and kept the weight off for at least 1 year. Women in the NWCR expend 2,445 calories per week and men expend 3,293 calories per week, the equivalent of walking 30 to 45 minutes every day.

Key behaviors identified by people in the registry were decreasing the amount of food they eat and their intake of fat to decrease their total caloric intake. In addition, all members of the registry increased their activity levels and maintained this increase.

The belief is that identifying the behaviors associated with weight gain, loss, and maintenance can lead to interventions that target these behaviors, ultimately helping to prevent type 2 diabetes. The Nurses' Health Study showed that in over 50,000 nurses followed for 6 years, television watching was positively associated with obesity and type 2 diabetes. In this study, for every 2 hours or more per day that a nurse watched television, there was a 23% increase in obesity and a 14% increase in the risk of developing type 2 diabetes. In addition, the time the nurs-

es spent sitting at work was positively associated with increased obesity and risk of type 2 diabetes. Conversely, each hour a day spent by the nurses engaging in brisk walking was associated with 24% less obesity and a 34% decrease in the incidence of type 2 diabetes. The study concluded that lifestyle changes could affect obesity and diabetes for nurses who watched television less than 10 hours a week and did 30 or more minutes a day of brisk walking.

The importance of physical activity was also emphasized in a prospective study of postmenopausal women in Iowa. Over 30,000 such women were followed over a 10-year period through the use of questionnaires regarding their physical activity, nutrition, and health status. Women who reported medium-to-high physical activity were thinner and had a lower waist-to-hip ratio. The most active women had one-half the risk of developing type 2 diabetes. Moderate-to-rigorous activity frequencies were combined for a physical activity index. This index was strongly negatively associated with the incidence of type 2 diabetes.

Thus, several studies have shown that weight loss, and then maintenance of that loss, and increased physical activity can significantly decrease the risk of type 2 diabetes.

Behavioral changes in adults

The challenge then becomes how to help people at risk to make critical behavior changes related to obesity. Regardless of the behavior being targeted, health care providers can use several strategies to help their at-risk patients. These include helping patients identify and remove cues related to overeating as well as reinforcing healthy eating patterns and physical activity. In addition, cognitive therapy may help patients correct negative thoughts when they don't reach their goals. This strategy can help patients avoid giving up on trying to change their eating behaviors.

STAGES OF CHANGE

This chart identifies stages of change and provides some examples of what an overweight or obese patient might say to indicate the stage of change he's in.

STAGE	STATEMENTS THAT INDICATE STAGE
Precontemplative	■ Fat is beautiful. ■ Being overweight is normal for me; everyone in my family is overweight. ■ Diets don't work; I've tried them all.
Contemplative	■ Being overweight may be harmful. ■ My sister lost 20 pounds; I wonder how. ■ My mother died from diabetes; was obesity the cause?
Action	■ Are there any diets that can help me? ■ I'll look in the phone book for an Overeater's Anonymous group. ■ I'll keep a record of everything I eat for 3 days.
Maintenance	■ I've lost 20 pounds, but the holidays are coming and I'm worried. ■ What would happen if I go off my meal plan on this cruise? ■ It's difficult not being able to eat all that everyone else does.
Identification	■ My health is important to me, and my meal plan is important for my health. ■ If I eat something that's high in calories, I increase my exercise. ■ Fatty food tastes so greasy it makes me ill.

Adapted from Prochaska, J.O. "Health Behavior Change Research: A Consortium Approach to Collaborative Science," *Annals of Behavior Medicine* 29(Suppl):4-6, 2005 with permission of the publisher.

Teaching obese patients how to identify the ABCs of overeating may be beneficial. "A" stands for the antecedent event(s) that leads to overeating, "B" represents the behavior that leads to overeating, and "C" stands for the consequences, cognitive and emotional, of overeating.

Behavioral treatment has specific characteristics. It's a goal-oriented strategy and those goals must be measurable. For example "lose weight" isn't a behavioral goal; however, a behavioral goal would be to "eat smaller portions of fatty foods at dinner 5 times per week." A behavioral goal is also process oriented. It states when, where, and how the behavior will be accomplished. For the best results, it focuses on small, rather than large, changes in behavior. In reviewing progress toward a goal with a patient who hasn't adopted a behavior, explore the barriers to adoption and remove them if possible, or change to a more realistic or feasible goal. In addition, screening the patient for depression is reasonable because depression can exacerbate overeating. Health care providers need to project the attitude that weight management is a set of skills that can be learned rather than a case of willpower.

Determining a person's readiness to change his behavior is a useful step in behavioral treatment. A good tool is the Prochaska Stages of Change model that describes the stages of behavior changes, including precontemplative, contemplative, action, maintenance, and identification. (See *Stages of change*.)

STRATEGIES FOR BEHAVIORAL CHANGES TO CHALLENGE OBESITY

To assist a patient in weight loss to combat obesity, various strategies can be used. These include:

- Daily self-monitoring of food, activity, and weight
  - Types, amounts, and caloric content of food eaten
  - Physical activity, amount, time, intensity
  - Later, add times, places, and feelings associated with eating
- Stimulus control
  - Shop from a list
  - Store food in hard-to-reach places
- Physical activity
  - Use positive cues
  - Keep exercise equipment handy
- Cognitive restructuring
  - Identify irrational thoughts
  - Unrealistic behaviors and goals
  - Self-criticism

Source: Wadden, T.A., and Butryn, M.L. "Behavioral Treatment of Obesity," *Endocrinology and Metabolism Clinics of North America* 32(4):981-1004, 2003.

A number of other strategies may also be used in the behavioral treatment of obesity. These include self-monitoring, nutrition education, stimulus control, slower eating, physical activity, problem solving, and relapse prevention. (See *Strategies for behavioral changes to challenge obesity*.)

Self-monitoring includes detailed daily logs of food intake, physical activity, and weight. The purpose of a daily log is to identify the types, amounts, and calories of foods that are eaten and to identify and remove hidden sources of fat and sugar, thereby reducing caloric intake by 500 to 1,000 calories per day. This self-monitoring behavior typi-

cally identifies caloric intake that patients aren't aware of, for example, the amount of juice or regular sodas they consume. Recording also helps to avoid the underestimation of what's being consumed. When monitoring exercise, patients can use pedometers. For sedentary persons, a goal of 6,000 to 7,000 steps a day is reasonable, whereas for more active persons, a goal of 10,000 steps a day could be targeted. The initial self-monitoring can be used to identify how much a patient walks per day for 1 week; then the patient can increase that amount by a set number of steps per day or week. In addition, finding a friend to walk with regularly can boost a patient's motivation and compliance.

The strategy of stimulus control helps avoid inappropriate eating. Stimulus control is involved in avoiding high-risk situations, such as buffets, thereby avoiding the temptation to overindulge. Another example of stimulus control is storing calorie-dense foods in hard-to-reach places, such as putting cookies in the freezer or on a shelf where the patient must use a chair to reach them. Other techniques used in stimulus control are to use smaller plates, remove serving dishes from the table, and clean plates immediately after eating.

Positive cues have been shown to increase physical activity behaviors. Cues such as keeping a calendar of activity in plain sight can remind patients of their progress toward goals. Physical activity affects weight loss and is also important in keeping the weight off. Therefore, it should be incorporated into any behavior treatment of obesity.

There are many barriers to increasing activity. One of these barriers is a lack of time. To overcome this barrier, patients can be encouraged to strategize how they can increase their activity levels in 10-minute increments. If a patient has been sedentary, the long-term goal would be to increase his activity to 30 minutes per day, 5 days per week. The ultimate goal (that varies among individuals), would be to increase activity level to 60 minutes, 5 days per week. The patient may start with short-term goals of 10 minutes, 3 days per week, and gradually progress. The intensity can be moderate to vigorous depending on the patient's fitness and desire; no extra benefit seems to derive from vigorous exercise.

Behavioral changes in children and adolescents

In the United States today, obesity and being overweight are more prevalent in children and youth than at any other time in our history. In addition, being overweight or obese is increasing in children worldwide. In dealing with children, the approaches differ from those for adults.

In randomized controlled trials with behavior therapy, there has been success in helping overweight children in such settings as camps and residential schools where food can be controlled and physical activity can be promoted. Some of the techniques used may also be helpful outside these settings. The techniques include contingency contracting (with non-food rewards for short-term goals), self-monitoring of caloric intake, praise, and stimulus control. Other strategies that are effective in overweight children are to set individualized treatment goals and approaches based on the child's age, degree of overweight, and co-morbidities, and to involve the family or caregivers in the planning and implementation of the treatment program. In addition, the health care team needs to consider the behavioral, psychological, and social correlates of weight gain. It's important that dietary changes and physical activity plans are feasible within the child's environment and that they foster health and growth and development.

Bariatric surgery

When patients are morbidly obese, bariatric surgery may be considered. This type of surgery has had consider-

able success in producing weight loss of greater than 50%. Its success isn't only in treating diabetes successfully, but also in preventing the disease. However, patients should have adequate psychological evaluation before this surgery and be prepared for the possible adverse effects. Dietary changes are also necessary. Surgeons with experience in the procedure should be used, and long-term follow-up is essential.

Medications for obesity

Only a select number of drugs are available to treat obesity, with varied and somewhat limited effects. One drug, orlistat (Xenical), acts by inhibiting the enzyme lipase, which in turn leads to impaired absorption of ingested fat. As a result, weight loss occurs, usually in the range of 11 to 22 lb (5 to 10 kg). In some patients, this weight loss isn't adequate to reduce the risk of co-morbidities. Although the drug is associated with few adverse effects, some patients do experience loose stools that require cessation of therapy. In addition, two situations may occur with this medication. One, if the patient eats a high-fat diet, diarrhea develops, then the patient learns to decrease his fat intake while on the medication. Two, the patient may stop taking the medication altogether because of this adverse effect. In addition, patients have difficulty maintaining the weight loss 2 to 3 years after stopping therapy.

Another drug that may be used is sibutramine (Meridia). This drug acts to inhibit the reuptake of serotonin and catecholamines at nerve endings, thus helping to decrease appetite and increase heat metabolism. Sibutramine is associated with hypertension and tachycardia and thus limits its widespread use in patients.

RECOMMENDATIONS FOR PREVENTION

As the incidence of diabetes increases in the United States and worldwide, strategies to prevent this serious disease

AVAILABLE RESOURCES FOR
DIABETES PREVENTION

Below is a list of resources that can be useful when implementing strategies to assist communities, groups, or individuals to make the behavioral changes necessary to prevent type 2 diabetes.

Task Force on Community Preventive Services
"The Guide to Community Preventive Services: What Works to Promote Health?" (2005)
Available from: Oxford University Press
198 Madison Avenue
New York, NY 10016
800-451-7556
212-726-6000
www.oup.com/us

U.S. Department of Health and Human Services
"Steps to a Healthier U.S.: A Program and Policy Perspective"
Available from: U.S. Department of Health and Human Services
200 Independence Avenue SW Room 615
Washington, DC 20201
202-619-0257
www.hhs.gov

Hankinson, S.F., et al., eds. "Healthy Women, Healthy Lives: A Guide to Preventing Disease from the Landmark Nurses' Health Study" (2001)
Available from: Simon and Schuster
866 3rd Avenue
New York, NY 10022

"The LEARN Program for Weight Management" by K.D. Brownell
Available from: American Health Publishing
Dept. 80
Dallas TX 75261-0430
817-545-4500
Available at: *www.thelifestylecompany.com*
Also available at: *www.amazon.com*

Texas Diabetes Council
"Diabetes Medical Nutrition Therapy and Prevention Algorithm"
Texas State Department of Health Services
Available at: *www.tdk.state.tx.us/diabetes/healthcare/standards.htm*

Weight-control Information Network Newsletter
"Preventing Childhood Obesity: A Multipronged Approach"
Weight-control Information Network
WIN Notes, Summer 2001
1-866-WIN-4627

AVAILABLE RESOURCES FOR

DIABETES PREVENTION *(continued)*

National Center for Chronic Disease Prevention and Health Promotion
"State Programs in Action: Exemplary Work to Prevent Chronic Disease and Promote Health"
      National Center for Chronic Disease Prevention and Health Promotion
      4770 Bufor Highway, NE Mail stop K-40
      Atlanta, GA 30341-3717
      404-488-5401
Available at: *www.cdc.gov/nccdphp*

National Diabetes Education Program
Flyer for lay audience:
"Get Real! You Don't Have to Knock Yourself Out to Prevent Diabetes."
For community:
"Making a Difference: The Business Community Takes on Diabetes. The National Diabetes Education Program: A Diabetes Community Partnership Guide."
For health care professionals:
"Small Steps, Big Rewards: Your Game Plan for Preventing Type 2 Diabetes."
Available at: www.ndep.nih.gov.

become more critical for health care providers. Whereas medications and bariatric surgery have been successful in selected patients, maintained weight reduction and increased physical activity remain strategies that can be applied to all individuals at risk for type 2 diabetes.

In employing these lifestyle strategies, practitioners should remember that behaviors relating to weight and physical activity are highly individualized. The natural model of behavior provides a framework for prevention. This model poses that people are influenced by internal biological and psychological forces, and function within an environment of family, friends, and small groups with which there's frequent contact. Beyond the small groups, the individual's behavior is influenced by his culture, including the systems and groups he belongs to or believes in. Beyond the culture, behavior is also influenced by the community he lives in and the policies that govern

these communities. Thus, if diabetes prevention strategies are to be effective, all of these influences should be considered.

In general, the ADA has issued the following guidelines for prevention of type 2 diabetes:
● A need for individuals at high risk to become aware of the positive effects of weight loss and physical activity
● Counseling about weight loss and increased physical activity for those with impaired glucose tolerance or impaired fasting glucose
● Continued follow-up and counseling to maintain success
● Monitoring every 1 to 2 years for the possible development of diabetes
● Close monitoring and, if necessary, treatment for cardiovascular risk factors such as smoking, hypertension, and dyslipidemia. For other resources, see *Available resources for diabetes prevention.*

The ADA also suggests that drug therapy not be used as a preventive strategy until it can be determined to be cost-effective.

In addition, such resources as the National Diabetes Education Program, sponsored by the National Institutes of Health and the Centers for Disease Control and Prevention, can be helpful. This Web site (*www.ndep.nih.gov*) provides free, non-copyrighted materials that are available in various languages and can be used in various settings. A particularly useful tool is the health care provider's tool kit, "Small steps, big rewards: Your game plan for preventing type 2 diabetes."

Selected references

American Diabetes Association. "Diagnosis and Classification of Diabetes Mellitus," *Diabetes Care* 28(Suppl 1):S37-S49, January 2005.

American Diabetes Association. "Screening for Type 2 Diabetes," *Diabetes Care* 28(Suppl 1):S11-S14, January 2004.

American Diabetes Association, National Institute of Diabetes and Kidney Diseases. "The Prevention or Delay of Type 2 Diabetes," *Diabetes Care* 26(Suppl 1):S47-S54, 2004.

Andersen, R.E., et al. "Can Inexpensive Signs Encourage the Use of Stairs? Results from a Community Intervention," *Annals of Internal Medicine* 129(5): 363-69, September 1998.

Bjaras, G., et al. "Strategies and Methods for Implementing a Community-based Diabetes Prevention Program in Sweden," *Health Promotion International* 12(2):151-60, June 1997.

Bjaras, G., et al. "Walking Campaign: A Model for Developing Participation in Physical Activity? Experiences from Three Campaign Periods of the Stockholm Diabetes Prevention Program," *Patient Education and Counseling* 42(1):9-14, January 2001.

Brownell, K.D. *The LEARN Program for Weight Management.* Dallas: American Health Publishing Co., 2000.

Buchanan, T.A., et al. "Preservation of Pancreatic Beta-cell Function and Prevention of Type 2 Diabetes by Pharma-cological Treatment of Insulin Resistance in High-risk Hispanic Women," *Diabetes* 51(9):2796-803, September 2002.

Chiasson, J.L., et al. "Acarbose for the Prevention of Type 2 Diabetes Mellitus: The STOP-NIDDM Randomised Trial," *Lancet* 359(9323):2072-2077, June 2002.

Daniel, M., et al. "Effectiveness of a Community-directed Diabetes Prevention and Control in a Rural Aboriginal Population in British Columbia, Canada," *Social Science Medicine* 48(6):815-32, March 1999.

Daniels, S.R., et al. "Overweight in Children and Adolescents: Pathophysiology, Consequences, Prevention, and Treatment," *Circulation* 111(15):1999-2012, April 2005.

"Diabetes Prevalence" [Online]. International Diabetes Federation; 2005. *www.idf.org/home.*

Diabetes Prevention Program Research Group. "Costs Associated with the Primary Prevention of Type 2 Diabetes Mellitus in the Diabetes Prevention Program," *Diabetes Care* 26(1):36-47, January 2003.

Diabetes Prevention Program Research Group. "The Diabetes Prevention Program (DPP): Description of Lifestyle Intervention," *Diabetes Care* 25(12): 2165-171, December 2002.

Diabetes Prevention Program Research Group. "Reduction in the Incidence of Type 2 Diabetes with Lifestyle Intervention or Metformin," *New England Journal of Medicine* 346(6):393-403, February 2002.

Eisenberg, D., and Bell, R.L. "The Impact of Bariatric Surgery on Severely Obese Patients with Diabetes," *Diabetes Spectrum* 16(4):240-45, October 2003.

Epping-Jordan, J.E., et al. "Preventing Chronic Disease: Taking Stepwise Action," *Lancet* 366(9497):1667-671, November 2005.

Fisher, E.B., et al. "Behavioral Science Research in the Prevention of Diabetes," *Diabetes Care* 25(3):599-606, March 2002.

Folsom, A.R., et al. "Physical Activity and Incident Diabetes Mellitus in Postmenopausal Women," *American Journal of Public Health* 90(1):134-38, January 2000.

Holcomb, J.D., et al. "Evaluation of Jump Into Action: A Program to Reduce the Risk on Non-insulin Dependent Diabetes Mellitus on Schoolchildren on the Texas-Mexico Border," *Journal of School Health* 68(7):282-89, September 1998.

Hu, F.B., et al. "Television Watching and Other Sedentary Behaviors in Relation to Risk of Obesity and Type 2 Diabetes Mellitus in Women," *JAMA* 289(14):1785-791, April 2003.

Inzucchi, S.E., and Sherwin, R.S. "Applying the Lessons of the DPP to Clinical Practice," *Clinical Diabetes* 21(2):91-92, June 2003.

Jakicic, J.M. "Exercise in the Treatment of Obesity," *Endocrinology and Metabolism Clinics of North America* 32(4):967-80, December 2003.

Kaiser, T., and Sawicki, P.T. "Acarbose for the Prevention of Diabetes, Hypertension and Cardiovascular Events? A Critical Analysis of the STOP-NIDDM Data," *Diabetologia* 47(3):575-80, March 2004.

Kaufman, F.R. *Diabesity: The Obesity Epidemic that Threatens America — and What We Must Do To Stop It.* New York: Bantam Books, 2005.

Miller, S.T., et al. "Shaping Environments for Reductions in Type 2 Diabetes Risk Behaviours: A Look at CVD and Cancer Interventions," *Diabetes Spectrum* 15(3):176-82, July 2002.

National Diabetes Fact Sheet. Centers for Disease Control and Prevention, 2005. *www.cdc.gov/diabetes/pubs*

Pan, X.R., et al. "Effects of Diet and Exercise in Preventing NIDDM in People with Impaired Glucose Tolerance: The Da Qing IGT and Diabetes Study," *Diabetes Care* 20(4):537-44, April 1997.

Plodkowski, R.A., and St. Jeor, S.T. "Medical Nutrition Therapy for the Treatment of Obesity," *Endocrinology and Metabolism Clinics of North America* 32(4):935-66, December 2003.

Prochaska, J.O. "Health Behavior Change Research: A Consortium Approach to Collaborative Science," *Annals of Behavioral Medicine* 29(Suppl):4-6, 2005.

Satterfield, D.W., et al. "Community-based Lifestyle Interventions to Prevent Type 2 Diabetes," *Diabetes Care* 26(9):2643-52, September 2003.

Simmons, D., et al. "A Pilot Diabetes Awareness and Exercise Programme in a Multiethnic Workforce," *New Zealand Medical Journal* 109(1031):373-76, October 1996.

Simmons, D., et al. "A Pilot Urban Church-based Programme to Reduce Risk Factors for Diabetes Among Western Samoans in New Zealand," *Diabetic Medicine* 15(2):136-41, February 1998.

Teufel, N.I., and Ritenbaugh, C.K. "Development of a Primary Prevention Program: Insight Gained in the Zuni Diabetes Prevention Program," *Clinical Pediatrics* 37(2):131-41, February 1998.

Trevino, R.P., et al. "Bienestar: A Diabetes Risk-factor Prevention Program," *Journal of School Health* 68(2):62-67, February 1998.

Tuomilehto, J., et al. "Prevention of Type 2 Diabetes Mellitus by Changes in Lifestyle Among Subjects with Impaired Glucose Tolerance," *New England Journal of Medicine* 344(18):1343-350, May 2001.

Wadden, T.A., and Butryn, M.L. "Behavioral Treatment of Obesity," *Endocrinology and Metabolism Clinics of North America* 32(4):981-1003, December 2003.

Wing, R.R., and Hill, J.O. "Successful Weight Loss Maintenance," *Annual Review of Nutrition* 21:239-41, 2001.

World Health Organization Study Group on Diet Nutrition and Prevention of Noninfectious Diseases. *Diet, Nutrition, and the Prevention of Chronic Diseases: Report of a Joint WHO/FAO Expert Group.* Geneva, Switzerland: World Health Organization 2003.

Part

2

TREATING DIABETES MELLITUS

Nutritional therapy

Good nutrition is a vital human need that changes throughout the life cycle and is essential to a person's well-being. Indeed, food is an integral part of our lifestyles: for many, it's the essence of socialization, centered around major life events, traditions, and pastimes. A person's nutrition also affects his health and illness status. Commonly, individuals with poor nutrition experience a prolonged or complicated recovery from illness.

According to the U.S. Surgeon General, 8 out of the 10 leading causes of death in the United States are related to food intake. Unfortunately, preventive measures involving nutrition may not be emphasized as strongly as those related to managing a specific disease process. To improve a patient's quality of life, continuous supportive measures of good health and nutrition must be implemented along with lifestyle changes.

NUTRITION AND DIABETES

Diabetes is a disease process characterized by an imbalance between the supply and demand of insulin. A pancreatic hormone secreted by the beta cells of the islets of Langerhans, insulin is essential for the metabolism of glucose. By enhancing the transport of glucose across the cell membrane, insulin regulates blood glucose levels. To maintain optimal blood glucose control and well-being, individuals with diabetes must make significant permanent changes in lifestyle. Although these changes may seem daunting, they're essential in slowing down or decreasing the development of diabetes-related complications. These lifestyle changes include proper nutrition, adequate exercise, appropriate dietary management, and weight reduction and maintenance. They provide a simple, cost-effective means of improving insulin sensitivity, reducing glucose and lipid levels and, ultimately, successfully treating and managing diabetes. (See *Goals of nutritional therapy*.)

Glycemic index

The primary goal of nutritional management of diabetes focuses on maintaining blood glucose levels as close to normal levels as possible. The glucose response to carbohydrates is a key indicator in glucose control. Indeed, studies have shown that certain carbohydrates elicit a higher glucose response than others. Thus, in an effort to determine what foods will cause a greater increase in glucose levels, carbohydrates have been ordered and ranked according to how high glucose levels rise after the intake of specific carbohydrates; this measurement system is termed the *glycemic index*. The index examines the increase in glucose after ingestion of a 50-g source of a carbohydrate in comparison with the rise in levels after ingestion of a 50-g portion of white bread, which serves as the index food. The response in glucose level to the index food (the white bread) is considered to be 100%. How high glucose levels increase after ingestion of a specific food determines whether that food is categorized as a low- or high-index food.

Having a low- or high-index value doesn't necessarily classify the food as being a healthy choice. Carrots, for example, have a high glycemic index but are a much healthier choice than potato chips, which have a low glycemic index and offer little nutritional value.

Also, the glycemic index value is calculated for individual foods and doesn't consider the glucose response for foods eaten in combination. The following range serves as a guideline for assessing glycemic index:

- 55 or less: low
- between 56 and 69: medium
- 70 or greater: high.

Selecting foods with a lower glycemic index may help control the rise in glucose values after meals. Low glycemic foods also promote a sense of fullness and facilitate weight loss. Although some controversy exists over its use in meal planning, overall, selecting foods with a low glycemic index is useful in improving insulin sensitivity and controlling glucose levels.

Glycemic load

How foods are ingested also affects glucose response. The glycemic response to a carbohydrate depends on the type of carbohydrate as well as the amount consumed. This concept is referred to as *glycemic load*. Glycemic load is the glycemic index of a food divided by 100 and multiplied by its amount of carbohydrates: glycemic load = glycemic index/100 × net carbohydrates.

When using this formula to calculate glycemic load, it's important to consider the net carbohydrates as the total amount of carbohydrates in a serving minus its dietary fiber content. The following range is a guideline for assessing glycemic load:

- 10 or less: low
- between 11 and 19: medium

GOALS OF NUTRITIONAL THERAPY

For the patient with diabetes, nutrition is a key component of care. Regardless of the type of diabetes and other therapies, the nutritional goals are the same. These goals include:

- optimal metabolic outcomes
  - blood glucose levels that are as close to normal as possible
  - serum lipid profiles and blood pressure levels within acceptable ranges (to reduce the risk of macrovascular disease)
- treatment and prevention of chronic complications through adjustments in nutrient intake and lifestyle
- improvement in health through physical activity and healthy food choices
- individualization of the patient's needs involving:
  - cultural and personal preferences
  - lifestyle patterns
  - desire and motivation to change.

- 20 or greater: high.

The recommended daily guideline for glycemic load is:

- less than 80: low
- greater than 120: high.

The average person takes in about 100 glycemic load units, or a glycemic load of 80 to 180 each day. Although the glycemic index for some foods remains undetermined, the general rule is that foods with a low glycemic index usually have a low glycemic load. Although individual responses may be vary, meal planning centered on the glycemic index and glycemic load ultimately benefits the patient with diabetes by keeping glucose levels within normal range. (See *Glycemic index and glycemic load of common foods*, pages 54 and 55.)

(Text continues on page 56.)

GLYCEMIC INDEX AND GLYCEMIC LOAD OF COMMON FOODS

The glycemic index and glycemic load values of selected common foods are listed in the chart below.

TYPE	ITEM	GLYCEMIC INDEX	GLYCEMIC LOAD
Breads and cereal			
	All-Bran cereal	42	8
	Cheerios	74	15
	Corn flakes	81	21
	Life cereal	66	16
	Shredded wheat	75	15
	Sourdough wheat bread	54	15
	Whole wheat bread	71	9
	White wheat bread	70	10
Fruit (fresh and juice)			
	Apples	38	6
	Apple juice	40	11
	Bananas	52	12
	Cantaloupe	65	4
	Grapes	46	8
	Oranges	42	5
	Orange juice	50	12
	Peaches	42	5
	Pears	38	4
	Pineapple	59	7
	Strawberries	40	1
	Watermelon	72	4

GLYCEMIC INDEX AND GLYCEMIC LOAD
OF COMMON FOODS *(continued)*

Type	Item	Glycemic index	Glycemic load
Beans			
	Chick	28	8
	Kidney	28	7
	Red lentils	26	5
	Navy	38	12
	Pinto	39	10
Potatoes and vegetables			
	Beets	64	5
	Carrots	47	3
	Green peas	48	3
	Sweet corn	54	9
	New potatoes	57	12
	Sweet potatoes	61	17
Miscellaneous foods			
	Couscous	65	23
	Fettuccine	40	18
	Linguine	52	23
	Macaroni	47	23
	Parboiled rice	47	17
	Pearled barley	25	11
	Peanuts	14	1
	Spaghetti	42	20
	Popcorn	72	8
	Sucrose (table sugar)	68	7
	White rice	64	23
	Wild rice	57	18

Exchange list program

In addition to using glycemic index and glycemic load when planning meals for the patient with diabetes, another concept involves the exchange list program, which counts carbohydrates. Developed by the American Diabetes Association and the American Dietetic Association, the exchange list program helps to identify carbohydrate-containing foods (based on calories and macronutrients), thus controlling glucose levels and promoting portion control. The program also tailors nutritional management to the individual.

Divided into specific sections or categories, the exchange list includes carbohydrates, meat and meat substitutes, and fats. (See *Exchange list categories of selected foods.*) Food choices may not be exchanged among lists, except for carbohydrate exchanges, which include starch, fruits, milk, and other carbohydrates.

Carbohydrate exchanges

The carbohydrate exchanges consist of starches, fruits, nonstarchy vegetables, sweets, desserts, and other carbohydrates, such as milk and milk products. Each item on the list is equivalent to one exchange and may be substituted for any other. One starch exchange is equivalent to:
- 15 g carbohydrate
- 3 g protein
- 0 to 1 g fat
- 80 calories.

The fruit component of the carbohydrate exchange is equivalent to:
- 15 g carbohydrate
- 0 g protein
- 0 g fat
- 60 calories.

Fruit choices (2 to 3 servings) should include whole, fresh fruits because they're high in fiber and are generally filling. Juices without added sugar are also allowed.

Fresh or frozen nonstarchy vegetables (2 to 3 servings) are also recommended because they're rich in carbohydrates, vitamins, protein, and fiber, as well as being low in sodium. Canned vegetables should be drained and rinsed with water before cooking. The nonstarchy vegetable component of the exchange list is equivalent to:
- 5 g carbohydrate
- 2 g protein
- 0 g fat
- 1 to 4 g fiber
- 25 calories.

Milk and milk products are considered part of the carbohydrate group. These items provide calcium and protein; however, some also may contain fat. The fat-free and low-fat milk component of the carbohydrate exchange is equivalent to:
- 12 g carbohydrate
- 8 g protein
- 0 to 3 g fat
- 90 calories.

The reduced-fat milk component is equivalent to:
- 12 g carbohydrate
- 8 g protein
- 5 g fat
- 120 calories.

The whole milk component is equivalent to:
- 12 g carbohydrate
- 8 g protein
- 8 g fat
- 150 calories.

Individuals with diabetes shouldn't deprive themselves by completely omitting sweets or desserts. The key is moderation, and these items may be included as a part of the meal.

Meat and meat substitutes exchanges

The meat and meat substitutes exchanges are subdivided according to fat content: lean, medium-fat, or high-fat. The serving size — 3 oz of cooked meat (about the size of a deck of cards) — consists of 21 g protein. However, the fat content dictates the amount of cal-

(Text continues on page 62.)

EXCHANGE LIST CATEGORIES OF SELECTED FOODS

The chart below highlights the major food categories of the exchange list program and lists some of the common foods in each category.

TYPE	ITEM	SERVING SIZE
Carbohydrate group		
Starches		
Bread	Bagel or English muffin	½ (1 oz)
	Bread (whole wheat, rye, white)	1 slice
	Reduced-calorie bread	2 slices
	Hamburger bun	½ (1 oz)
	Pita bread (6″ diameter)	½
Cereal	Bran	½ cup
	Oatmeal or Cream of Wheat	½ cup
	Puffed cereal	1½ cups
	Shredded wheat	1 biscuit
Miscellaneous starches	Rice: white or brown (cooked)	⅓ cup
	Couscous	⅓ cup
Peas, beans, lentils	Baked beans	⅓ cup
	Cooked peas	½ cup
	Lentils	½ cup
Starchy vegetables	Corn	½ cup
	Mixed vegetables	1 cup
	Potato: baked or broiled	1 small (3 oz)
	Yam or sweet potato	½ cup
	Winter squash	1 cup
Soups	Bean	½ cup
	Broth-base	1 cup

(continued)

EXCHANGE LIST CATEGORIES OF SELECTED FOODS

(continued)

TYPE	ITEM	SERVING SIZE
Soups *(continued)*	Cream-base	1 cup
Crackers and snacks	Animal crackers	8
	Graham crackers	3
	Melba toast	4
	Matzo	¾ oz
	Popcorn (low-fat or nonfat)	3 cups
	Rice or popcorn cakes	2
	Pretzel sticks	¾ oz
Other starches (occasional use or as part of a planned meal or snack)	Angel food cake	1 ½" slice
	Frozen yogurt	½ cup
	Fat-free frozen yogurt	⅓ cup
	Gelatin (sugar sweetened)	½ cup
	Ice cream (fat-free)	½ cup
	Sherbet	¼ cup
	Biscuit	1 small
	Chow mein noodles	½ cup
	French fries	16 to 25
	Corn muffin	1 (2 oz)
	Pancake (4" diameter)	1
	Plain donut	1 small
Fruits	Apple	1 small
	Apricots	4 medium
	Banana	½ (4 oz)
	Blueberries	¾ cup

EXCHANGE LIST CATEGORIES OF SELECTED FOODS
(continued)

Type	Item	Serving size
Fruits (continued)	Cantaloupe	⅓ small
	Cherries	12 large
	Fresh figs	2 medium
	Grapefruit	½ large
	Grapes	17 small
	Nectarine	1 small
	Orange	1 small
	Papaya	½ medium
	Peach	1 medium
	Pear	½ large
	Pineapple	¾ cup
Nonstarchy vegetables	Artichoke	½ cup
	Asparagus (cooked)	½ cup
	Broccoli (raw)	1 cup
	Cabbage (cooked)	½ cup
	Carrots (raw)	1 cup
	Celery (raw)	1 cup
	Mushrooms (raw)	1 cup
	Spinach (cooked)	½ cup
	Tomato (raw)	1 cup
Milk and milk products	Milk (fat-free, ½%, 1%, 2%)	1 cup
	Dry milk powder (fat-free)	⅓ cup
	Buttermilk	1 cup
	Yogurt (plain)	⅔ cup

(continued)

EXCHANGE LIST CATEGORIES OF SELECTED FOODS
(continued)

Type	Item	Serving size
Milk and milk products (continued)	Yogurt (fat-free)	⅔ cup
	Soy milk (plain)	1 cup
	Milk (whole)	1 cup
	Evaporated whole milk	½ cup
Meat and meat substitutes group		
Lean meats	Poultry without skin	1 oz
	Fish (fresh or frozen)	1 oz
	Tuna, salmon, or mackerel (canned, drained)	1 oz
	Beef, USDA select or choice, fat trimmed (rib, ground round)	1 oz
	Lamb (roast, chop, leg)	1 oz
	Pork (tenderloin, center)	1 oz
	Veal (roast, lean chop)	1 oz
	Cheese (less than 3 g fat per ounce)	1 oz
	Cottage cheese (fat-free, low-fat, regular)	¼ cup
	Parmesan cheese	2 tbs
	Egg substitute	¼ cup
	Egg whites	2
	Hot dog	1 small
	Luncheon meat (fat-free, low-fat, less than 3 g fat per ounce)	1 oz
Medium-fat meats	Poultry with skin	1 oz
	Fried fish	1 oz
	Ground meat (beef, chicken)	1 oz
	Lamb (rib roast)	1 oz

EXCHANGE LIST CATEGORIES OF SELECTED FOODS
(continued)

Type	Item	Serving size
Medium-fat meats *(continued)*	Veal cutlet	1 oz
	Sausage (less than 5 g fat per ounce)	1 oz
	Cheese (feta, mozzarella)	1 oz
	Ricotta cheese	¼ cup
	Egg	1
	Tofu (soybean curd)	½ cup
High-fat meats	Pork spareribs, ground pork	1 oz
	Bacon	3 slices
	Sausage (Polish, bratwurst)	1 oz
	Luncheon meats (bologna, salami)	1 oz
	Peanut butter	1 tbs (counts as 1 meat and 2 fats)
Fat group		
Monounsaturated fats	Avocado	2 tbs
	Olives (black or ripe)	8 large
	Peanuts	10 large
	Peanut butter (smooth, crunchy)	½ tbs
	Oil (canola, olive, peanut, sesame)	1 tsp
Polyunsaturated fats	Margarine	1 tsp
	Mayonnaise	1 tsp
	Nondairy cream substitute	¼ cup
	Salad dressing (regular)	1 tbs
Saturated fats	Butter	1 tsp
	Coconut, shredded	2 tbs

(continued)

EXCHANGE LIST CATEGORIES OF SELECTED FOODS
(continued)

Type	Item	Serving size
Saturated fats (continued)	Cream cheese	1 tbs
	Gravy	2 tbs
	Half-and-half (light cream)	2 tbs
Free foods groups		
	Water	Unlimited
	Carbonated and flavored water	
	Coffee (regular or decaffeinated)	
	Diet soft drinks (sugar-free)	
	Tea (regular or decaffeinated)	
	Butter flavoring (fat-free)	
	Garlic	
	Herbs	
	Pepper and spices	
	Bouillon and fat-free broth	
	Flavored gelatin	
	Sugar substitutes (aspartame, saccharin)	
	Barbecue sauce	1 to 2 tbs
	Dill pickles	1½ large
	Jam or jelly (low-sugar or light)	1 to 2 tbs
	Pancake syrup (sugar-free)	1 to 2 tbs

ories each exchange provides. For example:

● very lean or lean meat — 1 serving provides 0 to 3 g fat and 35 to 55 calories

● medium-fat meat — 1 serving provides approximately 5 g fat and 75 calories

● high-fat meat — 1 serving provides 8 to 13 g fat and 100 or more calories.

Understandably, lean meat choices are recommended because they're lower in saturated fat, cholesterol, and calories; if high-fat meat is consumed, servings should be limited to no more than three times per week so as not to affect cholesterol levels.

Preferred methods of preparation include baking, boiling, grilling, broiling, steaming, and roasting. Nonstick vegetable sprays are preferred over fats; if fats are used, the amount must be counted in the total daily allowance. Additionally, starches used in meal preparation (bread crumbs, flour) also must be counted.

Fat exchanges

The fat component of the exchange list is divided into three subcategories: monounsaturated, polyunsaturated, and saturated fats. Monounsaturated and polyunsaturated fats are recommended over saturated fats because the latter contain transfats, which may contribute to cardiac disease. Fats are high in calories, thus serving sizes should be monitored carefully when following the exchange list. One fat exchange is equivalent to 5 g fat and 45 calories.

Free foods exchanges

The exchange lists also include free foods, some of which may be incorporated into the meal plan in unlimited amounts, such as sugar substitutes, carbonated water, coffee, diet soft drinks, lemon juice, garlic, herbs, vinegar, and mustard. Other exchanges on this list are limited to a maximum of three servings per day, each of which provides approximately 20 calories, such as fat-free cream cheese, fat-free or reduced fat mayonnaise, light jelly or jam, catsup, pickles, and soy sauce. These choices should be spaced throughout the day to inhibit a sudden rise in glucose levels.

NUTRITIONAL MANAGEMENT GUIDELINES

An abundant food supply along with adequate fortification, preparation, and storage of nutrients contributes to maintaining optimal health secondary to appropriate dietary intake. Adhering to dietary guidelines for optimal weight, however, sometimes leads to excesses and imbalances that may contribute to the development and progression of preventable diseases. Exceeding the body's requirement of nutrient intake is linked with such diseases as cancer, hypertension, cardiac disease, and diabetes.

Historically, recommended dietary allowances (RDAs) emphasized appropriate nutrient levels that were sufficient to prevent diseases related to inadequate dietary intake. Today, this focus has changed, incorporating measures that meet this need as well as strategies to avoid nutritional excess. New standards, the dietary reference intake (DRI), incorporate updated RDAs and target nutrient-based requirements to promote optimal health. Each individual guideline included in the DRI establishes goals specific to the person's age and gender. The guidelines also focus on meeting nutritional needs to reduce the risk of chronic diseases such as diabetes.

Nutritional therapy planning and meal planning are integral to the nutritional management of patients with diabetes.

Nutritional therapy planning

Nutritional therapy planning for patients with diabetes requires a multidisciplinary approach. Typically, a registered dietitian is involved who's knowledgeable and skilled in integrating nutrition therapy with diabetes management. In addition, other team members, such as the patient's primary health care provider, diabetes educator, and nurses, must have a working knowledge base about the link between nutritional therapy and diabetes so that they can provide added support to the patient.

Nutritional therapy focuses on a well-balanced meal plan to maintain glucose levels close to normal levels. The patient's energy or caloric intake should be sufficient to maintain his targeted goal weight. His meal intake should be consistent, and his dietary intake of carbohydrates, fats, and protein should remain within the recommended daily guidelines, which include:
- 11% to 18% of calories from protein
- 25% to 30% of calories from fat
- 45% to 65% of calories from carbohydrates.

The patient with diabetes doesn't have to eat foods in combination with others to support digestion or weight loss; indeed, he can enjoy a wide variety of foods. By understanding the basic concepts related to nutrient intake, you can help to promote healthy dietary patterns in patients with diabetes.

✳ **ALERT** *Always remember that regulating blood glucose to achieve near normal levels is the priority. Therefore, nutritional strategies that limit hyperglycemia after a meal can minimize possible complications. Be aware that carbohydrates — both the amount consumed and the type ingested — influence blood glucose levels.*

Food sources
Dietary guidelines for patients with diabetes focus on selecting foods from the five major food groups, within the recommended guidelines. Through making balanced choices, such as whole grains, fruits, and vegetables, the patient with diabetes can meet the minimum daily requirements without excess.

In patients with diabetes, low-carbohydrate diets aren't recommended. Although carbohydrates play a major role in elevating blood glucose levels after meals, they're also an important source of energy, water-soluble vitamins, minerals, and fiber. The National Academy of Sciences, Food, and Nutrition Board recommends that about 45% to 65% of total calories be derived from carbohydrate sources. An additional argument against low-carbohydrate diets stems from the needs of the brain and central nervous system for glucose as their primary energy source. Therefore, in patients with diabetes, total carbohydrate restriction shouldn't fall below 130 g/day.

Alcohol
Alcohol may be permitted in moderation. The current recommendation is two drinks per day for men and one drink per day for women. Serving size is essential: one serving of wine is equivalent to a 5-oz glass, one serving of light beer is equal to a 12-oz glass, and one serving of 80-proof distilled spirits is equivalent to 1½ oz.

Vitamins and minerals
Vitamins aren't manufactured by the body; they must be provided through the intake of foods and supplementation. They're required by the body to promote biochemical reactions within the cells. Deficiencies occur when the intake is inadequate; high intakes may result in toxicity. Examples of fat-soluble vitamins include:
- vitamin A
- vitamin D
- vitamin E
- vitamin K.

Water-soluble vitamins include:
- vitamin C
- B vitamins (B_1, B_2, B_6, B_{12}, biotin, folate, niacin, and pantothenic acid).

Minerals are provided in the diet mainly by plant sources, and some may be found in drinking water. Routine vitamin and mineral supplementation in the individual who doesn't have deficiencies isn't recommended. Although there's no proven harm in supplementing the diet with a multiple vitamin-mineral source, dose levels are suggested at no higher than 100% of the RDA.

The safety and benefit of supplements haven't been proven; in fact, increased doses may predispose the individual to toxicity. A diet that's well balanced and tailored to the specific needs of the individual provides a sufficient source of vitamins and minerals.

Dietary supplements

Dietary supplements, as defined by the U.S. Food and Drug Administration (FDA), are products intended to serve as a supplement to the diet that contains any of the following ingredients: vitamins, minerals, herbs or other botanicals, amino acids, or other dietary substances, such as metabolites or extracts. The use of supplements may be related to a belief that health status is improved when they're included in the diet.

Originally designed to target deficiencies, supplements haven't been found to improve normal health status. Although labeling on supplement packing claims to improve health, the FDA mandates the inclusion of a statement that it hasn't evaluated these claims.

Some evidence suggests that patients with poor glycemic control and a deficiency in water-soluble micronutrients may benefit from dietary supplements, but standards don't justify them. Choosing a variety of foods gives the body the necessary vitamins and minerals and, combined with glycemic control, can negate the need for additional supplementation to maintain health.

Meal planning

Patients with diabetes may be overwhelmed by the information related to nutritional therapy. The need to monitor intake, determine serving sizes, and make appropriate food choices can be difficult to comprehend and implement. Commonly, the patient needs a great deal of assistance with this planning to avoid being overwhelmed, to increase knowledge, and to boost confi-

dence; this will result in compliance, ultimately, producing success.

Using the food guide pyramid

An important tool in meal planning that incorporates variety and balance is the Food Guide Pyramid. (See *Food Guide Pyramid*, page 66.)

The pyramid is a graphic representation of dietary guidelines that incorporates the concept of balance. Although it supports choosing a wide variety of foods from among the five food groups, it doesn't indicate appropriate serving sizes. Portions must be tailored to the patient, specific to his individual caloric requirements. Additionally, some foods offer more benefits than others. For example, fats and oils — illustrated on the pyramid by a very narrow band — are recommended for use sparingly. However, some fats are beneficial and should be encouraged in the diet. The meat and beans section of the pyramid doesn't include fish, which is rich in omega-3 fatty acids; nor does it limit high-fat, saturated meats.

Most recently, the Harvard School of Public Health developed the Healthy Eating Pyramid, which incorporates daily exercise and weight control at the base of the pyramid, signifying its relationship between food intake and physical activity, as well as the concepts of variety and balance. For example, rather than listing starches as a food choice, this pyramid focuses on a recommendation of what starches should be included in the balance of nutrients eaten. Whole grains and fiber share the allotted slot with plant oils, which are low in saturated fat. Amounts of these are equally recommended, as are vegetables and fruits. Dairy, calcium, nuts, and legumes are included, as well as a recommendation to drink alcohol in moderation. At the apex of the pyramid is red meat and butter along with white rice, bread, pasta, and potatoes — all recommended for use sparingly.

FOOD GUIDE PYRAMID

The revised MyPyramid combines the *2005 Dietary Guidelines for Americans* by the U.S. Department of Agriculture and the U.S. Department of Health and Human Services. MyPyramid was designed to make Americans aware of the health benefits of following nutrition guidelines and to promote healthy food choices based on individual preferences.

For a 2,000-calorie diet, you need the amounts below from each food group. To find the amounts that are right for you, go to *MyPyramid.gov.*

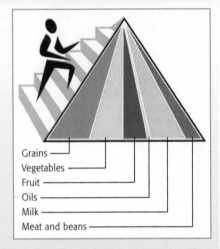

Grains
Vegetables
Fruit
Oils
Milk
Meat and beans

Grains
Make half your grains whole.
Eat at least 3 oz of whole-grain cereals, breads, crackers, rice, or pasta every day.
1 oz is about 1 slice of bread, about 1 cup of breakfast cereal, or ½ cup of cooked rice, cereal, or pasta.
Eat 6 oz every day.

Vegetables
Vary your veggies.
Eat more dark-green veggies, such as broccoli, spinach, and other dark leafy greens.
Eat more orange vegetables, such as carrots and sweet potatoes.
Eat more dry beans and peas, such as pinto beans, kidney beans, and lentils.
Eat 2½ cups every day.

Fruits
Focus on fruits.
Eat a variety of fruit.
Choose fresh, frozen, canned, or dried fruit.
Limit fruit juices.
Eat 2 cups every day.

Milk
Get your calcium-rich foods.
Go low-fat or fat-free when you choose milk, yogurt, and other milk products.
If you don't or can't consume milk, choose lactose-free products or other calcium sources, such as fortified foods and beverages.
Get 3 cups every day; for kids ages 2 to 8, it's 2 cups.

Meat & beans
Go lean with protein.
Choose low-fat or lean meats and poultry.
Bake it, broil it, or grill it.
Vary your protein routine – choose more fish, beans, peas, nuts, and seeds.
Eat 5½ oz every day.

Find your balance between food and physical activity.
- Be sure to stay within your daily calorie needs.
- Be physically active for at least 30 minutes most days of the week.
- About 60 minutes a day of physical activity may be needed to prevent weight gain.
- For sustaining weight loss, at least 60 to 90 minutes a day of physical activity may be required.
- Children and teenagers should be physically active for 60 minutes every day, or most days.

Know the limits on fats, sugars, and salt (sodium).
- Make most of your fat sources from fish, nuts, and vegetable oils.
- Limit solid fats like butter, margarine, shortening, and lard, as well as foods that contain these.
- Check the Nutrition Facts label to keep saturated fats, trans fats, and sodium low.
- Choose food and beverages low in added sugars. Added sugars contribute calories with few, if any, nutrients.

DEVELOPING A MEAL PLAN

Developing a meal plan can be overwhelming for the patient with diabetes. Use these tips to help him develop a plan tailored to his needs:
- Keep likes and dislikes of foods in mind.
- Include breakfast, lunch, dinner, and snacks in the plan.
- Prepare a schedule, and plug in favorite foods.
- Use a sample meal plan to develop an individual plan.
- Create a list of foods centered around each meal, helping to keep choices varied.
- Keep the list of foods readily available so replacing items is simpler.
- Never shop when hungry, and avoid food aisles with unhealthy food choices.
- Read food labels to determine nutritional content.

Lastly, the food guide pyramid empowers individuals to choose what foods they prefer, in the correct proportions, which in turn may help them adhere to a prescribed meal plan. (See *Sample meal plan: Food pyramid*, page 266.)

Considering individual preferences

Use of a pyramid is an effective strategy in teaching variety and balance to the patient with diabetes as it allows the patient to visualize appropriate food choices and amounts necessary to maintain optimal wellness. Most importantly, individualizing meals addresses the patient's food preferences and lifestyle, which promotes adherence and positive outcomes. It's easier to revise unhealthy habits when the meal plan fits within the patient's established behaviors and lifestyle patterns. The patient with diabetes should be encouraged to make time on a weekly basis to plan his meals, including all his food preferences.(See *Developing a meal plan*.)

Also, dietary change should evolve gradually because it's much easier to incorporate it one step at a time, giving the patient some sense of control. Realistic goals must be developed to successfully manage nutrition for a chronic disease such as diabetes. Providing an individualized plan of nutritional management may help him achieve the goals of weight loss and maintenance and glucose control.

Choosing meal plans

When choosing a meal plan, the patient should choose from a variety of preferred foods (in appropriate portions) to help promote proper intake of nutrients within each food group with the goal of getting the patient's blood glucose levels within normal levels. Providing several options helps empower the patient and support his adherence to a treatment plan that focuses on the nutritional management of diabetes.

Various meal plans may be used to meet the individual's needs. One basic plan involves calorie counting. (See *Sample meal plan: Calorie-based*, page 267.)

Other meal plan options include exchange lists, carbohydrate counting, and "rate your plate." Each targets the ability of the patient with diabetes to incorporate various portion-controlled, healthy food choices to manage diabetes, improve his blood glucose levels, and lose excess weight.

Exchange lists

Exchange lists for meal planning, developed by the American Dietetic Association and the American Diabetes Associ-

WHAT'S IN A PORTION?

A major key to nutritional therapy planning is ensuring that the amount of food to be eaten is of the proper size. To help patients understand serving sizes (or portions), use these hints:

■ Use measuring spoons, measuring cups, or a food scale to determine the right amount.

■ Check the nutritional label on the food package to determine the size of one serving.

■ After measuring a serving size of cereal, pasta, or rice and pouring it into a bowl or plate, note the level to which the bowl or plate is filled; then use that same bowl or plate filled to the same level the next time you eat cereal, pasta, or rice.

■ Measure out 1 cup of milk (typically one serving) and pour it into a glass. Note the level of filling, and use that same size glass filled to the same level the next time you drink a serving of milk.

■ Be aware that meat shrinks after cooking. Typically, a 4-oz piece of raw meat weighs about 3 oz after cooking; if the meat has a bone, then about 2 oz are lost during cooking.

■ Use your body to help estimate serving sizes:
  – 1 serving of meat or meat substitute is about the size of the palm of your hand or a deck of cards.
  – 1 small piece of fruit or ½ cup of fruit, vegetables, or rice is about the size of a small fist.
  – 1 oz of meat or cheese is approximately the size of the thumb.
  – 1 tsp is about the size of the tip of the thumb..

ation, help to shape a meal plan based on the specific nutritional needs of the patient to maintain optimal health. Food choices and portion control are emphasized. (See *What's in a portion?*)

The exchange lists indicate a variety of foods that are specific to individual preferences. (See *Sample meal plan: Exchange lists*, page 268.)

Carbohydrate counting

Carbohydrate counting focuses on incorporating foods that fit within a predetermined daily allotment of carbohydrates. High-fiber choices are encouraged, with a recommendation of between 25 and 50 g of fiber each day. Other food choices, such as meats and meat substitutes, nonstarchy vegetables, and fats, are permitted within acceptable guidelines. (See *Sample meal plan: Carbohydrate counting*, page 269.)

Rate your plate

The "rate your plate" meal planning tool focuses on portion control. It also presents a visualization of meal planning within recommended guidelines. Individuals are instructed to draw an imaginary line through the center of the plate, dividing it into sections. About one-fourth of the plate is designated to a starchy food choice, one-fourth to protein, and the remaining half to nonstarchy vegetables. (See *Meal planner: Rate your plate*.)

NUTRITIONAL MANAGEMENT GOALS FOR TYPE 1 DIABETES

In patients with type 1 diabetes, insulin secretion is absent; therefore, patients must administer insulin to regulate blood glucose levels. Because glucose levels increase after eating, consis-

MEAL PLANNER: RATE YOUR PLATE

"Rate your plate" is a quick and easy way for the patient with diabetes to visualize and ensure that he's making healthy food choices. It involves drawing an imaginary line through the center of the plate. Then on one of the two halves, the patient draws another imaginary line across to split that section into two.

- One-fourth of the plate should contain grains or starches.
- One-fourth of the plate should contain protein.
- The remaining one-half of the plate should be filled with nonstarchy vegetables.

To round out the meal, the patient adds a glass of nonfat milk and a small roll or piece of fruit.

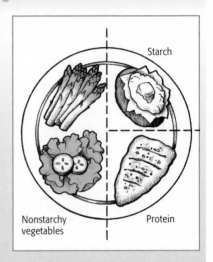

Starch

Nonstarchy vegetables

Protein

---

tency in timing, size, and composition of meals must correlate with insulin doses to keep glucose levels within normal range. (See *Recommended goals for type 1 diabetes*, page 70.) Once a sound diet has been established, insulin therapy can then be individualized according to the meal plan, with adjustments made accordingly. (See chapter 7, Insulin therapy, for more information.)

Maintaining a regular meal plan may also help control the rise in glucose levels following a meal and the fall in glucose levels that occurs between meals. Additionally, portion control and consistency in the amount of foods that contain carbohydrates correlates with insulin action and improved glucose levels.

Understanding caloric requirements

The caloric need of a person with type 1 diabetes is no different from that for a nondiabetic person. For both, needs are determined by the patient's weight, age, gender, activity level, and genetic background. Typically, the patient and practitioner decide on an appropriate calorie level based on the optimal weight that the patient can achieve and maintain. For example, a small-framed woman who exercises regularly may ingest between 1,200 and 1,600 calories daily. A medium-framed man who rarely exercises may ingest between 1,600 and 2,000 calories daily. For a large-framed woman who has a physically active job, between 2,000 and 2,400 may be a realistic target. Caloric intake should be evenly distributed throughout the course of a patient's day and be consistent with his insulin therapy. (See *Distributing calories evenly*, page 71.)

Calories are derived from the intake of specific nutrients. Recommendations for the daily allowance of carbohydrates, fat, and protein intake might be:

RECOMMENDED GOALS FOR TYPE 1 DIABETES

The American Diabetes Association has developed nutritional therapy recommendations specific to the patient with type 1 diabetes. These goals include:

- an individualized meal plan that incorporates the patient's usual intake and lifestyle
- consistent intake of carbohydrates, correlating meal times with the times of insulin action (when fixed insulin regimens are used)
- blood glucose monitoring before the premeal insulin dose and after eating with adjustments in insulin doses for the total amount of carbohydrates ingested (when patients are receiving intensive insulin therapy)
- maintenance of weight with prevention of weight gain
- insulin dosage adjustments to prevent hypoglycemia when patients deviate from their usual eating or exercise plan, with the possible addition of carbohydrates for unplanned exercise.

- 55% to 65% calories from carbohydrates
- 25% to 30% calories from total fats
- 11% to 18% calories from protein.

Carbohydrates

The body's primary source of energy, carbohydrates are classified as either simple or complex, depending on the number of single sugar molecules they contain. Simple carbohydrates include monosaccharides (such as glucose and ribose) and disaccharides (such as lactose and maltose), which are composed of one and two saccharide molecules,

respectively. Complex carbohydrates include polysaccharides, which are found in starch, glycogen, and fiber.

The amount of carbohydrates taken in should be specific to the needs of the individual. One serving provides approximately 15 g of a carbohydrate. The recommended intake of carbohydrates required to meet the energy needs of the body is estimated at 130 g/day. Therefore, the total carbohydrate content of a meal is a major consideration in maintaining glucose levels for optimal wellness in the patient with diabetes.

Carbohydrate sources include breads, pasta, rice, fruit, vegetables, milk, and legumes. As a primary energy source, carbohydrates provide 4 kcal/g.

Fiber — a blend of nondigestible polysaccharides — historically has been classified as either *soluble* or *insoluble*. Providing texture to plant foods, insoluble fiber may be found in the skin of fruits, the covering of seeds, the shell of corn kernels, and in bran, which is the outer layer of grains. Wheat bran, whole grains, dried peas and beans (legumes), and vegetables are excellent sources of insoluble fiber. Recent evidence supports phasing out the terms soluble and insoluble because certain foods provide both benefits. Fiber increases the weight of stools, thereby facilitating evacuation. It has also been credited with lowering cholesterol and glucose levels. For patients with diabetes, the recommended daily fiber intake is between 25 and 50 g/day.

Fats

Dietary fat is also used as a source of energy, supplying 9 kcal/g and playing a role in caloric consumption. Fat has more than twice as many calories as carbohydrates or protein. Fats (or lipids) may be subcategorized as either *saturated* (animal fats, dairy products, coconut, palm or palm kernel oil, and hardened shortenings, which increase cholesterol levels) or *unsaturated* (vegetable fats,

DISTRIBUTING CALORIES EVENLY

To maintain blood glucose levels with insulin, the patient with type 1 diabetes needs to eat consistently throughout the day.

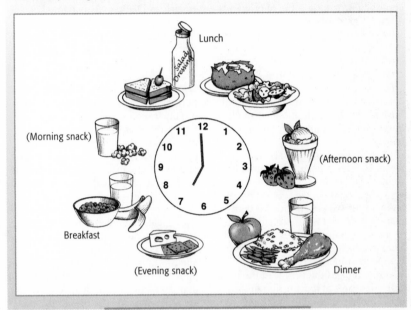

which are liquid at room temperature and lower cholesterol levels). They're emulsified in the stomach and stay there longer than carbohydrates and proteins, leading to a feeling of fullness. Fats are then digested and absorbed in the small intestine.

Nutritional recommendations emphasize that saturated fat should be restricted to less than 10% of total daily intake and that total fat intake should be limited to less than 30% of daily caloric intake. If fat intake falls within this target range, the patient with diabetes can maintain glucose levels at near normal ranges. Sources of fats include oils from seeds, grains, butter, cream, and cheese.

Educating patients with diabetes about the myth that fat-free foods are better choices is also important when teaching about caloric intake. The patient must understand that some fat-free foods still contain calories that count just as much as those with fat; some fat-free foods replace the "fat" with carbohydrates.

When discussing fats, it's also important to touch on cholesterol. Not an essential component of our diets, cholesterol is synthesized in the liver from glucose or saturated fatty acids. An increase in fiber in the diet enhances the excretion of bile acids and decreases cholesterol levels. It's recommended that cholesterol intake be limited to 200 mg to 300 mg daily. Sources of cholesterol are animal products, most abundantly organ meats as well as egg yolks and dairy products containing fat.

Protein

Dietary protein intake is an essential component in maintaining glucose control. The caloric value of protein is 4 kcal/g. The body makes more than 1,000 different proteins through a combination of 22 building blocks, also known as *amino acids*. They may be classified as *complete* (with sufficient amounts and proportion of all essential amino acids, coming from animals) or *incomplete* (deficient in one or more amino acids, coming from plant proteins).

The recommended dietary intake for protein is 0.8 g per kilogram of body weight. Such sources of protein as dairy, eggs, meat, and cheese (derived from animal sources) are considered complete proteins, whereas proteins from vegetables, grains, and beans (derived from plant sources) are considered incomplete proteins.

Protein digestion begins in the stomach, with most of it occurring in the small intestine. Proteins are then absorbed through the mucosa of the small intestine with the assistance of vitamin B_6. Proteins function to replace and support the growth of new tissue, regulate fluid balance, work with the immune system, and provide energy as needed. (However, excessive intake of protein can be stored as fat.)

If a person doesn't take in enough protein, the breakdown of amino acids for energy occurs. This breakdown then causes a negative nitrogen balance (when protein breakdown exceeds protein synthesis), which causes the kidneys to excrete excessive nitrogenous waste.

NUTRITIONAL MANAGEMENT GOALS FOR TYPE 2 DIABETES

When a patient is diagnosed with type 2 diabetes, he's typically overweight.

Therefore, moderate weight loss is recommended to aid in improving blood glucose and lipid levels and regulating blood pressure. Although the amount of weight loss varies with each individual, the ultimate goal is to achieve a reasonable (not necessarily ideal weight). The American Diabetes Association has developed specific goals related to nutritional therapy for patients with type 2 diabetes. (See *Recommended goals for type 2 diabetes.*)

Obesity and type 2 diabetes

Seriously affecting health and wellness, obesity (excess adipose tissue or body fat) contributes to the development of type 2 diabetes. In the United States, approximately one-third of people are obese, and the number of obese people developing type 2 diabetes is growing by about 6% every year.

Obesity is related to physiologic, psychological, and environmental factors, as well as genetic predisposition, and is also associated with increased morbidity and mortality. Individuals who are morbidly obese (with a weight of greater than 100% over their ideal body weight) are at 12 times greater risk for premature death than those who aren't obese.

Approximately 80% to 95% of the rise in type 2 diabetes incidence is directly related to those who have *central* obesity (excess body fat in the abdomen), which contributes to insulin resistance. Obesity-triggered insulin resistance leads to abnormal glucose levels and diabetes, as well as to hypertension and an increased risk of abnormal lipid levels, cardiac disease, and stroke. Target outcomes for these patients aim to reduce weight, maintain glucose levels close to normal range, and reduce the risk of diabetes complications.

Nutritional management for the overweight patient with type 2 diabetes begins with a focused assessment. This includes a review of the individual's understanding of diabetes, along with his readiness to learn and his willingness to incorporate lifestyle changes. It's also important to evaluate his baseline vital signs, height, weight, body mass index (BMI), and lipid levels. Total body fat measurement is used not only to diagnose obesity but to design a meal plan specific to the patient's individual needs. BMI is based on a person's weight in kilograms divided by his height in meters, squared: BMI = weight (kg)/height (meters)^2.

To define obesity, use these guidelines:
- BMI 18.5 to 24.9 kg/m^2 = normal
- BMI 25 to 29.9 kg/m^2 = overweight
- BMI greater than 30 kg/m^2 = obesity
- BMI greater than 40 kg/m^2 = morbid obesity.

A BMI of 27 kg/m^2, or a body weight of 120% of ideal weight, is classified as the threshold at which insulin resistance begins to impair glucose disposal, putting the patient at increased risk for developing abnormally high levels of glucose (or hyperglycemia) and hyperlipidemia.

Nutritional management for weight loss

In patients with type 2 diabetes, weight loss, through physical activity and dietary management, is the single most effective measure for improving insulin sensitivity, improving glucose and lipid levels, and decreasing blood pressure. Nutritional management for the patient with type 2 diabetes should foster an approach that's individualized to the patient. A meal plan low in calories and fat and high in dietary fiber can typically result in a target weight loss of 1 to 2 lb (0.5 to 1 kg) per week

While designing an appropriate meal plan for the overweight patient with type 2 diabetes, it's also important to be sensitive to the patient's feelings, attitudes, and behaviors related to food intake (a critical component to successful weight loss). Previously unsuccessful attempts at weight loss may trigger feelings of failure and may cause a rebound effect causing the individual to increase

RECOMMENDED GOALS FOR TYPE 2 DIABETES

The American Diabetes Association has developed nutritional therapy recommendations specific to the patient with type 2 diabetes. These goals include:
- increased activity and exercise to promote better glucose control and decrease insulin resistance and cardiovascular risk
- lifestyle changes that lead to decreased caloric intake and increased physical activity, resulting in a greater expenditure of energy for individuals who are overweight and insulin resistant
- reduction in dietary intake of carbohydrates, saturated fats, cholesterol, and sodium to achieve a decrease in glucose, lipid, and blood pressure that can be maintained
- moderate caloric restriction involving a reduction of carbohydrate and total fat intake in conjunction with an increase in exercise for those who are excessively overweight.

his food intake. Further, change isn't always easy, especially when it comes to dietary changes; thus, working closely with the patient to identify, face, and, ultimately, modify his eating behaviors should result in a weight-loss meal plan that achieves target weight and glucose control.

Increasing physical activity

Successful weight loss with nutritional management also must incorporate increased physical activity, tailored to the individual. So, when teaching glucose control measures, encourage the patient to incorporate exercise into his daily routine and coordinate the amount and level of physical activity with his food intake. Physical activity:

● facilitates weight loss by burning calories

● improves glucose levels and supports glycemic control with improved metabolism and increased muscle mass

● enhances the body's response to insulin and decreases glucose levels, thereby decreasing the risk of complications of diabetes.

Additionally, regular exercise may lower triglyceride levels and increase high-density lipoprotein levels.

Although the greatest benefits of an exercise plan are seen in the early stages of type 2 diabetes (when insulin resistance is the major presenting abnormality), the overall advantages are also evident. In addition to improving insulin sensitivity, exercise reduces the risk of heart disease in overweight patients with type 2 diabetes.

To promote not only improved glucose levels but weight loss as well, the patient should exercise a minimum of 30 to 60 minutes, 3 to 5 days per week; this exercise regimen burns a minimum of 1,500 calories — a significant amount for achieving weight loss secondary to increased physical activity.

Exercise must be enjoyable so that the individual will participate and continue. Cost may be a factor for some, however, such as when a person decides to join a health club or gym. If this isn't possible, free alternatives include brisk walking or bike riding — both effective strategies in glucose management.

The patient with diabetes must be able to exercise in comfort. Footwear should be properly fitted and comfortable. The patient also needs to perform meticulous foot care to prevent possible complications.

Before exercising, the individual with diabetes should be encouraged to drink at least two glasses of water. He should also drink water during and after exercise whether or not he feels thirsty, because the body needs adequate hydration during periods of physical activity.

A warm-up and cool-down period also is recommended.

ALERT *Testing blood glucose levels before exercising is essential in the patient with diabetes. If glucose levels are above 300 mg/dl, the patient shouldn't exercise. If glucose levels are below 100 mg/dl, he should eat a small snack because physical activity will lower the levels further. Also encourage the patient to bring a snack and a cell phone (in case he needs help) with him when exercising, because physical activity may also cause hypoglycemia.*

Planning an exercise regimen that focuses on enjoyment and safety is key to helping the patient achieve weight loss goals and improve glucose levels.

Controlling blood glucose levels

Another goal of nutritional management in patients with type 2 diabetes is to control blood glucose, thus decreasing the occurrence of elevated glucose levels, or hyperglycemia. Common signs and symptoms of hyperglycemia include:

● blurred vision

● elevated glucose levels

● glycosuria

● nausea and vomiting

● polydipsia

● polyphagia

● polyuria

● weakness and fatigue.

Common contributing causes of hyperglycemia include:

● too much food intake

● too little or no insulin or hypoglycemic agents

● stress

● illness or infection.

Screening blood glucose levels evaluates the effectiveness of nutritional therapy and diabetes management. When trying to minimize hyperglycemia and its related complications, individuals with type 2 diabetes should self-monitor their blood glucose levels as an adjunct to nutritional management.

Understanding caloric requirements

To maintain glycemic control, patients with type 2 diabetes should reduce their total number of daily calories by 500 to 1,000. Research has shown that maintaining a calorie-restricted diet for as little as 10 days demonstrates up to an 87% drop in glucose levels.

In patients with type 2 diabetes, it's important to establish the basal metabolic rate (BMR) — the minimum caloric energy requirement to sustain life. BMR is assessed under basal conditions: 12 hours after eating, following a restful sleep and with no exercise, activity, or emotional excitement. Optimal BMR supports adequate oxygen uptake during periods of rest and activity. To determine BMR, multiply an individual's healthy weight in pounds by 10 for women or by 11 for men. Use this formula to establish the number of calories an individual can safely ingest on a daily basis to maintain health. For example, for a male who weighs 160 lb (72.6 kg), the minimum number of calories required is 1,760 per day (160 lb × 11 calories/lb = 1,760 calories/day).

Another calorie-based weight loss treatment option is the very-low-calorie diet, which allows 800 or fewer calories per day, plus vitamin and mineral supplementation. This diet yields substantial weight loss with a rapid improvement in glucose and lipid levels. Glucose levels improve before significant weight loss occurs, implying that reducing calories is key in managing elevated glucose levels. However, there's disagreement regarding the plan's effectiveness as it doesn't promote long-term weight loss or establish real changes in the patient's dietary behaviors.

Meeting protein needs

In patients with type 2 diabetes, assessing daily protein intake is a key component in facilitating a successful weight loss. Between 11% and 18% of total daily calories should come from protein sources. The total daily allowance of protein is 0.8 g/kg of body weight to maintain the minimal daily protein requirements in a 3,000-calorie diet.

In nondiabetic patients, approximately 50 to 80 g of glucose is yielded after a person ingests 100 g of protein. However, this standard doesn't hold true for patients with type 2 diabetes. In the latter population, dietary protein doesn't produce this increase in glucose levels, possibly because of an increase in the secretion of insulin, especially when protein is included in a mixed meal.

A successful strategy is to incorporate protein into the diet within the recommended guidelines. Meeting daily protein requirements helps produce a steady weight loss of between 1 and 2 lb (0.5 and 1 kg) per week.

NUTRITIONAL THERAPY COVERAGE

Nutritional therapy is covered by third-party payers, including Medicare, under the category of medical nutritional therapy, defined as "nutritional diagnostic, therapy, and counseling services for the purpose of disease management, which are furnished by a registered dietitian or nutritional professional." These professionals must be enrolled as Medicare providers and must follow nationally recognized protocols such as those of the American Dietetic Association.

To qualify for services, the individual must meet the necessary diagnostic criteria and demonstrate medical necessity. In addition, the primary care physician or treating physician must order medical nutritional therapy.

Initially, the patient can receive 3 hours of medical nutritional therapy, with an additional 2 hours of follow-up in a year. If more time is needed, the treating physician must order the additional hours and substantiate that a change in the medical condition, diagnosis, or treatment plan has occurred that affects the nutritional therapy plan.

Selected references

"All About Diabetes" [Online]. Available at: *www.diabetes.org/about-diabetes.jsp.* [2005 October 19].

American Diabetes Association. "Diagnosis and Classification of Diabetes Mellitus," *Diabetes Care* 28(Suppl 1):S37-42, January 2005.

American Diabetes Association. "Standards of Medical Care in Diabetes," *Diabetes Care* 28(Suppl 1):S4-36, January 2005.

Chalmers, K.H. "Medical Nutrition Therapy," in Kahn, C.R., et al. *Joslin's Diabetes Mellitus,* 14th ed. Philadelphia: Lippincott Williams & Wilkins. 2005.

Counting Calories and Carbos. Princeton, N.J.: Novo Nordisk Pharmaceuticals, Inc., 2000.

"Diabetes: Your Diet's Role in Blood Sugar Control" [Online]. Available at: *www.mayoclinic.com/invoke.cfm? objectid=15BFEA7A-OFD3-4F24-B4F777100D.* [2005 October 19].

Dudek, S. *Nutrition Essentials for Nursing Practice,* 5th ed. Philadelphia: Lippincott Williams & Williams, 2006.

Franz, M., and Bantle, J., eds. *American Diabetes Association Guide to Medical Nutrition Therapy for Diabetes. American Diabetes Association Clinical Education Series.* Alexandria, Va.: American Diabetes Association, 1999.

Franz, M., ed. *Diabetes Management Therapies: A Core Curriculum for Diabetes Education,* 4th ed. Chicago: American Association of Diabetes Educators, 2001.

"Glycemic Index, Glycemic Load, Satiety, and the Fullness Factor" [Online]. Available at: *www.nutritiondata.com/ glycemic-index.html.* [2005 October 24].

"Health Eating: Make It Happen" [Online]. Available at: *www.diabetes.org/ weightloss-and-exercise/weightloss/ healthy-eating.jsp.* [2005 October 19].

"Making the Decision to Lose Weight" [Online]. Available at: *www.diabetes. org/weightloss-and-exercise/weightloss/ getting-motivated.jsp.* [2005 October 19].

"Meal Improvement: Rate Your Plan—A Guide to Eating and Diabetes" [Online]. Available at: *www.diabetes.org/ all-about-diabetes/chan-eng/i3/i3p3. htm* [2005 November 4].

Mendosa, D. "Glycemic Values of Common American Foods" [Online]. Available at: *www.mendosa.com/ common_foods.htm* [2005 October 5].

Mendosa, D. "Revised International Table of Glycemic Index (GI) and Glycemic Load (GL) Values" [Online]. Available at: *www.mendosa.com/gilists.htm* [2005 October 24].

"MyPyramid" [Online]. Available at: *www.mypyramid.com* [2005 October 19].

National Guideline Clearinghouse. "Nutrition Practice Guidelines for Type 1 and Type 2 Diabetes Mellitus" [Online]. Available at: *www.guideline.gov/ summary/summary.aspx?ss=15&doc_id =3296&nbr=2522* [2005 October 29].

"Part B Medicare Benefits for Medical Nutrition Therapy" [Online]. Available at: *www.diabetes.org/ for-health-professionals-and-scientists/ recognition/dsmt-mntfaqs.jsp.*

"Portion Control, or How Much Food is Enough?" [Online]. Available at: *www.diabetes.org/weightloss-and-exercise/weightloss/portioncontrol.jsp* [2005 October 19].

"Rate Your Plate" [Online]. Available at: *www.diabetes.org/nutrition-and-recipes/nutrition/rate-your-plate.jsp* [2005 November 4].

Rendell, M. "Advances in Diabetes for the Millennium: Nutritional Therapy of Type 2 Diabetes," *Medscape General Medicine* 6(3s): 2004. Available at: *www.medscape.com/veiwprogram/3378.*

"Small Steps for Your Health" [Online]. Available at: *www.diabetes.org/utils/printthispage.jsp ?PageID=WEIGHTLOSS3_294975* [2005 October 19].

"What are the Lifestyle Measures for Managing Type 2 Diabetes?" [Online]. Available at: *www.umm.edu/ patiented/articles/what_lifestyle_ measures_managing_type_2_diab.* [2005 October 29].

"What I Need to Know About Eating and
    Diabetes" [Online]. Available at:
    *www.diabetes.niddk.nih.gov/dm/pubs/
    eating_ez/eating.pdf* [2005 November
    1].
"What is the Glycemic Index?" [Online].
    Available at: *www.glycemicindex.
    com/main.htm* [2005 October 24].
"Who Gets Type 2 Diabetes?" [Online].
    Available at: *www.umm.edu/patiented/
    articles/who_gets_type_2_diabetes_
    000060_3.htm* [2005 October 29].

Drug therapy

Although pharmacologic therapy for diabetes is wide ranging, insulin is typically the first-line treatment for type 1 diabetes. With the development of insulin analogs, insulin is also being used in patients with type 2 diabetes. Pharmacologic treatment options for type 2 diabetes range from the first-generation sulfonylurea agents of the 1970s to the newly released incretin mimetics and various forms of insulin therapy.

However, despite this wide array of available agents, the percentage of patients achieving the American Diabetes Association's target glycosylated hemoglobin (HbA_{1c}) of 7.0% (having an average blood glucose level of approximately 170 mg/dl) has decreased over the past 10 years, from 44.5% in the National Health and Nutrition Examination Survey of 1988–1994 to 35.8% in 1999–2000.

For the millions of people living with diabetes, it's vital that health care providers and patients work collaboratively to use the appropriate pharmacologic agents to achieve blood glucose control and, ultimately, better quality of life.

ORAL ANTIDIABETIC AGENTS

Since their development and introduction in 1955, sulfonylureas (oral antidiabetic agents) have remained the mainstay of oral medication therapy in the treatment of type 2 diabetes in the United States — until the approval of metformin in 1995. Since that time, several new categories of antidiabetic agents have been made available for clinical use.

Currently, six chemical classes of oral medications are approved for the treatment of type 2 diabetes mellitus. In individuals with substantial capacity for insulin secretion, these agents may be used as monotherapy or in combination with one another, with insulin, or with the incretin mimetics. Some agents are also being studied and used for the prevention of type 2 diabetes and as treatment for insulin resistance associated with polycystic ovarian syndrome (PCOS).

Of those patients with diabetes who are on drug therapy, oral medication use accounts for 57% of the total number, followed by insulin therapy (16%), neither therapy (15%), and combination oral medication with insulin therapy (12%). (See *Pharmacologic treatment in adults with diabetes*.)

Additionally, recent studies have revealed some new trends in pharmacologic therapy for treating diabetes. Specifically, the percentage of patients treated with either oral medications or insulin therapy alone appears to be decreasing, while the use of combination therapy has increased. This trend may continue with the advent of additional oral and injectable medications with complementary actions.

PHARMACOLOGIC TREATMENT IN ADULTS WITH DIABETES

This chart illustrates the distribution of the various pharmacologic therapies for adults diagnosed with diabetes in the United States from 2001 to 2003.

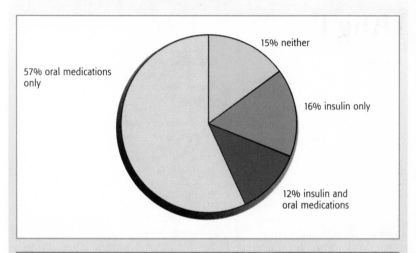

57% oral medications only

15% neither

16% insulin only

12% insulin and oral medications

Source: The National Diabetes Information Clearinghouse, a service of the National Institute of Diabetes and Digestive and Kidney Diseases (NIDDK). National Diabetes Statistics fact sheet: general information and national estimates on diabetes in the United States, 2005. Bethesda, MD: U.S. Department of Health and Human Services, National Institutes of Health, 2005.

Classes of oral agents

The classes of oral agents that are currently approved for use in patients with type 2 diabetes include first- and second-generation sulfonylureas, alpha-glucosidase inhibitors, biguanides, thiazolidinediones, and meglitinide analogs (benzoic acid derivatives and D-phenylalanine derivatives). (See *Classes of oral antidiabetic agents*, page 80.)

General mechanism of action

Blood glucose regulation involves interplay among various processes, including intestinal absorption of glucose, pancreatic insulin secretion, hepatic glucose production, and peripheral glucose uptake by muscle cells and fat cells. If the normal functioning of these tissues gets interrupted, blood glucose regulation is affected, leading to abnormally high blood glucose levels. This process is discussed more fully in chapter 2, Causes and pathophysiology.

It's well accepted that the causes of type 2 diabetes aren't limited to a single defect; rather, several factors contribute to the condition. Specifically, enhanced glucose absorption, decreased pancreatic insulin secretion, impaired insulin action with resulting insulin resistance, decreased peripheral glucose uptake, and increased hepatic glucose output combine to elevate blood glucose levels.

To address these separate concerns, several pharmacologic therapies have been developed. Each of the various

CLASSES OF ORAL ANTIDIABETIC AGENTS

The chart below identifies the six major classes of oral antidiabetic agents and examples of drugs for each class.

DRUG CLASS	DRUGS CURRENTLY AVAILABLE
Sulfonylureas	
First-generation	Tolbutamide (Orinase)
	Chlorpropamide (Diabinese)
	Acetohexamide (Dymelor)
	Tolazamide (Tolinase)
Second-generation	Glyburide (Micronase, DiaBeta)
	Micronized glyburide (Glynase)
	Glipizide (Glucotrol)
	Glipizide GITS (Glucotrol XL)
	Glimepiride (Amaryl)
Biguanides	Metformin (Glucophage, Glucophage XR)
Thiazolidinediones	Pioglitazone (Actos)
	Rosiglitazone (Avandia)
Benzoic acid derivative	Repaglinide (Prandin)
D-phenylalanine derivative	Nateglinide (Starlix)
Alpha-glucosidase inhibitors	Acarbose (Precose)
	Miglitol (Glyset)

classes of oral antidiabetic medications target a specific defect associated with the pathophysiology of the disease. (See *Where agents act to control type 2 diabetes.*)

The United Kingdom Prospective Diabetes Study (UKPDS) showed that type 2 diabetes is a progressive disease. Beta cell function decreases with the duration of diabetes, initially resulting in increases in postprandial glucose levels, followed later by rises in fasting glucose values. Therefore, periodic upgrading of pharmacologic therapy is necessary; thus, the patient with type 2 diabetes may encounter a variety of oral and injectable medications.

In 2005, two injectable agents, exenatide and pramlintide, received FDA approval for use as adjunctive therapy. The two classes of drugs are:

● amylin analogue — pramlintide (Symlin)
● incretin mimetic — exenatide (Byetta).

Pramlintide is approved for use with insulin therapy and can also be administered to patients receiving metformin or sulfonylureas therapy; exenatide, an incretin mimetic, is approved for use with oral antidiabetic agents. These agents mimic the effects of hormones normally released during food ingestion and enhance insulin secretion at physi-

WHERE AGENTS ACT TO CONTROL TYPE 2 DIABETES

The different drug classes act in different ways to control type 2 diabetes. Here's how they work:

- sulfonylureas (beta cell stimulator) – stimulate pancreatic secretion of insulin
- biguanides – reduce hepatic glucose production; increase peripheral glucose utilization
- thiazolidinediones – reduce insulin resistance in the periphery and possibly in the liver
- benzoic acid derivative (beta cell stimulator) – stimulates pancreatic secretion of insulin for a short time
- D-phenylalanine derivative (beta cell stimulator) – stimulates pancreatic secretion of insulin for a short time
- alpha-glucosidase inhibitors – prevent breakdown of sucrose and complex carbohydrates in the small intestine, prolonging absorption.

This illustration highlights the major mechanism of action for each class of medications used to treat type 2 diabetes.

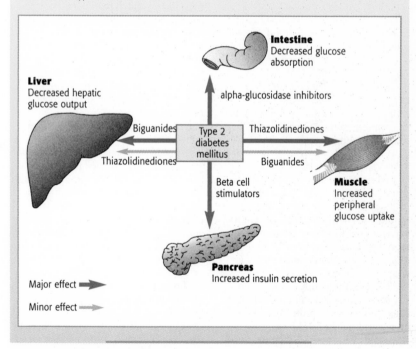

ologic concentrations. Most important-ly, they stimulate glucose-dependent insulin secretion that, along with other mechanisms of action, affects postpran-dial blood glucose levels.

SULFONYLUREAS
Sulfonylureas are classified as either first- or second-generation, based on three distinguishing characteristics. (See *Examples of first- and second-generation sulfonylureas*, page 82.)

EXAMPLES OF FIRST- AND SECOND-GENERATION SULFONYLUREAS

Sulfonylureas are categorized as first- or second-generation agents.

First-generation agents include:
- acetohexamide
- chlorpropamide
- tolazamide
- tolbutamide.

Second-generation sulfonylureas include:
- glimepiride
- glipizide
- glipizide GITS
- glyburide
- micronized glyburide.

First, sulfonylureas are categorized based on their potency. The second-generation sulfonylureas are approximately 100 times more potent than the first-generation drugs. Second, these drugs are distinguished based on their potential for adverse effects, with the first-generation sulfonylureas having much greater potential for adverse effects. Third, the first- and second-generation drugs differ in their binding to serum proteins; this also affects their risk of drug interactions.

Mechanism of action
Called *secretogogues*, sulfonylureas stimulate pancreatic secretion of insulin by binding to a regulatory protein (referred to as the sulfonylurea receptor) found on the pancreatic beta cells' surface. The binding of these receptors results in closure of voltage-dependent potassium adenosine triphosphate (KATP) channels, helping cell membrane depolarization and the influx of calcium into the cell. Insulin is then secreted and released at lower glucose thresholds than normal. The increased circulating insulin concentration, even in the presence of insulin resistance, results in a lowering of blood glucose levels.

A proposed secondary mechanism of action — a decrease in insulin resistance — has also been studied. It ap-

pears, however, that the effects of sulfonylureas on peripheral tissues are most likely related to a reduction in glucose toxicity, secondary to lower blood glucose concentrations.

Sulfonylureas are rapidly and completely absorbed and unaffected by food, with the exception of short-acting glipizide. Most sulfonylureas are metabolized in the liver to active or inactive metabolites, with the exception of chlorpropamide, which is partially excreted unchanged in the urine. Glyburide and, to a lesser degree, glipizide are significantly excreted through the liver; therefore, caution should be taken when prescribing sulfonylureas in patients with significant liver disease. In patients with renal deficiency, caution and close attention to dose adjustment must be given to agents with active metabolites, or a parent drug that's excreted through the kidneys.

The efficacy of sulfonylurea monotherapy in lowering HbA_{1c} levels has been shown to be equal to or better than that of any other class of oral medications. Generally, sulfonylureas lower the HbA_{1c} level by 1.5% to 2.0%. Fasting blood glucose levels may be lowered by about 50 to 60 mg/dl.

Adverse effects
The most significant adverse effect of sulfonylurea agents is hypoglycemia,

which is likely to occur with insufficient or improperly timed carbohydrate intake, excessive or poorly timed exercise, or in those who have experienced weight loss, resulting in a decrease in insulin resistance. The risk of hypoglycemia varies among the sulfonylurea agents and is increased with glyburide and chlorpropamide. It's generally accepted that glyburide has twice the risk of the other second-generation sulfonylurea agents. This is because of glyburide's increased duration of binding to sulfonylurea receptors, resulting in increased fasting hyperinsulinemia.

Chlorpropamide's prolonged half-life of 24 to 48 hours and duration of 72 hours places elderly patients and those with renal insufficiency at higher risk. Because of the possibility of severe and prolonged hypoglycemia with these agents, patients experiencing hypoglycemia may require hospitalization for ongoing observation and treatment.

Other adverse effects of sulfonylureas include headache, photosensitivity, facial flushing, nausea, vomiting, heartburn, rash, pruritus, cholestasis, jaundice, hemolytic anemia, and thrombocytopenia. In addition, all sulfonylureas have been associated with weight gain, which may result from the decrease in glycosuria achieved by the drug's lowering of blood glucose levels. If the patient doesn't reduce his caloric intake, calories previously lost through glycosuria are stored as fat.

ALERT *Sulfonylureas have also been reported to produce a disulfiram-type reaction if combined with alcohol. Disulfiram (Antabuse) produces an extremely unpleasant reaction when even a small amount of alcohol is ingested. The patient may experience flushing, throbbing in the head and neck, headache, respiratory difficulty, nausea, vomiting, thirst, chest pain, palpitations, tachycardia, hypotension, vertigo, syncope, weakness, blurred vision, and confusion. Inform patients taking sulfonylureas of this potential reaction, and caution them about alcohol use.*

One concern that has surrounded sulfonylureas since the University Group Diabetes Program in the early 1970s is the increase in cardiovascular risk. However, recent studies, including the UKPDS, have shown a stronger trend toward reduced cardiovascular events with sulfonylureas. A decrease in microvascular complications also has been associated with sulfonylurea therapy.

Dosing considerations

As insulin secretogogues, sulfonylureas act to lower blood glucose levels. To reduce the risk of significant hypoglycemia, therapy is usually initiated with a short-acting sulfonylurea given at a low dose. Blood glucose testing should be used to monitor response to sulfonylurea therapy and the dose titrated upward gradually. Although maximum doses are listed for each drug, it's generally accepted that the maximum response to therapy is reached at approximately one-half of the listed maximum dosage.

Although sulfonylureas can be combined with other antidiabetic agents, combining two sulfonylurea agents isn't recommended. (Combination therapy is discussed later in this chapter.)

Primary failure rates (drug isn't succesful) occur with all oral antidiabetic medications. With appropriate patient choice, it's estimated that primary failure rates with sulfonylureas can be reduced to 15%. Appropriate patient choice factors include age older than 40, weight between 110% and 160% of ideal body weight, duration of diabetes less than 5 years, either insulin naive or controlled on less than 40 units/day, and fasting blood glucose levels under 200 mg/dl. Secondary failure rates have been reported to be 10% per year or higher.

(Text continues on page 86.)

SUMMARY OF FIRST-GENERATION SULFONYLUREAS

This chart summarizes key information about the first-generation sulfonlyureas.

	TOLBUTAMIDE	CHLORPROPAMIDE
Pharmacokinetics	Onset: 1 hr Peak: 4–6 hr Half-life: 5–7 hr Duration: 6–12 hr	Onset: 1 hr Peak: 3–4 hr Duration: 60 hr
Metabolism	Totally metabolized to an inactive form in the liver; inactive metabolite excreted via the kidney	Metabolized in the liver; half-life 36 hr
Distribution	Crosses placenta; enters breast milk	Crosses placenta; enters breast milk
Excretion	Excreted in urine	Excreted in urine and bile
Adverse reactions	*Cardiovascular:* Increased risk of cardiovascular mortality *Dermatologic:* Allergic skin reactions, eczema, pruritus, erythema, urticaria, photosensitivity *GI:* Anorexia, nausea, vomiting, epigastric discomfort, heartburn *Hematologic:* Hypoglycemia, leukopenia, thrombocytopenia, anemia *Hypersensitivity:* Fever, eosinophilia, jaundice	*Cardiovascular:* Possible increased cardiovascular mortality *Endocrine:* Syndrome of inappropriate antidiuretic hormone (SIADH) *GI:* Anorexia, nausea, vomiting, epigastric discomfort, heartburn *Hematologic:* Hypoglycemia, leukopenia, thrombocytopenia, anemia *Hypersensitivity:* Allergic skin reaction, eczema, pruritus, erythema, urticaria, photosensitivity, fever, jaundice
Interactions	■ Increased risk of hypoglycemia with insulin, sulfonamides, chloramphenicol, salicylates, monoamine oxidase inhibitors (MAOIs), rifampin, gemfibrozil, anticoagulants, azole antifungals, histamine-2 antagonists, magnesium salts, methyldopa, probenecid, tricyclic antidepressants, and alternative therapies, including juniper berries, celery, ginseng, garlic, fenugreek, coriander, and dandelion root ■ Decreased drug effectiveness with diazoxide (of both drugs, if taken concurrently) ■ Increased risk of hyperglycemia with thiazides; other diuretics ■ Increased risk of hypoglycemia and hyperglycemia with alcohol	■ Increased risk of hypoglycemia with insulin, sulfonamides, urine acidifiers, chloramphenicol, salicylates, probenecid, MAOIs, rifampin, and alternative therapies, including juniper berries, ginseng, garlic, fenugreek, coriander, dandelion root, and celery ■ Decreased effectiveness with diazoxide (of both drugs, if taken concurrently) ■ Increased risk of hyperglycemia with urine alkalinizers, thiazides, and other diuretics ■ Increased risk of hypoglycemia or hyperglycemia with alcohol; disulfiram reaction possible

ACETOHEXAMIDE	TOLAZAMIDE
Onset: 1 hr Peak: 2–4 hr Half-life: 6–8 hr Duration: 12–24 hr	Onset: Varies Peak: 4–6 hr Half-life: 7 hr Duration: 12–24 hr
Metabolized in the liver	Metabolized slowly in the liver; metabolite active but less potent than parent compound
Enters breast milk	Crosses placenta; enters breast milk
Excreted in urine	Excreted in urine
Cardiovascular: Possible increased risk of cardiovascular mortality *Dermatologic:* Allergic skin reaction, eczema, pruritus, erythema, urticaria, photosensitivity *Endocrine:* SIADH *GI:* Anorexia, nausea, vomiting, epigastric discomfort, heartburn, hunger, weight gain *Hematologic:* Hypoglycemia, leukopenia, thrombocytopenia, anemia *Hypersensitivity:* fever; jaundice	*Cardiovascular:* Potential for increased cardiovascular mortality *Dermatologic:* Allergic skin reaction, eczema, pruritus, erythema, urticaria, photosensitivity *GI:* Anorexia, nausea, vomiting, epigastric discomfort, heartburn *Hematologic:* Hypoglycemia, leukopenia, thrombocytopenia, anemia *Hypersensitivity:* Fever, eosinophilia, jaundice
■ Increased risk of hypoglycemia with insulin, sulfonamides, urine acidifiers, chloramphenicol, salicylates, MAOIs, clofibrate, and alternative therapies, including juniper berries, ginseng, garlic, fenugreek, coriander, dandelion root, and celery ■ Decreased effectiveness with beta-adrenergic blockers (may also mask signs of hypoglycemia); rifampin; diazoxide (decreased effects of both if taken concurrently) ■ Increased risk of hyperglycemia with thiazides, other diuretics, phenytoin, nicotinic acid, sympathomimetics ■ Increased risk of hypoglycemia or hyperglycemia with alcohol; disulfiram reaction possible	■ Increased risk of hypoglycemia with insulin, sulfonamides, chloramphenicol, salicylates, MAOIs, and alternative therapies, including juniper berries, ginseng, garlic, fenugreek, coriander, dandelion root, and celery ■ Decreased effectiveness with diazoxide (of both drugs, if taken concurrently) ■ Increased risk of hyperglycemia with thiazides, and other diuretics ■ Increased risk of hypoglycemia or hyperglycemia with alcohol; disulfiram reaction possible

(continued)

	TOLBUTAMIDE	CHLORPROPAMIDE
Contraindications and precautions	■ Allergy to sulfonylureas; type 2 diabetes complicated by severe illness, type 1 diabetes, significant hepatic or renal dysfunction ■ Use cautiously with uremia, thyroid or endocrine disorders, glycosuria, hyperglycemia associated with primary renal disease, lactation ■ *Pediatrics:* Safety and efficacy not established ■ *Geriatrics:* May have increased sensitivity; start with lower initial dose, monitor for 24 hr and titrate according to response	■ Allergy to sulfonylureas; type 2 diabetes complicated by severe illness, type 1 diabetes, significant hepatic or renal dysfunction, lactation ■ Use cautiously with uremia, thyroid or endocrine disorders, glycosuria, hyperglycemia associated with primary renal disease ■ If severe GI distress occurs, give as divided doses before breakfast and evening meal ■ *Pediatrics:* Safety and efficacy not established ■ *Geriatrics:* Monitor and titrate dose

First-generation agents
Tolbutamide
Tolbutamide (Orinase), like others in this category, stimulates insulin release from functioning pancreatic beta cells. Other actions may include increased insulin binding to receptors or an increased number of receptors. It's the least potent of the first-generation sulfonylureas and has the shortest half-life. These factors, along with its complete metabolism in the liver to an inactive form, make it especially useful in patients with kidney disease. (See *Summary of first-generation sulfonylureas*, pages 84 to 87.)

Chlorpropamide
Chlorpropamide (Diabinese) is indicated as an adjunct to diet and exercise in patients with type 2 diabetes. Similar in action to tolbutamide, it can also increase the effects of antidiuretic hormone.

Chlorpropamide has the longest duration of the sulfonylureas; as such, caution must be used in elderly patients and those with decreased renal function. If severe hypoglycemia occurs as a result of overdose, I.V. administration of glucose should be given and the patient monitored for as long as 3 to 5 days. Other concerns with the use of chlorpropamide include a risk of hyponatremia due to increased effects of antidiuretic hormone. Chlorpropamide also has produced disulfiram-like reactions when taken concomitantly with alcohol.

Acetohexamide
Acetohexamide (Dymelor) stimulates the release of insulin from pancreatic beta cell. Possibly improving insulin receptor binding and number of receptors, acetohexamide has significant uricosuric (excretion of uric acid) activity.

Tolazamide
Tolazamide (Tolinase) is the last of the first-generation sulfonylureas. Like the others, its main action is to stimulate the release of insulin from pancreatic beta cells. It may also improve insulin binding to receptors and increase their numbers. Tolazamide has been found to be as effective as tolbutamide, but with less severe adverse effects.

ACETOHEXAMIDE

- Allergy to sulfonylureas, type 2 diabetes complicated by severe illness, type 1 diabetes, significant hepatic or renal dysfunction, lactation
- Use cautiously with uremia, thyroid or endocrine disorders, glycosuria, hyperglycemia associated with primary renal disease
- *Pediatrics:* Safety and efficacy not established
- *Geriatrics:* Start with lower initial dose; monitor effects for 24 hr and titrate

TOLAZAMIDE

- Allergy to sulfonylureas, type 2 diabetes complicated by severe illness, type 1 diabetes, significant hepatic or renal dysfunction
- Use cautiously with uremia, thyroid or endocrine disorders, glycosuria, hyperglycemia associated with primary renal disease, lactation
- *Pediatrics:* Safety and efficacy not established
- *Geriatrics:* Start with a lower initial dose; monitor effects for 24 hr and titrate

Second-generation agents

Second-generation sulfonylureas are preferred for use today over the first-generation agents for several reasons. First, the potency of the second-generation drugs is 50 to 200 times more than that of first-generation sulfonylureas. As a result, patients take fewer milligrams of the medication, which lessens the risk of adverse effects. Second, these agents have less potential for disulfiram-type reactions. Overall, the second-generation sulfonylureas have shorter half-lives than the first-generation agents, potentially lessening the risk of prolonged hypoglycemia. Other drug-specific characteristics of the second-generation sulfonylureas, such as improved insulin binding of glyburide or delayed release formulations, also make them the more preferred choice. (See *Summary of second-generation sulfonylureas*, pages 88 to 91.)

Glyburide and micronized glyburide

Glyburide (Micronase, DiaBeta, Glynase PresTab) stimulates insulin release from pancreatic beta cells. Secondary actions may include improved insulin binding to receptors or increased numbers of receptors. The micronized form of glyburide, Glynase PresTab, has quicker absorption and a corresponding quicker onset than the nonmicronized form. Glyburide has a prolonged duration, which increases the risk of hypoglycemia. As stated previously, it has twice the risk of hypoglycemia as other sulfonylureas.

Glipizide and glipizide GITS

Although glipizide may be given once daily or in divided doses, glipizide GITS (Gastrointestinal Therapeutic System) (Glucotrol, Glucotrol XL) is designed for once-daily dosing only. The agent is packaged in a wax matrix medium that allows for delayed release. Patients must be instructed to always swallow the tablet whole. They also should be informed that the wax matrix, appearing as a pill, will be excreted in their bowel movement. They should be assured that this doesn't mean that the medication wasn't absorbed.

(Text continues on page 90.)

SUMMARY OF SECOND-GENERATION SULFONYLUREAS

This chart summarizes key information related to second-generation sulfonylureas.

GLYBURIDE (MICRONIZED) AND GLYBURIDE (NONMICRONIZED)

Pharmacokinetics	***Micronized glyburide (Glynase PresTab)*** Onset: 1 hr Peak: 2-3 hr Half-life: biphasic 3.2 + 10 Duration: 12–24 hr ***Nonmicronized glyburide (Micronase and DiaBeta)*** Onset: 1 hr Peak: 4 hr Half-life: 10 hr Duration: 12–24 hr
Metabolism	24% absorbed; completely metabolized in the liver to nonactive derivatives
Distribution	Crosses placenta; enters breast milk
Excretion	Excreted in urine and bile 50% by each route
Adverse reactions	*Central nervous system:* Drowsiness, tinnitus, fatigue, asthenia, nervousness, tremor, insomnia *Cardiovascular:* Possible increased cardiovascular mortality *Dermatologic:* Allergic skin reaction, eczema, pruritus, erythema, urticaria, photosensitivity *Endocrine:* Hypoglycemia *GI:* Anorexia, nausea, vomiting, epigastric discomfort, heartburn, diarrhea *Hematologic:* Leukopenia, thrombocytopenia, anemia *Hypersensitivity:* Fever, eosinophilia, jaundice
Interactions	■ Increased risk of hypoglycemia with sulfonamides, chloramphenicol, salicylates, clofibrate, and alternative therapies, including juniper berries, ginseng, garlic, fenugreek, coriander, dandelion root, and celery ■ Decreased effectiveness with diazoxide (of both drugs, if taken concurrently) ■ Increased risk of hyperglycemia with rifampin, thiazide diuretics ■ Increased risk of hypoglycemia or hyperglycemia with alcohol

GLIPIZIDE AND GLIPIZIDE GITS

Onset: 1–1.5 hr
Peak: 1–3 hr
Half-life: 2–4 hr
Duration: 10–24 hr

GLIMEPIRIDE

Onset: 2–3 hr
Peak: 2–3 hr
Half-life: 5.5–7 hr
Duration: 24 hr

Metabolized in the liver to inactive metabolites	Metabolized by oxidative biotransformation to two major metabolites
Crosses placenta; enters breast milk	Crosses placenta; enters breast milk
Excreted primarily in urine; secondarily in bile	Excreted in urine (60%) and bile (40%)

Cardiovascular: Increased risk of cardiovascular mortality
Central nervous system: Drowsiness, asthenia, nervousness, tremor, insomnia, tinnitus, fatigue
Dermatologic: Allergic skin reactions, eczema, pruritus, erythema, urticaria, photosensitivity
Endocrine: Hypoglycemia, syndrome of inappropriate antidiuretic hormone (SIADH)
GI: Anorexia, nausea, vomiting, epigastric discomfort, heartburn, diarrhea
Hematologic: Leukopenia, thrombocytopenia, anemia
Hypersensitivity: Fever, eosinophilia, jaundice

Cardiovascular: Possible increased risk of cardiovascular mortality
Central nervous system: Drowsiness, asthenia, nervousness, tremor, insomnia
Dermatologic: Allergic skin reactions, eczema, pruritus, erythema, urticaria, photosensitivity
Endocrine: Hypoglycemia, SIADH
GI: Anorexia, nausea, vomiting, epigastric discomfort, heartburn, diarrhea
Hematologic: Leukopenia, thrombocytopenia, anemia
Hypersensitivity: Ffever, eosinophilia, jaundice
Other: Diuresis, tinnitus, fatigue

■ Increased risk of hypoglycemia with insulin, sulfonamides, chloramphenicol, salicylates, and alternative therapies, including juniper berries, ginseng, garlic, fenugreek, coriander, dandelion root, and celery
■ Decreased effectiveness with diazoxide (of both drugs, if taken concurrently)
■ Increased risk of hyperglycemia with rifampin, thiazide diuretics
■ Increased risk of hyperglycemia and hypoglycemia with alcohol

■ Increased risk of hypoglycemia with androgens, anticoagulants, azole antifungals, chloramphenicol, fenfluramine, fluconazole, gemfibrozil, histamine-2 blockers, magnesium salts, monoamine oxidase inhibitors, methyldopa, probenecid, salicylates, sulfinpyrazone, sulfonamides, tricyclic antidepressants, urinary acidifiers, and alternative therapies, including juniper berries, ginseng, garlic, fenugreek, coriander, dandelion root, and celery
■ Decreased effectiveness with diazoxide (of both drugs, if taken concurrently)

(continued)

SUMMARY OF SECOND-GENERATION SULFONYLUREAS
(continued)

GLYBURIDE (MICRONIZED) AND GLYBURIDE (NONMICRONIZED)

Contraindications and precautions	■ Allergy to sulfonylureas, type 2 diabetes complicated by severe illness, diabetic ketoacidosis, sole therapy for type 1 diabetes or pregnancy complicated by diabetes, significant hepatic or renal dysfunction, uremia ■ Use cautiously with lactation, thyroid or endocrine disorders, glycosuria, hyperglycemia associated with primary renal disease, labor and delivery (if used during pregnancy, drug should be discontinued at least 1 month before delivery) ■ *Pediatrics:* Safety and efficacy not established ■ *Geriatrics:* Monitor for 24 hr and titrate dose upward as indicated after at least 1 week

Glimepiride

Sometimes referred to as the third generation of sulfonylureas, glimepiride (Amaryl) is indicated for type 2 diabetes not controlled by diet and exercise alone. Its main action is to increase pancreatic beta cell secretion of insulin, and it also may be given in combination with metformin or insulin to improve glucose control. Its once-daily dosing makes it attractive to some patients.

ALPHA-GLUCOSIDASE INHIBITORS

Alpha-glucosidase inhibitors are another group of oral antidiabetic agents used as treatment. Acarbose (Precose) and miglitol (Glyset) are currently the only agents in this drug class for treating diabetes. (See *Summary of alpha-glucosidase inhibitors*, page 92.)

Mechanism of action

Alpha-glucosidase inhibitors don't target a specific defect related to the pathophysiology of type 2 diabetes; rather, they work to delay intestinal carbohydrate absorption. Obtained from the fermentation process of microorganisms, alpha-glucosidase inhibitors competitively inhibit the alpha-glucosidase enzyme in the brush border of the proximal small intestinal endothelium from breaking down disaccharides and more complex carbohydrates. As a result of this inhibition, intestinal carbohydrate absorption is delayed, which suppresses postprandial blood glucose elevations.

When compared to sulfonylureas or metformin, the efficacy of acarbose and miglitol is significantly less, with an average HbA_{1c}-lowering effect of approximately 0.5% to 1%. As expected, given their mechanism of action, the greatest effect is on postprandial glucose levels.

GLIPIZIDE AND GLIPIZIDE **GITS**	GLIMEPIRIDE
	■ Possible decreased hypoglycemic effect with beta-adrenergic blockers, calcium channel blockers, cholestyramine, corticosteroids, diazoxide, estrogens, hydantoins, hormonal contraception, isoniazid, nicotinic acid, phenothiazines, rifampin, sympathomimetics, thiazide diuretics, thyroid agents, urinary alkalizers ■ Increased risk of hyperglycemia with rifampin, thiazide diuretics
■ Allergy to sulfonylureas, type 2 diabetes complicated by severe illness, sole therapy for type 1 diabetes, ketoacidosis, significant hepatic or renal dysfunction, uremia ■ Use cautiously with thyroid or endocrine disorders, glycosuria, hyperglycemia associated with primary renal disease, labor and delivery (if used during pregnancy, discontinue use at least 1 month before delivery), lactation	■ Allergy to sulfonylureas, type 2 diabetes complicated by severe illness, sole therapy for type 1 diabetes, ketoacidosis, significant hepatic or renal dysfunction, uremia, use cautiously with thyroid or endocrine disorders, glycosuria, hyperglycemia associated with primary renal disease, labor and delivery (if used during pregnancy, discontinue use at least 1 month before delivery), lactation ■ *Pediatrics:* Safety and efficacy not established ■ *Renal patients:* Monitor and titrate dose carefully; lower doses possibly sufficient

One study showed a 38 mg/dl reduction in 2-hour postprandial blood glucose levels. In another study, the effect on fasting blood glucose results was small, with only a 5.4 mg/dl reduction in fasting blood glucose levels reported. Acarbose has demonstrated approximately one-half of the blood glucose lowering effect of the sulfonylurea tolbutamide. Although some studies have claimed the efficacy of acarbose to be equal to that of sulfonylureas and metformin, they didn't always use the proper dose of the comparison drug; thus, the results are questionable.

Adverse effects

Flatulence and other GI adverse reactions, such as diarrhea and abdominal pain, commonly lead to discontinuation of the drugs. At high doses, the drugs may elevate liver enzyme levels.

Alpha-glucosidase inhibitors, however, do have some beneficial effects. They're essentially nonsystemic and aren't associated with weight gain, a problem common in several other classes of antidiabetic agents. In addition, when given as monotherapy, acarbose and miglitol aren't associated with hypoglycemia. It's important to note, however, that when combination therapy with a secretogogue is given, hypoglycemia can occur. In this case, the patient must be treated with a monosaccharide, such as glucose tablets or milk, because alpha-glucosidase inhibitors will delay the absorption of other sources of carbohydrates.

Additional benefits of acarbose include small reductions in triglycerides and reductions in postprandial insulin levels. The decrease in postprandial hyperglycemia also may have potential cardiovascular benefits.

SUMMARY OF ALPHA-GLUCOSIDASE INHIBITORS

This chart summarizes key information for the two alpha-glucosidase inhibitors used to treat type 2 diabetes.

	ACARBOSE	MIGLITOL
Pharmacokinetics	Onset: Rapid Peak: 1 hr Half-life: 2 hr Duration: 6 hr	Onset: Rapid Peak: 2–3 hr Half-life: 2 hr Duration: Short
Metabolism	Less than 2% absorbed, metabolized in the intestine	Not metabolized
Distribution	Very little	Very little
Excretion	Feces; small amount in urine	Unchanged via urine and feces
Adverse reactions	*Endocrine:* Hypoglycemia *GI:* Abdominal pain, flatulence, diarrhea, anorexia, nausea, vomiting *Hematologic:* Leukopenia, thrombocytopenia, anemia	*Dermatologic:* Rash *Endocrine:* Hypoglycemia (in combination with other drugs) *GI:* Abdominal pain, flatulence, diarrhea, anorexia, nausea, vomiting
Interactions	■ Increased risk of hypoglycemia with alternative therapies, including juniper berries, ginseng, garlic, fenugreek, coriander, dandelion root, and celery ■ Effects of acarbose decreased when taken with digestive enzymes or charcoal ■ Possible decreased digoxin levels if taken concurrently; monitor patient closely	■ Increased risk of hypoglycemia with alternative therapies, including juniper berries, ginseng, garlic, fenugreek, coriander, dandelion root, and celery ■ Effects of drug decreased when taken with digestive enzymes or charcoal ■ Possible decreased digoxin levels if taken concurrently; monitor patient closely ■ Decreased bioavailability with propranolol, ranitidine
Contraindications and precautions	■ Hypersensitivity to acarbose, type 1 diabetes, diabetic ketoacidosis (DKA), cirrhosis, inflammatory bowel disease and other bowel conditions or predisposition to intestinal obstruction ■ Use cautiously with renal insufficiency, lactation ■ Combination therapy with sulfonylureas: blood glucose levels may be much lower; monitor closely because lower doses may be required	■ Hypersensitivity to miglitol, type 1 diabetes, DKA, cirrhosis, inflammatory bowel disease and other bowel conditions or predisposition to intestinal obstruction ■ Use cautiously with renal insufficiency, lactation ■ Combination therapy with sulfonylureas: blood glucose levels may be much lower; monitor closely because lower doses may be required

Dosing considerations

Although these agents are approved for monotherapy and combination therapy with sulfonylureas, monotherapy is rarely used because of the agents' lower efficacy. Alpha-glucosidase inhibitors may be given with sulfonylureas, metformin, or insulin to optimize glyvemic control. The drug is administered with the first bite of each meal. If the patient develops hypoglycemia, he must be instructed to ingest a carbohydrate that contains glucose or fructose (such as glucose tablets or milk) instead of carbohydrates that contain sucrose (such as table sugar) because these agents prevent absorption. Monitoring of the patient's 2-hour postprandial blood glucose level is key to evaluating the effectiveness of this class of drugs.

BIGUANIDES: METFORMIN

Metformin, in its original form (Glucophage) and extended release form (Glucophage XR), is the only agent in the biguanide class of antidiabetic agents. Used for decades internationally, metformin wasn't approved for use in the United States until the mid-1990s. The delay in metformin's release was due to a previous biguanide — phenformin — that was removed from the market in the mid-1970s because of its high risk of fatal lactic acidosis. In comparison to phenformin, metformin's risk of lactic acidosis is 10 to 20 times lower and is mainly a concern only in patients with renal insufficiency, chronic pulmonary disease, or heart failure. Metformin is commonly the initial drug of choice for patients with type 2 diabetes, especially in those who are obese.

Mechanism of action

Although metformin's exact mechanism of action remains unknown, its predominant effect is thought to decrease hepatic gluconeogenesis in the presence of insulin, improving fasting blood glucose levels. A secondary effect of improved insulin action occurs in peripheral muscle tissue; thus, metformin is also considered an insulin sensitizer. This secondary effect is likely due to a phenomenon that results from a lowering of glucotoxicity, not a direct effect of metformin itself. It also may be related to the drug's ability to lower free fatty acids (FFAs) and the mild anorexia and resulting weight loss that some patients taking metformin experience. (See *Summary of biguanides: Metformin*, page 94.)

Metformin's efficacy has the ability to lower HbA_{1c} levels 1% to 2%, similar to that of sulfonylureas. Studies with metformin have shown fasting blood glucose level reductions of approximately 52 to 58 mg/dl.

Several factors affect the choice of metformin. First, by increasing insulin sensitivity, metformin improves other factors that lead to increased cardiovascular risk. For example, unlike agents that stimulate beta cell secretion, circulating insulin levels tend to decline with metformin, leading to possible cardiovascular benefit. Second, decreases in low-density lipoprotein by cholesterol (LDL-C) of 8%, reductions of fasting triglycerides of 16%, and increases of high-density lipoprotein cholesterol (HDL-C) of 2% have also been reported. Decreases in antifibrinolytic factor plasminogen activator inhibitor-1 have been observed, and positive effects on vascular reactivity or endothelial function also have been reported. In the UKPDS, metformin was shown to significantly lower the rate of myocardial infarction (MI) and all-cause mortality. Patients receiving metformin had a 32% reduction in any diabetes-related end point, 42% fewer diabetes-related deaths, and a 36% reduction in all-cause mortality. More specifically, as compared to the conventional group, the risk of MI was reduced by 39% and all macrovascular end points by 30%.

In addition to its positive cardiovascular effects, metformin's appetite-suppressive effect helps the patient to

SUMMARY OF BIGUANIDES: METFORMIN

This chart summarizes key information related to metformin therapy.

METFORMIN	
Pharmacokinetics	**Metformin** Onset: not related to dose Peak: 2–2.5 hr Half life: 6.2 hr Duration: 10–16 hr **Metformin (Glucophage XR)** Onset: not related to dose Half-life: 17.6 hr Duration: up to 24 hr
Metabolism	**Metformin** Metabolized in liver
Distribution	Crosses placenta; enters breast milk
Excretion	Excreted unchanged in urine
Adverse reactions	*Endocrine:* Hypoglycemia, lactic acidosis *GI:* Anorexia, nausea, diarrhea, vomiting, epigastric discomfort, heartburn *Hypersensitivity:* Allergic skin reactions, eczema, pruritus, erythema, urticaria
Interactions	■ Increased risk of hypoglycemia with cimetidine, furosemide, digoxin, amiloride, vancomycin, and alternative therapies, including juniper berries, ginseng, garlic, fenugreek, coriander, dandelion root, and celery ■ Increased risk of lactic acidosis with glucocorticoids, alcohol ■ Increased risk of acute renal failure and lactic acidosis with iodinated contrast media
Contraindications and precautions	■ Allergy to metformin, type 1 diabetes, type 2 diabetes complicated by serious illness, serious hepatic or renal impairment, uremia, thyroid or endocrine disease, glycosuria, hyperglycemia associated with primary renal disease, labor and delivery (if used during pregnancy, drug should be discontinued at least 1 month before delivery) ■ Use with caution in elderly patients ■ *Pediatrics:* Safety and efficacy not established

either maintain his weight or lose weight; this has been shown with monotherapy and combination therapy. Metformin is also associated with a much lower rate of hypoglycemia than the sulfonylureas. In women with insulin resistance and PCOS, metformin has improved ovulatory function. Recent findings have also shown that metformin can decrease the progression from impaired glucose tolerance to type 2 diabetes.

Adverse effects

The most common adverse effect of metformin is GI intolerance, including nausea, abdominal pain, and diarrhea. Another adverse effect is a metallic taste in the mouth. Reports indicate that up to 50% of patients experience GI distress, which is commonly related to the total dose and the rapidity of upward titration. Adverse effects can be minimized by giving metformin with food and increasing the dose slowly — for example, starting with 500 mg and increasing by 500 mg every 1 to 2 weeks until the full dose is reached. Discontinuing metformin therapy because of adverse GI adverse effects is uncommon.

As mentioned, phenformin (because of its high risk of lactic acidosis) is no longer available for use in the United States. The risk of lactic acidosis with metformin is about 100 times less than with phenformin — about 1 in every 30,000 patients. Symptoms include anorexia, nausea, vomiting, abdominal pain, difficulty breathing, and severe muscle weakness.

Metformin is contraindicated in patients at risk for lactic acidosis, including those with renal insufficiency who have a serum creatinine level greater than or equal to 1.5 (in men) or greater than or equal to 1.4 (in women), or a creatinine clearance of less than 60 ml/minute. This agent also should be avoided in patients who have or are at risk for liver disease, such as alcoholics or binge-drinkers, and in patients with heart failure, pulmonary disease, metabolic acidosis, or dehydration. Caution should also be used in patients older than age 80. As a precaution, metformin should be withheld during acute injury, surgery, or administration of contrast media.

Dosing considerations
Metformin is approved for and commonly initiated as monotherapy for type 2 diabetes; however, the UKPDS revealed that beta cell failure continues in patients taking this drug. Metformin is also approved for use in combination therapy with various sulfonylureas, thiazolidinediones, and insulin. Fixed combination agents containing metformin include Metaglip, Avandamet, and ACToplus met.

An extended-release form of metformin, Glucophage XR, is available as a once-daily dose. The risk of diarrhea with extended-release metformin appears to be similar to that of metformin, based on a comparison of trials of both formulations. Trials with extended-release metformin also showed an unexplained increase in triglyceride levels that wasn't seen in trials with metformin. The only real benefit of extended-release metformin appears to be the once-daily dosing.

THIAZOLIDINEDIONES
In 1997, the first agent in a new classification of oral antidiabetic agents, known as thiazolidinediones (TZDs), was introduced in the United States. Troglitazone (Rezulin) was the first drug approved in this class, followed by two others in 1999, called rosiglitazone (Avandia) and pioglitazone (Actos). Although troglitazone was removed from the market in 2000 following reports of rare idiosyncratic hepatocellular injury, rosiglitazone and pioglitazone remain in widespread use without evidence of similar problems. (See *Summary of thiazolidinediones*, page 96.)

Mechanism of action
Although the unique mechanism of action of TZDs isn't completely understood, it's known that they bind to PPAR-gamma nuclear receptors, which affect gene regulation in adipocytes (fat cells). These genes regulate carbohydrate and lipid (fatty acid) metabolism. It appears that elevated FFA levels increase insulin resistance. TZD agents lower serum FFA levels by approximately 20% to 40%, resulting in improved insulin-stimulated glucose uptake in skeletal muscle. Thus, the main effect of TZDs is a decreased insulin resistance in peripheral tissues through interaction with adipocytes. This interaction may be mediated by leptin, FFAs, tumor necrosis factor, adiponectin, and resistin. Hepatic glucose production also may be decreased at the highest doses.

SUMMARY OF THIAZOLIDINEDIONES

This chart highlights key information about the two agents in the thiazolidinedione (TZD) drug class.

	PIOGLITAZONE	ROSIGLITAZONE
Pharmacokinetics	Onset: Rapid Peak: 2–4 hr Half-life: 3–7 hr Duration: n/a	Onset: Rapid Peak: 1.3–3.5 hr Half-life: 3–4 hr Duration: n/a
Metabolism	Mainly hepatic	Mainly hepatic
Distribution	Crosses placenta; enters breast milk	Crosses placenta; enters breast milk
Excretion	Urine and feces	Urine and feces
Adverse reactions	*Cardiovascular:* Fluid retention *Central nervous system:* Headache, pain, myalgia *Endocrine:* Hypoglycemia, hyperglycemia, aggravated diabetes *GI:* Diarrhea, hepatic injury *Respiratory:* Sinusitis, upper respiratory infection, rhinitis *Other:* Infections, fatigue, tooth disorders	*Central nervous system:* Headache, pain *Endocrine:* Hypoglycemia, hyperglycemia *GI:* Diarrhea, hepatic injury *Respiratory:* Sinusitis, upper respiratory infection, rhinitis *Other:* Infections, fatigue, accidental injury, edema
Interactions	■ Increased risk of hypoglycemia with alternative therapies, including juniper berries, ginseng, garlic, fenugreek, coriander, dandelion root, and celery ■ Decreased effectiveness with hormonal contraceptives; ovulation and risk of pregnancy	■ Increased risk of hypoglycemia with alternative therapies, including juniper berries, ginseng, garlic, fenugreek, coriander, dandelion root, and celery ■ Decreased effectiveness with hormonal contraceptives; ovulation and risk of pregnancy
Contraindications and precautions	■ Allergy to any TZD, type 1 diabetes and diabetic ketoacidosis (DKA), lactation ■ Advanced heart failure; liver failure, don't give if aspartate aminotransferase (AST) > 2.5 times the upper limit of normal	■ Allergy to any TZD, type 1 diabetes and DKA, lactation ■ Advanced heart failure; liver failure, don't give if AST > 2.5 times the upper limit of normal ■ *Pediatrics:* Safety and efficacy not established

TZDs don't function as secretogogues that stimulate beta cell production of insulin; they enhance the responsiveness and efficacy of the beta cells by decreasing glucose and FFAs. Elevated FFAs are associated with lipotoxicity, which leads to beta cell death. A reduction in FFA levels improves beta cell function by decreasing this lipotoxicity, increasing beta cell function by up to 60%. Results of the UKPDS reported that this increase in

PIOGLITAZONE AND MIs

Recently, researchers found that pioglitazone helps to reduce the risk of myocardial infarction (MI) in patients with type 2 diabetes who had a history of MIs. The study subjects included those who had an MI at least 6 months before the study. The major variable in the study was the addition of pioglitazone. In the study group that was given the drug, the risk of recurrent MI was reduced by 28%.

The study also found that adding the drug resulted in a 37% reduction in the risk of acute coronary syndrome and an overall reduction (19%) in the risk of a major coronary event, stroke, or condition necessitating an invasive heart procedure. Based on the results, the researchers recommended adding pioglitazone to the patient's regimen to decrease the risk of cardiac complications.

beta cell function is maintained for at least 2 years.

When comparing patients taking TZDs with those taking other antidiabetic agents, such as sulfonylureas or metformin, TZDs appear to be slightly less effective, possibly because of the significant rate of TZD nonresponders. However, when comparing those who do respond, these agents demonstrated a lowering of HbA_{1c} equivalent to that of sulfonylureas and metformin. Further, TZDs show greater efficacy than alpha-glucosidase inhibitors.

The TZDs rosiglitazone and pioglitazone are approved for use in combination with other oral agents and with insulin. Triple combination therapy with Glucovance (glyburide and metformin) and rosiglitazone also is approved for use.

One of the most striking findings is that these agents have been found to raise HDL-C by up to 13%. Indeed, rosiglitazone actually surpasses pioglitazone in its ability to increase the most protective HDL subtype, HDL-2, whereas pioglitazone performs better with triglycerides and LDL-C. Although effects on LDL-C have been variable, TZDs tend to shift the LDL-C from small, dense more atherogenic particles to larger, less atherogenic molecules. (See *Pioglitazone and MIs*.)

In addition to affecting lipid levels, TZDs also lower cardiovascular risk markers, including:
- slightly reducing blood pressure
- positively affecting plasminogen activator inhibitor
- decreasing C-reactive protein
- improving endothelial function
- decreasing smooth-muscle proliferation
- decreasing carotid intimal media thickness.

Adverse effects

Adverse effects of TZDs include weight gain, mainly in peripheral, subcutaneous sites. TZDs are associated with a reduction in visceral fat stores, which are more closely linked with insulin resistance. Edema may occur, although edema and weight gain are more common in patients receiving insulin therapy along with the TZD. Anemia also has been reported. Although the liver injury that prompted the removal of troglitazone from the market hasn't been associated with rosiglitazone and pioglitazone, the U.S. Food and Drug Administration (FDA) continues to recommend baseline and periodic measurement of liver function. TZDs should be used with extreme caution in patients with advanced heart failure and those with liver impairment.

Dosing considerations

TZDs are approved for use as monotherapy along with diet and exercise or as combination therapy with sulfonylureas, metformin, or insulin. However, these drugs increase plasma volume, which may lead to fluid retention and heart failure. Therefore, they should be used cautiously in patients with cardiovascular risk factors. Rosiglitazone may be administered once daily or in two divided doses. Pioglitazone may administered once daily.

MEGLITINIDE ANALOGS

Meglitinide analogs, also referred to as *nonsulfonylurea secretogogues*, include the benzoic acid derivative repaglinide (Prandin) and the D-phenylalanine derivative, nateglinide (Starlix). These agents differ from sulfonylureas in their more rapid onset and shorter duration of action, which allows for dosing at each meal. Patients take the medication only if they're going to eat; specifically, they're instructed to "take a meal, take a dose; skip a meal, skip a dose." (See *Summary of meglitinide analogs*.)

Mechanism of action

The mechanisms of action of repaglinide and nateglinide are similar to each other and to the sulfonylureas, all of them interacting with voltage-dependent KATP channels on beta cells. The end result is increased beta cell insulin secretion and lowered blood glucose levels.

The short half-lives of repaglinide and nateglinide have two significant consequences. First, postprandial glucose elevations are moderated by the rapid, increased insulin release immediately upon eating. This is important, as control of postprandial glucose is an integral part of optimal diabetes care. In addition to the harmful effects of elevated postprandial glucose levels on overall diabetes management, studies have shown that elevated postprandial glucose levels may be associated with a greater risk of cardiovascular disease.

Yet, studies haven't assessed the long-term efficacy of meglitinides in decreasing microvascular and macrovascular risk.

Second, because insulin secretion isn't as prolonged as with sulfonylureas, there's less insulin being secreted in the late postprandial phase. This potentially lessens the risk of hypoglycemia between meals, which could benefit individuals with erratic mealtimes.

Repaglinide and nateglinide have some identified differences in action and efficacy. Nateglinide appears to have little stimulatory effect on insulin when taken during a fasting state; thus, it may enhance meal-stimulated insulin release more than other secretogogues. It may also have less potential for hypoglycemia than repaglinide. Nateglinide does have a more simplified dosing regimen and is preferred in patients with renal compromise. In terms of ability to decrease HbA_{1c} levels, studies have shown repaglinide to be comparable to sulfonylureas and metformin, whereas nateglinide fared less well. Studies have shown little difference with either agent, as compared to sulfonylureas, on postprandial blood glucose levels.

Adverse effects

Similar to other secretogogues, adverse effects of meglitinides include hypoglycemia and weight gain; however, these effects may be less pronounced as a result of their short half-life. One drawback of their use may be their frequent dosing schedule with each meal. Another factor is their increased cost compared with sulfonylureas.

Dosing considerations

Meglitinides are approved for use as monotherapy and combination therapy with metformin and TZDs. Use of combination therapy may result in improved glycemic control; however, combination therapy with a sulfonylurea is simply a duplication of therapy, providing no additional glycemic benefit.

SUMMARY OF MEGLITINIDE ANALOGS

This chart highlights key information related to drugs belonging to the class of meglitinide analogs.

	REPAGLINIDE	NATEGLINIDE
Pharmacokinetics	Onset: Rapid Peak: 1 hr Half-life: 1 hr Duration: 2–3 hr	Onset: Rapid Peak: 1 hr Half-life: 1.5 hr Duration: 4 hr
Metabolism	Hepatic; metabolized to inactive metabolite	Hepatic
Distribution	Crosses placenta; may enter breast milk	Crosses placenta; may enter breast milk
Excretion	Feces and urine; less than 1% of parent drug excreted via kidney	Feces and urine; 16% of parent drug excreted via kidney
Adverse reactions	*Central nervous system:* Headache, paresthesia *Endocrine:* Hypoglycemia *GI:* Nausea, diarrhea, constipation, vomiting, dyspepsia *Respiratory:* Upper respiratory infection, sinusitis, rhinitis, bronchitis	*Central nervous system:* Headache, paresthesia, dizziness *Endocrine:* Hypoglycemia (low risk) *GI:* Nausea, diarrhea, constipation, vomiting, dyspepsia *Respiratory:* Upper respiratory infection, sinusitis, rhinitis, bronchitis
Interactions	■ Increased risk of hypoglycemia with gemfibrozil; risk is severe if gemfibrozil and itraconazole are combined; alternative therapies, including juniper berries, ginseng, garlic, fenugreek, coriander, dandelion root, and celery	■ Increased risk of hypoglycemia with alcohol, salicylates, nonsteroidal anti-inflammatory drugs, beta-adrenergic blockers, monoamine oxidase inhibitors
Contraindications and precautions	■ Hypersensitivity to repaglinide, type 1 diabetes, diabetic ketoacidosis (DKA) ■ Use cautiously in patients with renal or hepatic impairment, lactation ■ *Pediatrics:* Safety and efficacy not established	■ Hypersensitivity to nateglinide, type 1 diabetes, DKA ■ Use cautiously in patients with renal or hepatic impairment, lactation ■ *Pediatrics:* Safety and efficacy not established

AMYLIN ANALOG: PRAMLINTIDE

Pramlintide is an injectable agent and is synthetic version of the human hormone amylin that's secreted by pancreatic beta cells in response to hyperglycemia. In concert with insulin, amylin is a glucoregulatory peptide hormone that's released into the portal vein and enters the systemic circulation in response to the ingestion of a carbohydrate-containing meal. These two pancreatic beta cell hormones coordinate the rate of glucose appearance and disappearance in the circulation, therefore

COMPARISON OF PLASMA AMYLIN LEVELS

In the graph shown here, amylin levels are decreased in patients with both type 1 and type 2 diabetes who use insulin. Decreases in amylin secretion affect diabetes control because of the loss of its effects on glucagon release, gastric emptying, appetite, and hepatic glucose production.

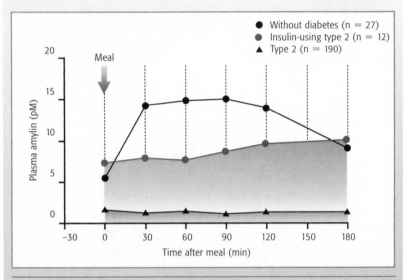

Adapted with permission from Amylin Pharmaceuticals, Inc., San Diego, California.

managing the postprandial rise of blood glucose levels.

Amylin works in combination with insulin through several different mechanisms:
- suppression of glucagon release, leading to decreased hepatic glucose output
- regulation of the rate of gastric emptying
- modulation of appetite and satiety
- suppression of hepatic glucose production.

In type 1 diabetes, circulating amylin is absent; in type 2 diabetes, postprandial circulating amylin concentrations are decreased. Without adequate concentrations of circulating amylin during the postprandial period, blood glucose levels are elevated and demonstrate an exaggerated response to carbohydrate intake. (See *Comparison of plasma amylin levels*.)

Mechanism of action

Suppression of inappropriate glucagon release is a major function of amylin. In both type 1 and type 2 diabetes, inappropriate secretion of glucagon has been identified as an important contributing factor to elevated postprandial glucose elevations and increased hepatic glucose output. Injected pramlintide suppresses inappropriate glucagon secretion, leading to suppression of output from the liver.

Another function of amylin is to reduce the rate of gastric emptying from the stomach to the small intestine. In diabetes, insulin deficiency is commonly accompanied by this accelerated rate of emptying resulting in elevated postprandial glucose levels. By affecting the rate of gastric emptying, pramlintide can modify postprandial glucose elevations.

A third function by which amylin affects blood glucose levels is through increased satiety and reduced food intake. Weight reduction and preventing weight gain are significant issues for most patients with type 2 diabetes and for some with type 1 because of the effects of insulin and oral diabetes therapies. Through increased satiety and reduced food intake, pramlintide's potential outcomes include improved postprandial hyperglycemia and modestly improved HbA_{1c} levels. Specifically, studies of pramlintide's clinical effectiveness have shown:

● reduction in postprandial blood glucose by 50 to 100 mg/dl
● modest reduction in HbA_{1c} by 0.4% to 0.8%
● modest reduction in weight by 2 to 3 lb (0.5 to 1 kg)
● reduction in postprandial triglycerides.

Adverse effects

Because amylin affects the rate of gastric emptying, the most common adverse effects include nausea, vomiting, abdominal pain, and decreased appetite. Nausea may occur less frequently when there's a gradual introduction of the medication to the patient's regimen. Also, because of the drug's effect on the GI system, it should be used cautiously with oral antidiabetic agents because it may cause changes in drug absorption. Hypoglycemia may occur because it's used in conjunction with insulin. Close monitoring of the patient's blood glucose level should be done to adjust insulin dosage appropriately. Other adverse effects include headache, fatigue, dizziness, and coughing.

Dosing considerations

Pramlintide is indicated as an adjunct treatment for patients with type 2 diabetes who use mealtime insulin, but have failed to achieve target blood glucose levels (despite optimal insulin therapy) with or without combination therapy (sulfonylurea and metformin). It's also indicated as adjunctive therapy for patients with type 1 diabetes who take mealtime insulin, but who also haven't achieved target blood glucose levels. (See *Summary of new hormonal agents*, pages 102 and 103.)

Appropriate patient selection is vital to the safe, effective use of pramlintide. The health care provider should perform a thorough review of the patient's self-monitoring data, HbA_{1c} results, current medication regimen, body weight, and history of hypoglycemic episodes.

To that end, certain individuals shouldn't use pramlintide therapy. These include pediatric patients as well as patients with:

● poor compliance with current treatment regimen
● poor compliance with self-monitoring
● HbA_{1c} levels greater than 9%
● history of recurrent, severe hypoglycemia requiring assistance
● hypoglycemia unawareness
● confirmed diagnosis of gastroparesis or use of medications that stimulate motility.

There are several additional factors to be considered before initiating pramlintide therapy. These factors are detailed in the FDA-approved *Symlin Medication Guide*, which accompanies the medication. The health care provider and patient should be thoroughly familiar with this information before initiating therapy.

Pramlintide's impact as a treatment option for the patient with type 1 or type 2 diabetes, who's taking mealtime insulin, remains to be seen. The complexity surrounding the dosing regimen, the demands on the health care provider and patient, and the cost of the

SUMMARY OF NEW HORMONAL AGENTS

This chart highlights two new hormonal agents developed for use as adjunct therapy in patients with diabetes.

	PRAMLINTIDE	EXENATIDE
Pharmacokinetics	Onset: 20 min Peak: Unknown Half-life: 48 min Duration: Unknown	Onset: Rapid Peak: 2.1 hr Half-life: 2.4 hr Duration: 10 hr
Metabolism	Kidney	Kidney
Distribution	Unknown whether enters breast milk	Unknown whether enters breast milk
Excretion	Renal	Renal
Adverse reactions	■ Local, systemic allergy ■ Nausea, anorexia; tolerance usually develops	■ Decreased drug levels or delayed absorption with digoxin, lovastatin, lisinopril, acetaminophen ■ With drugs dependent on threshold concentrations, exenatide could slow absorption of oral drugs because of slowed gastric emptying effects ■ Some antibiotics, contraceptives should be taken 1 hr before exenatide injection ■ Can't be mixed with insulin in a syringe
Interactions	■ Not to be taken with drugs that alter GI motility or agents that slow intestinal absorption of nutrients ■ Delayed gastric emptying may affect oral medications taken with or up to 2 hr following pramlintide ■ Increased risk of hypoglycemia with insulin, oral antidiabetic agents, angiotensin-converting enzyme inhibitors, disopyramide, fibrates, fluoxetine, monoamine oxidase inhibitors, pentoxifylline, propoxyphene, salicylates, and sulfonamide antibiotics	Hypoglycemia, in combination with sulfonylureas *GI:* Nausea, vomiting, diarrhea, dyspepsia; tolerance to GI effects usually occurs in 1–2 weeks *Other:* Jittery feeling, dizziness, headache
Contraindications and precautions	■ Known hypersensitivity to pramlintide or components; children ■ Severe gastroparesis; hypoglycemia unawareness or recurrent, severe hypoglycemia; lactation (unknown whether excreted in breast milk) ■ Reduce rapid/short insulin dose by 50%	■ Known hypersensitivity ■ Type 1 diabetes or diabetic ketoacidosis ■ End-stage renal disease, severe renal impairment or severe GI disease *Pediatrics:* Not currently approved for use in children

SUMMARY OF NEW HORMONAL AGENTS *(continued)*

PRAMLINTIDE	EXENATIDE
■ Can't be mixed with insulin ■ Inject in abdomen or thighs; site must be more than 2" (5.1 cm) from insulin injection site *Pediatrics:* Not studied for use in children	

agent may limit its widespread use. The drug demands that the health care provider be well versed in its safety and efficacy; currently, its use is mainly limited to endocrinologists. Appropriate candidates for pramlintide therapy should be identified through a careful screening process. After proper patient selection, education, and implementation of pramlintide therapy have been accomplished, the potential benefits in terms of postprandial glucose levels, satiety, and weight control may be significant.

INCRETIN MIMETIC: EXENATIDE

Exenatide (Exendin-4; Byetta) is an injectable synthetic form of glucagon-like peptide-1 (GLP-1), a hormone found in the saliva of the Gila monster. It's the first in a new class of agents used to treat type 2 diabetes, called incretin mimetics. Incretin hormones have generated much interest since they were discovered in the 1960s. It was found that oral glucose elicited a greater secretory response than I.V. glucose. Oral administration indicated that factors in the digestive system must have an effect on pancreatic insulin secretion. In fact, it has since been shown that about 60% of postprandial insulin secretion is a result of this "incretin effect" that's impaired in patients with type 2 diabetes mellitus.

The two peptide hormones credited with this effect are released from the brush border of the small intestine. K-cells (glucose-dependent insulinotropic peptide) of the jejunum and L-cells (GLP-1) of the ileum are released in response to food ingestion. After they're released, these hormones are rapidly metabolized. Of the two, GLP-1 has been of special interest because of its multiple glucoregulatory effects that go beyond just beta cell stimulation. These effects include:

● enhanced glucose-dependent first phase insulin secretion
● suppression of inappropriate postprandial glucagon secretion
● enhanced satiety, thereby reducing food intake
● slowed rate of gastric emptying, limiting postprandial glucose elevations.

Mechanism of action

Exenatide's physiologic actions are triggered as it binds to the GLP-1 receptor found in many organs, including the pancreas and brain. It stimulates insulin secretion from pancreatic beta cells in a glucose-dependent manner. Specifically, exenatide stimulates insulin secretion when the glucose concentration is elevated; its actions decline when the glucose lowers, which helps prevent hypoglycemia.

Exenatide also suppresses glucagon secretion from the pancreatic alpha cells in a glucose-dependent manner. It suppresses glucagon secretion after eating and it reduces glucagon suppression during hypoglycemia. Patients with type 2 diabetes commonly have inappropriately elevated glucagon levels, which result in increased hepatic glucose output and elevated postprandial blood glucose levels.

Through its effect on the receptors in the brain, exenatide produces feelings of satiety, leading to a reduction of food intake. Over time, this can induce weight loss, which is important for patients with type 2 diabetes, most of whom are overweight or obese.

Exenatide also affects the rate of gastric emptying. It has been shown that gastric emptying is commonly accelerated in type 2 diabetes, resulting in rapid rises in postprandial blood glucose levels. In contrast, exenatide slows the rate of gastric emptying, which allows for slower delivery and absorption in the small intestine. The result is slower absorption of carbohydrates into the circulation, with a decrease in postprandial blood glucose elevations. Lastly, GLP-1 may play a role in the maintenance of pancreatic beta cell health. In animal studies, GLP-1 administered to healthy rodents resulted in islet neogenesis, beta cell proliferation, and an increase in beta cell mass. It has also been shown to preserve islet integrity and reduce apoptosis in human islets. Like pramlintide, exenatide has been shown to reduce postprandial blood glucose levels, modestly reduce HbA_{1c} levels, and reduce weight. Specifically, studies of exenatide have produced these results:

- reduction in postprandial blood glucose by 50% to 80%
- modest reduction of HbA_{1c} by 0.5% to 1%
- modest reduction of weight by 2 to 6 lb (1 to 3 kg).

Adverse effects

Because exenatide affects the rate of gastric emptying, the most common adverse effects include nausea, vomiting, diarrhea, acid stomach, and decreased appetite. If nausea occurs, it usually decreases with continued use of exenatide. Hypoglycemia may occur because it's used in conjunction with oral antidiabetic agents. Blood glucose level should be monitored and drug dosages adjusted accordingly. Other adverse effects include headache, dizziness, and feeling jittery.

Dosing considerations

Exenatide is indicated as adjunctive therapy for patients whose type 2 diabetes isn't adequately controlled with metformin or a combination of metformin and sulfonylurea. Currently, it isn't approved for monotherapy.

Exenatide should be taken twice per day, within 1 hour before meals; it shouldn't be taken after meals. If a dose is missed, the patient should wait until the next scheduled dose. Appropriate injection sites include the abdomen, thighs, and arms. Pens should be refrigerated between doses, but exenatide shouldn't be frozen. Patients should discard the pens 30 days after the first use.

Because of its multiple effects on type 2 diabetes control, exenatide has the potential to significantly affect multiple treatment options. First, its glucose-dependent effects on both insulin secretion and glucagon suppression help to alter postprandial blood glucose levels without significantly increasing the risk of hypoglycemia. Second, exenatide promotes weight loss — a major issue for patients with type 2 diabetes — by increasing satiety and slowing gastric emptying. A third potential benefit is the preservation of beta cell functioning. In addition, the simple dosing of the drug and its few adverse effects, such as nausea, make it relatively safe.

A main drawback of exenatide is that it's an injectable, which is why some patients and health care providers are slower to accept this therapy. Cost is also a valid concern; some patients who may benefit most may not be able to afford the drug. These and other factors may influence the acceptance of incretin mimetic therapy.

DIABETES TYPE 2 TREATMENT ALGORITHM

With so many drug therapies available, choosing the right one can be challenging. This algorithm can help you assist your patients with type 2 diabetes.

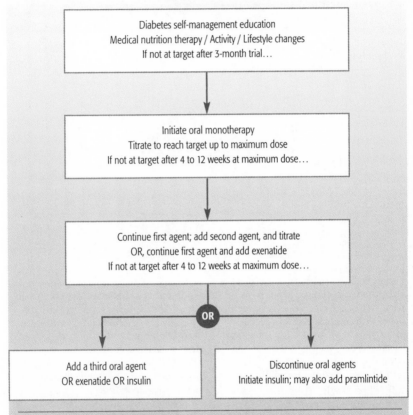

Adapted from American Association of Diabetes Educators, *Core Concepts: The Art & Science of Diabetes Education.* Chicago: American Association of Diabetes Educators, 2003, with permission of the publisher.

CHOOSING AN APPROPRIATE THERAPY

Because there are so many drug options available for managing type 2 diabetes, choosing one to help achieve your patient's treatment goals can seem daunting. However, algorithms exist that can help with this choice. (See *Diabetes type 2 treatment algorithm.*)

Monotherapy

The appropriate choice of a specific therapeutic agent for the patient with type 2 diabetes is based on several factors. First, therapy should match disease progression. For example, if type 2 diabetes is of recent onset, and if the patient displays characteristics of insulin resistance, therapy with an insulin sen-

CHOOSING THE RIGHT MONOTHERAPY

——————•——————

The chart below highlights some important patient characteristics that influence the selection of a drug used as a single agent for treating type 2 diabetes.

PATIENT CHARACTERISTICS	APPROPRIATE AGENT
Lean	Sulfonylureas
Obese Dyslipidemias Insulin resistant Elevated fasting blood glucose levels	Metformin
Postprandial hyperglycemia	Acarbose and miglitol Repaglinide and nateglinide
Renal impairment Insulin resistant	Thiazolidinediones
Glucotoxicity	Insulin

Adapted from American Association of Diabetes Educators, *Core Concepts: The Art & Science of Diabetes Education.* Chicago: American Association of Diabetes Educators, 2003, with permission of the publisher.

sitizer, such as metformin or a TZD, is an appropriate choice. Metformin is particularly appropriate if the patient is overweight and experiences elevated fasting blood glucose levels related to increased hepatic glucose output. If the patient is contraindicated for metformin, pioglitazone or rosiglitazone would be appropriate agents. Patients with elevated postprandial blood glucose levels are best managed with secretogogues or alpha-glucosidase inhibitors.

To appropriately match the patient's therapy to his disease state, his diabetes history must be established. Such factors as his weight, whether he's newly diagnosed or new to drug therapy, allergies, comorbidities, and laboratory findings, including fasting and postprandial blood glucose level results and HbA_{1c} and insulin and lipid levels, should be assessed.

Depending on the agent chosen, assessment of hepatic and renal function should be performed before initiating therapy (and periodically) as indicated. Finally, the patient's ability to pay for the medication must be discussed, along with his ability to understand how to properly take the medication and his willingness to comply.

For a guide to making appropriate decisions regarding monotherapy, see *Choosing the right monotherapy.*

Combination therapy

If lifestyle modifications and monotherapy don't work for the patient with type 2 diabetes, combination therapy is given. Indeed, although it may be used as initial therapy, combination therapy is typically determined by disease progression.

Results of the UKPDS revealed that most patients with type 2 diabetes will eventually require multiple oral agents

APPROVED COMBINATION THERAPIES

The following combinations of agents are approved by the U.S. Food and Drug Administration for use in combination therapy in patients with diabetes.

AGENT	MAY BE COMBINED WITH:
Metformin	Sulfonylurea, repaglinide, nateglinide, pioglitazone, acarbose, rosiglitazone, insulin
Miglitol	Sulfonylurea, insulin
Acarbose	Sulfonylurea, metformin, insulin
Pioglitazone (triple therapy)	Sulfonylurea, insulin, metformin, repaglinide, combination product (sulfonylurea plus metformin)
Rosiglitazone (triple therapy)	Metformin, sulfonylurea, repaglinide, insulin, combination product (sulfonylurea plus metformin)
Repaglinide	Pioglitazone, rosiglitazone, metformin
Nateglinide	Metformin

From Peragallo-Dittko, V. PowerPoint presentation sponsored by Novo Nordisk Pharmaceuticals Inc., 2003.

or other therapies to reach and maintain their target goals. The study revealed that after 3 years, only 50% of patients' type 2 diabetes was adequately controlled with a single drug; by 9 years, the percentage decreased to 25%.

Clinical trials examining combination therapy of oral agents have demonstrated additive HbA_{1c} reductions. Dual- and triple-combination therapies, using agents with different mechanisms of action and target tissues, have been shown to improve overall glycemic control, lower overall drug dosing (in some instances), and minimize adverse effects.

The most commonly used combination of agents is a sulfonylurea with an insulin sensitizer, usually metformin. This combination offers high potency, low cost, and lower potential for weight gain. Other combinations include a sul-

fonylurea with a TZD, although both agents may cause weight gain; and metformin combined with a TZD — although they're both insulin sensitizers, they target insulin resistance in different tissues, and metformin may also help counteract the weight gain associated with TZDs.

When prescribing combination therapy, it isn't appropriate to use two drugs from the same class or two drugs that target the same physiologic defect. This would duplicate therapy, which would increase cost and the potential for adverse reactions (particularly hypoglycemia). Although FDA-approved, the use of nonsulfonylureas and alpha-glucosidase inhibitors in combination provides decreased potency, increased cost, and increased potential for adverse reactions. (See *Approved combination therapies*.)

APPROVED FIXED-COMBINATION AGENTS

The following fixed-combination agents are approved by the U.S. Food and Drug Administration.

AGENT	COMBINATION AGENTS AND STRENGTHS
Glucovance	Glyburide and metformin 1.25 mg glyburide/250 mg metformin 2.5 mg glyburide/500 mg metformin 5 mg glyburide/500 mg metformin
Avandamet	Rosiglitazone and metformin 1 mg rosiglitazone/500 mg metformin 2 mg rosiglitazone/500 mg metformin 4 mg rosiglitazone/500 mg metformin
Metaglip	Metformin and glipizide 2.5 mg glipizide/250 mg metformin 2.5 mg glipizide/500 mg metformin 5 mg glipizide/500 mg metformin
ACTOplus met	Pioglitazone and metformin 15 mg pioglitazone/500 mg metformin 15 mg pioglitazone/850 mg metformin
Avandaryl	Rosiglitazone and glimepiride 4 mg rosiglitazone/1 mg glimepiride 4 mg rosiglitazone/2 mg glimepiride 4 mg rosiglitazone/4 mg glimepiride

From Peragallo-Dittko, V. PowerPoint presentation sponsored by Novo Nordisk Pharmaceuticals Inc., 2003.

Fixed-combination agents

Several fixed-combination medications are currently FDA-approved and available. (See *Approved fixed-combination agents*.)

Although fixed-combination agents are less expensive (one copay instead of two) and may potentiate increased compliance (fewer tablets to take), it's important to note that decreasing one copay may not offset the cost of newer drug combinations and their potential impact on health insurance premiums. Although it has been shown that compliance increases with the use of just one agent, it's difficult to predict that a patient will comply with the drug regimen solely because it's a fixed-combination agent.

The efficacy of combining two agents into one tablet as a fixed-dose combination also remains undetermined. Some unpublished, retrospective data suggest that glyburide and metformin tablets (Glucovance) lower HbA_{1c} levels better than metformin and glyburide taken as separate agents.

One disadvantage of fixed-dose combinations is that they don't allow for the specific needs of individual patients. For instance, most patients taking metformin require 2,000 mg/day. If the patient was receiving Avandamet which contained 500 mg metformin and 4 mg rosiglitazone, he would need to take 4 tablets of the fixed-combination to obtain 2,000 mg of metformin. However, the patient would also then receive 16 mg of rosiglitazone, possibly leading to an inappropriately high dose of the rosiglitazone (usual dose is 4 to 8 mg/day). So, although combining agents has been cited as a benefit, the true effects may vary among patients and between the prescribed combined agents.

INITIATING INSULIN THERAPY

Despite lifestyle modifications and the use of oral antidiabetic agents, insulin therapy will eventually be included in the treatment regimen of about 50% of patients with type 2 diabetes. Because insulin therapy is commonly viewed as a last resort, it has led some health care providers to coin the term *psychological insulin resistance*, which describes the reluctance of patients and health care providers to initiate insulin therapy earlier in the course of treatment.

According to the American Diabetes Association and the National Institute of Diabetes and Digestive and Kidney Diseases, studies have indicated that earlier initiation of insulin therapy may be one way of helping to preserve beta cell function. In general, guidelines indicate that, in addition to initiating insulin therapy when primary failure of oral antidiabetic agents occurs, insulin therapy should also be given when the patient experiences secondary failure of monotherapy or combination therapy. Treatment with insulin therapy is discussed further in chapter 7.

USING ANTIPLATELET THERAPY

It's well documented that diabetes can put a person at increased risk for macrovascular diseases. Indeed, coronary artery disease, cerebrovascular disease, and peripheral vascular disease are the most common, serious, and costly of the chronic complications experienced by patients with diabetes. An-

tiplatelet therapy is one of a number of interventions aimed at addressing the platelet and clotting-factor abnormalities usually found in patients with diabetes, thus reducing the risks associated with developing macrovascular disease.

Antiplatelet therapy has proven effective for both primary prevention and secondary prevention of macrovascular disease. Primary prevention targets those with diabetes or prediabetes who don't have diagnosed macrovascular disease but who are at increased risk. Antiplatelet therapy with aspirin has been shown to decrease MI by about 30% and stroke by 20%.

Secondary prevention is useful for those who have a positive history for macrovascular disease (acute coronary syndrome, stroke, peripheral vascular disease). Antiplatelet therapy with aspirin has been shown to decrease recurrent cardiac events in patients with diabetes.

Based on the positive outcomes associated with aspirin therapy, the American Diabetes Association recommends that people with diabetes older than age 30 (who have evidence of macrovascular disease) undergo daily antiplatelet therapy with aspirin for secondary prevention, unless contraindicated. Aspirin therapy should also be considered for primary prevention in high-risk individuals older than age 30.

Despite an increase in aspirin use since 1997 (with apparent success), it continues to be underused; less than one-half of adults older than age 35 with type 2 diabetes take aspirin daily. Aspirin use was noted to be lower in young adults ages 25 to 49, in women ages 35 to 64, and in individuals without diagnosed cardiovascular disease.

ALERT *Keep in mind that aspirin therapy shouldn't be used in patients younger than age 21 because of the increased risk of Reye's syndrome.*

Aspirin exerts its antiplatelet effect by blocking prostaglandin synthesis; specifically, it irreversibly inhibits prostaglandin cyclo-oxygenase. This effect lasts for the life of the platelet and prevents the formation of the platelet-aggregating substance thromboxane A_2. At somewhat higher doses, aspirin irreversibly inhibits the formation of prostaglandin 12 (prostacyclin), which inhibits platelet aggregation and has arterial vasodilating properties.

Selected references

Ahmann, A.J., and Riddle, M.C. "Current Oral Agents for Type 2 Diabetes," *Postgraduate Medicine* 111(5); 32-34, 37-40, 43-46, May 2002.

American Diabetes Association. "Aspirin Therapy in Diabetes," *Diabetes Care* 26(Suppl 1):S87-88, January 2003.

American Diabetes Association. "Standards of Medical Care in Diabetes," *Diabetes Care* 28(Suppl 1):S4-36, January 2005.

American Diabetes Association and National Institute of Diabetes and Digestive and Kidney Diseases. "The Prevention or Delay of Type 2 Diabetes," *Diabetes Spectrum* 15(3):147-57, 2002.

Bloomgarden, Z.T. "Thiazolidinediones," *Diabetes Care* 28(2):488-93, February 2005.

Buse, J. "Current Therapies and the Incretin Advantage for Achieving Tight Glycemic Control," Incretin-based Therapies: Achieving Better Glycemic Control in Type 2 Diabetes, pps. 24-33, August 2005.

Buse, J. "Understanding Tight Glycemic Control: Benefits and Barriers," Incretin-based Therapies: Achieving Better Glycemic Control in Type 2 Diabetes, pps. 5-11 August 2005.

Byetta Patient Information Guide. "Get a Few Solid Answers About Byetta and Your Type 2 Diabetes" [Online]. Available at: *www.pharmacistelink.com/product/highlights/pdfs/byetta_patient-guide.pdf* [2006 March 6].

Canadian Diabetes Association Clinical Practice Guidelines Expert Committee. "Pharmacologic Management of Type 2 Diabetes" [Online]. Available at: *www.diabetes.ca/cpg2003/downloads/pharmacologic.pdf* [2005 November 22].

Centers for Disease Control and Prevention. "National Diabetes Fact Sheet, 2005" [Online]. Available at: *www.cdc.gov/diabetes/pubs/factsheet05.htm*.

Chiquette, E., et al. "A Meta-analysis Comparing the Effect of Thiazolidinediones on Cardiovascular Risk Factors," *Archives of Internal Medicine* 164(19):2097-104, October 2004.

"Core Concepts: The Art & Science of Diabetes Education." Chicago: American Association of Diabetes Educators, 2003.

Cornell, S. "Diabetes 101: Medication Management in Type 2 Diabetes," in AADE Program Book (pp. 70-75). Chicago: American Association of Diabetes Educators, 2005.

DeFronzo, R.A., et al. "Effects of Exenatide (Exendin-4) on Glycemic Control and Weight Over 30 Weeks in Metformin-Treated Patients with Type 2 Diabetes," *Diabetes Care* 28(5):1092-100, May 2005.

Drucker, D. "The Incretin Effect in Glucose Metabolism," Incretin-based Therapies: Achieving Better Control in Type 2 Diabetes, pp. 12-23, August 2005.

Egede, L.E., et al. "The Prevalence and Pattern of Complementary and Alternative Medicine Use in Individuals with Diabetes," *Diabetes Care* 25(2):324-29, February 2002.

Eurich, D.T., et al. "Improved Clinical Outcomes Associated With Metformin in Patients With Diabetes and Heart Failure," *Diabetes Care* 28(10):2345-351 October 2005.

European Diabetes Working Party for Older People 2004. "Clinical Guidelines for Type 2 Diabetes Mellitus" [Online]. Available at: *www.eugms.org/document?action=get_document&id=4* [2005 November 22].

Geil, P., and Hieronymus, L. "Oral Medications for Type 2 Diabetes," *Diabetes Self-Management* 22(4):6, 8-10, 12, July-August 2005.

"The Glucoregulatory Effects of Glucagon-Like Peptide-1 (GLP-1)," Scientific Monograph. Amylin Pharmaceuticals, 2004.

Haines, S. "Pharmacological Strategies to Achieve Optimal Glycemic Control," in AADE Program Book (pps. 300-308). Chicago: American Association of Diabetes Educators, 2005.

Heine, R.J, et al. "Exenatide versus Insulin Glargine in Patients with Suboptimally Controlled Type 2 Diabetes: A Randomized Trial," *Annals of Internal Medicine* 143(8):559-69, October 2005.

Holmboe, E.S. "Oral Antihyperglycemic Therapy for Type 2 Diabetes," *JAMA* 287(3):373-76, January 2002.

Inzucchi, S.E. "Oral Antihyperglycemic Therapy for Type 2 Diabetes: Scientific Review," *JAMA* 287(3):360-72, January 2002.

Isley, W. L., and Oki, J.O. "Diabetes Mellitus, Type 2" [Online]. Available at: *www.emedicine.com/med/topic547.htm* [2005 November 28].

Karch, A. *Lippincott's Nursing Drug Guide.* Philadelphia: Lippincott Williams & Wilkins, 2005.

Kendall, D.M. "Postprandial Blood Glucose in the Management of Type 2 Diabetes: The Emerging Role of Incretin Mimetics," *Medscape Diabetes and Endocrinology* 7(2): 2005. Available at: *www.medscape.com/viewarticle/515693.*

Kendall, D., et al. "Effects of Exenatide (Exendin-4) on Glycemic Control Over 30 Weeks in Patients With Type 2 Diabetes Treated With Metformin and a Sulfonylurea" *Diabetes Care* 28(5):1083-1091, May 2005.

Koro, C.E., et al. "Glycemic Control From 1988 to 2000 Among U.S. Adults Diagnosed With Type 2 Diabetes: A Preliminary Report," *Diabetes Care* 27(1):17-20, January 2004.

Kimmel, B. & Inzucchi, S. "Oral Agents for Type 2 Diabetes: An Update," *Clinical Diabetes* 23(2):64-76, November 2005. *www.clinical.diabetesjournals. org/cgi/content/full/23/2/64.*

Moshang, J. "Type 2 Diabetes: Growing by Leaps and Bounds," *Nursing Made Incredibly Easy* 3(4):20-34, July-August 2005.

National Institute of Diabetes and Digestive and Kidney Diseases, National Institutes of Health. "National Diabetes Statistics" [Online]. Available at: *www.diabetes.niddk.nih.gov/dm/pubs/st atistics/* [2006 March 6].

Nesto, R., et al. "Thiazolidinedione Use, Fluid Retention, and Congestive Heart Failure: A Consensus Statement from the American Heart Association and American Diabetes Association," 27(1):256-63, January 2004.

"Oral Antidiabetic Therapy." (PowerPoint Presentation.) Princeton, N.J.: Novo Nordisk Pharmaceuticals, Inc., 2003.

PDR Concise Prescribing Guide. Montvale, N.J.: Thomson PDR, 2004.

Peragallo-Dittko, V. (PowerPoint Presentation.) Princeton, N.J.: Novo Nordisk Pharmaceuticals, Inc., 2003

Physician's Desk Reference, 59th ed. Montvale, N.J.: Thomson PDR, 2005.

Persell, S.D., and Baker, D.W. "Aspirin Use Among Adults With Diabetes: Recent Trends and Emerging Sex Disparities," *Archives of Internal Medicine* 164(22): 2492-499, December 2004.

Pharmacotherapy: A Pathophysiologic Approach, 5th ed. New York: McGraw-Hill Book Co., 2002.

Ramlo-Halsted, B.A., and Edelman, S.V. "The Natural History of Type 2 Diabetes: Practical Points to Consider in Developing Prevention and Treatment Strategies," *Clinical Diabetes* 18(2):80-84, Spring 2000.

Riddle, M.C., et al. "The Treat-to-Target Trial: Randomized Addition of Glargine or Human NPH Insulin to Oral Therapy of Type 2 Diabetic Patients," *Diabetes Care* 26(11):3038-3086, November 2003.

"The Role of the Hormone Amylin in Glucose Homeostasis," Scientific Monograph. Amylin Pharmaceuticals, 2004.

Salgo, P. (Moderator), Bode, B., et al. (Panelists). "The Type 2 Diabetes Challenge—Closing the Gap Between Recommended Standards and Real World Outcomes," in *Medical Crossfire* (Webcast) 5(12):4-17, July 2004.

Schernthaner, G., et al. "Efficacy and Safety of Pioglitazone versus Metformin in Patients with Type 2 Diabetes Mellitus: A Double-blind, Randomized Trial," *Journal of Clinical Endocrinology and Metabolism* 89(12):6068-6067, December 2004.

Schwartz, S., et al. "Insulin 70/30 Mix Plus Metformin versus Triple Oral Therapy in the Treatment of Type 2 Diabetes After Failure of Two Oral Drugs," *Diabetes Care* 26(8):2238-243, August 2003.

Sheehan, M.T. "Current Therapeutic Options in Type 2 Diabetes Mellitus: A Practical Approach," *Clinical Medicine & Research* 1(3):189-200, July 2003.

Siminerio, L. "Challenges, Opportunities, and Strategies for Moving Patients to Injectable Medications," Incretin-based Therapies: Achieving Better Glycemic Control in Type 2 Diabetes (pps. 34-44), August 2005.

Trecroci, D. "ACTOPlus Met Approved by the FDA for Type 2 Diabetes," *Diabetes Health* 14(11):24, November 2005.

Vinicor, F. "Macrovascular Disease," in *A Core Curriculum for Diabetes Education: Diabetes and Complications.* Edited by Franz, M. Chicago: The American Association of Diabetes Educators, 2003.

Wasmer, A.L. *New Drug Treatments for Diabetes,* 2nd ed. New York: R.A. Rapaport Publishing, Inc., 2004.

"What is Diabetes." (PowerPoint Presentation.) Princeton, N.J.: Novo Nordisk Pharmaceuticals, Inc., 2003.

White, J. and Campbell, R. "Pharmacologic Therapies for Glucose Management," in *A Core Curriculum for Diabetes Education: Diabetes Management Therapies.* Edited by Franz, M. Chicago: The American Association of Diabetes Educators, 2003.

7

Insulin therapy

Insulin is a hormone produced by the beta cells of the pancreas. It plays a critical role in transporting glucose in the blood to the cells and other body tissues where it's used for energy. It also plays a major role in metabolizing ingested carbohydrates, fats, and proteins. In nondiabetic individuals, insulin is secreted in appropriate amounts to meet the demands of increased glucose in the blood that occurs when food is metabolized. Patients with type 1 diabetes, however, have an absolute insulin deficiency — that is, the beta cells of the pancreas have been destroyed, resulting in the absence of insulin secretion. Therefore, these patients can't convert glucose into a usable form for cells to use, resulting in an increase in blood glucose levels, causing them to need insulin therapy.

Patients with type 2 diabetes have insulin resistance and impaired beta cell function — that is, the pancreas secretes some insulin but the body doesn't respond to it in the typical manner. Many patients with type 2 diabetes may require insulin therapy in conjunction with other antidiabetic drugs to maintain good glucose control.

Insulin is supplied in an injectable form that may be administered by several methods. Many different types of insulin are available, and they vary based on their time of onset, peak, and duration. Although a wide range of factors can influence the type of insulin thera-py prescribed, the choice typically is determined by the individual's lifestyle, the health care provider's preference and experience, and the patient's blood glucose levels. In most cases, insulin is self-administered. The information provided in this chapter will help you teach your patients with diabetes how to self-administer their own insulin therapy.

TYPES OF INSULIN

At one time, more than 20 types of insulin were available for use in the United States. The first insulin was produced from animals, such as cows (beef insulin) or pigs (pork insulin). However, these animal insulins are no longer available in the United States. Since the early 1980s, insulin has been manufactured by recombinant deoxyribonucleic acid technology in the laboratory, resulting in what's called human insulin. Advances in technology have also resulted in the development of insulin analogs. These analogs differ from human insulin in their amino acid structure, which alters the drug's onset and peak times.

Insulin is typically categorized according to the onset, peak, and duration of action as rapid-acting, short-acting, intermediate-acting, or long-acting. In addition, combination insulin is available in commercially prepared mixtures. (See *Comparing insulins*, page 114.)

COMPARING INSULINS

This chart highlights the major types of insulin and the most commonly used insulins.

Type of insulin	Appearance	Onset	Peak	Duration
Rapid-acting				
Insulin lispro (Humalog)	Clear	10–15 min	60–90 min	3–5 hr
Insulin aspart (NovoLog)	Clear	15 min	40–50 min	3–5 hr
Insulin glulisine (Apidra)	Clear	5–10 min	60–90 min	2–4 hr
Short-acting				
Regular (Humulin R, Novolin R)	Clear	30–60 min	2–3 hr	5–8 hr
Intermediate-acting				
NPH (Humulin N, Novolin N)	Cloudy	2–4 hr	4–10 hr	10–16 hr
Lente (Novolin L)	Cloudy	3–4 hr	4–12 hr	12–18 hr
Long-acting				
Insulin glargine (Lantus)	Clear	1 hr	None	24 hr
Insulin detemir (Levemir)	Clear	Bound to albumin	6–8 hr	24 hr+

Insulin also can be categorized as bolus or basal insulin. Bolus insulin is used to cover food intake at mealtimes. Bolus insulins usually include rapid-acting and short-acting insulins. These insulins attempt to mimic the normal increase in insulin secretion that occurs in nondiabetic individuals after ingesting a meal. Basal insulin includes the intermediate- and long-acting insulins. These insulins attempt to mimic usual insulin secretion that occurs between meals, during the night, and in fasting states.

Insulin is ordered in units and supplied in concentrations or strengths of 100 units per milliliter (U-100) or 500 units per milliliter (U-500). The U-100 insulin is the most common strength used in the United States. Use of U-500 insulin is rare and typically reserved for patients with severe insulin resistance who require extremely large doses of insulin.

✷ **ALERT** *In some foreign countries, such as Europe and Latin America, insulin may be supplied as 40 units per milliliter (U-40). Be sure to inform the patient of this variation if he'll be traveling to these areas.*

Rapid-acting insulins
As the name implies, rapid-acting insulins have an almost immediate onset of action. Three rapid-acting insulin analogs are available: insulin lispro

(Humalog), insulin aspart (NovoLog), and insulin glulisine (Apidra). These insulins are the drugs of choice for administration before meals. Lispro, aspart, and glulisine may be used in insulin infusion pump therapy.

All three rapid-acting insulins work similarly and should be taken at the beginning of a meal or immediately after a meal. The onset of action of these insulins occurs within 10 to 15 minutes; their peak of action is 1 to 2 hours — about the same time the stomach empties itself of food. Depending on the injection site, the effective duration of action is usually 3 to 4 hours, and the maximum duration of action is 4 to 6 hours. These insulin profiles mimic how normal digestion and insulin secretion would occur in a nondiabetic individual. The patient benefits from these insulins by having fewer episodes of postprandial hypoglycemia. Because of the short-acting characteristic of these insulins, a patient with type 1 diabetes who makes no insulin won't need additional basal insulin to achieve glycemic control.

ALERT *Rapid-acting insulins begin to act almost immediately after administration. Therefore, be sure to instruct patients that they need to eat immediately after taking their dose to prevent hypoglycemia.*

Short-acting insulins

Regular insulin (Humulin R, Novolin R) is the only short-acting insulin currently available. Regular insulin begins to act within 30 to 60 minutes after administration, with levels peaking in approximately 2 to 3 hours. Regular insulin has an effective duration of action of 3 to 6 hours and a maximum duration of 6 to 8 hours. Because of its slower onset of action, the patient must inject regular insulin ½ to 1 hour before meals so that the peak action of the drug occurs with the peak absorption time of a meal. Additionally, the patient is at risk for hypoglycemia 3 to 6 hours after a meal because of the drug's longer duration of action.

Regular insulin typically was the only insulin that could be given I.V. However, the development of insulin analogs has changed this scenario. Lispro and aspart may be administered I.V. and may also be mixed with normal saline or dextrose I.V. solutions.

Intermediate-acting insulins

Intermediate-acting insulins include isophane insulin suspension (NPH) (Humulin N, Novolin N) and lente (Humulin L, Novolin L) insulins. NPH insulin was first developed in the 1940s, and lente insulin was developed in the 1950s.

The formulation of this type of insulin is a suspension, which leads to a delay in absorption from subcutaneous sites. However, absorption of intermediate-acting insulins makes the onset and duration of effect inconsistent and highly variable with each patient.

NPH insulin has an onset of action of 2 to 4 hours and peaks in 6 to 10 hours. Its effective duration of action lasts from 10 to 16 hours, with a maximum duration of 14 to 18 hours. Lente insulin has an onset of action of 3 to 4 hours and peaks in 6 to 12 hours. Its effective duration of action lasts from 12 to 18 hours, with a maximum duration of 16 to 20 hours. Both insulins are considered basal insulins and help lower fasting and preprandial blood glucose levels. However, because of their prolonged action, they aren't useful in controlling postprandial blood glucose levels.

Long-acting insulins

Long-acting insulins, as the name implies, begin to work slowly and last for up to 24 hours. Insulin glargine (Lantus) and insulin detemir (Lemevir) are two examples of long-acting insulin preparations. Another example, ultralente (Humulin U), was recently discontinued by the manufacturer.

Studies have shown that insulin glargine provides a continuous level of insulin in a manner similar to that produced by the normal pancreas. However, unlike other insulins, glargine doesn't exert a peak effect. Subsequently, the risk of nighttime hypoglycemia is very low. Glargine has an onset of action of approximately 1 hour and an effective duration of action of 24 hours. Although the dose is typically administered at bedtime (daily), it may be injected at any time during the day as long as the drug is administered at approximately the same time each day. Because this is a basal insulin, the patient also commonly requires a rapid- or short-acting insulin preprandial to prevent postprandial hyperglycemia

ALERT *Warn patients not to mix insulin glargine in the same syringe with other drugs, including other types of insulin, because drug interactions can occur as a result of glargine's highly acidic nature.*

Insulin detemir differs from other insulins in that it remains soluble before and after injection. Additionally, its structure differs slightly from that of human insulin. This change in structure allows detemir to be reversibly bound to albumin. As a result, the drug is gradually released from the bound albumin, leading to a sustained and consistent absorption from the injection site, ultimately leading to less variation in blood glucose levels. Studies also show that fewer unexpected episodes of hyperglycemia and hypoglycemia occur with detemir, compared with NPH or insulin glargine. Insulin detemir is believed to be highly useful for patients who have wide fluctuations in blood glucose levels, those experiencing nocturnal hypoglycemia, or those who have difficulty managing their weight as blood glucose control improves.

Insulin detemir is similar to insulin glargine in that it's reported to have a relatively flat action profile. Its mean duration of action ranges from about 5.7 hours (at lowest dose) to 23.2 hours (at highest dose). When doses in the range of 0.2 to 0.4 units/kg were administered, more than one-half of the drug's maximum effect ranged from 3 to 4 hours up to 14 hours.

Like insulin glargine, insulin detemir shouldn't be mixed or diluted with other drugs (including other insulins) in a syringe because of the potential for possible drug interactions. Typically, the patient also requires a rapid- or short-acting insulin preprandial to prevent postprandial hyperglycemia.

ALERT *Insulin detemir isn't appropriate for use in an insulin infusion pump.*

Premixed formulations

Several insulins are available in premixed concentrations. These types of insulin can help patients who need basal and bolus insulins, but who have difficulty combining two different insulins in one syringe. Premixtures also help minimize the risk of errors from mixing two insulins in one syringe as well as decrease the number of steps necessary prior to injecting the insulin. All premixed insulins combine basal intermediate-acting insulin and bolus short-acting insulin.

The most commonly used premixture is 70/30, which includes 70% of an intermediate-acting insulin and 30% of a short-acting insulin. Examples of human insulin premixed formulations include Humulin 70/30 and Novolin 70/30. These two examples contain 70% NPH insulin and 30% regular insulin. Premixtures of rapid-acting insulin analogs are also available and are used by adding protamine suspension to the analog and then mixing it with the analog without the suspension; these insulins are Humalog 75/25, Humalog 50/50, and Novolog 70/30.

ALERT *Insulin analog premixtures shouldn't be given I.V. or via an insulin infusion pump. They*

also shouldn't be mixed with any other type of insulin.

Use of premixed formulations provides increased ease of preparation for certain patients, especially older adults and those with vision or manual dexterity problems. However, dosage adjustments for bolus and basal insulin are difficult with premixed formulations. For this reason, premixed formulations aren't recommended for patients with type 1 diabetes.

DEVICES FOR INSULIN ADMINISTRATION

A variety of devices are available for administering insulin. The choice of device is based on personal preference and the specific needs of the individual. Several products are also available to help patients who may have problems with vision or manual dexterity, which makes syringe preparation or injection more manageable.

Insulin

Insulin is commonly supplied in multi-dose vials marked with the specific type of insulin they contain. For example, regular insulin is marked with a large, bold, black R. Insulin is also available in prefilled cartridges of 1.5 ml or 3 ml of insulin (providing a total of 150 or 300 units of insulin, respectively) that work with specific delivery devices, such as insulin pens (discussed below), as well as disposable prefilled pens. (See *Insulin cartridges.*)

Syringes and needles

In the United States, insulin syringes are referred to as U-100 syringes. The type of syringe used needs to match the amount of insulin prescribed. Typically, patients use a 3/10 cc syringe if the dosage of insulin is 30 units or less; a ½ cc syringe if the dosage is 50 units or less; and a 1 cc syringe if the dosage is more than 50 units. (*See Insulin syringes,* page 118.)

Insulin syringes are supplied with an attached needle that can range in size from 28 to 31G, and in length from ⁵⁄₁₆″ to ½″. Typically, children use shorter needles because of less subcutaneous

INSULIN CARTRIDGES

These illustrations show examples of pre-filled cartridge units containing different types of insulin.

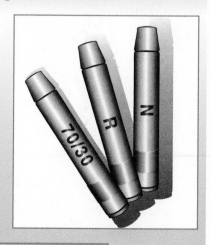

INSULIN SYRINGES

Typically, three different sizes of insulin syringes are available for use in patients with diabetes. They're illustrated below.

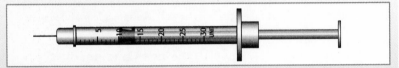

30-unit U-100 insulin syringe measuring 10 units

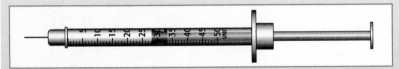

50-unit U-100 insulin syringe measuring 28 units

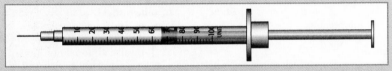

100-unit U-100 insulin syringe measuring 66 units

tissue; patients who are overweight typically require longer needles.

Insulin pens

If the patient has difficulty handling a syringe or preparing medication in a syringe, insulin pens may provide an easier alternative for injection. Similar to an old-fashioned ink pen, insulin pens are small, pocket-size delivery devices. They can be filled with a prefilled insulin cartridge. Some insulin pens contain a preset amount of insulin, and when the insulin is gone, the pen is discarded. (See *Disposable insulin pen.*)

Another type of insulin pen acts as a timer, showing the amount of time that has passed since the last dose of insulin, for up to 12 hours. The device indicates when the injection is complete and records the number of units of that injection in the memory of the device.

Insulin pens are convenient and accurate and are commonly used by individuals requiring multiple-dose regimens. A dial on the pen allows for forward or backward movement to deliver the specific dose ordered. The dial typically moves in 1- to 2-unit increments. In addition, the dial on many of the models exerts an audible clicking sound as the dial is moved. These "clicks" can help patients with vision problems dial the correct dose.

Several insulins are available for use with insulin pens, including regular, NPH, insulin lispro 70/30, insulin glargine, insulin detemir, insulin lispro 75/25, and aspart 70/30. However, because insulin is supplied in prefilled

DISPOSABLE INSULIN PEN

Insulin pens can be supplied with a prefilled cartridge containing insulin or as a disposable pen that contains a prefilled amount of insulin (as shown here). When the insulin is gone, the entire device can be discarded.

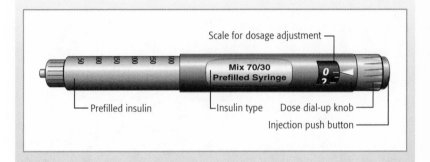

Scale for dosage adjustment

Mix 70/30
Prefilled Syringe

Prefilled insulin — Insulin type — Dose dial-up knob

Injection push button

cartridges, if more than one insulin is ordered, the patient must use separate injections. Also, the pens require the use of manufacturer-specific needles.

Insulin injectors

Insulin injectors, also known as *jet injectors*, are another type of device available for administering insulin. Rather than injecting the insulin through the skin into the subcutaneous tissue, an insulin injector produces a small stream of insulin that's dispersed under pressure through the skin and then into subcutaneous tissue. Jet injectors have no needles. (See *How a jet injector works*, page 120.)

Most jet injectors are easy to use and can be reused; however, the drawback is that they can cause bruising.

Insulin infusers

Using an insulin infuser involves placing a needle or catheter into the subcutaneous tissue. Usually, the needle or catheter is inserted into a site on the abdomen. There, it's secured and remains in place for 48 to 72 hours. The patient then prepares the syringe with the correct dose of insulin and administers the

insulin through the secured needle or catheter, thus minimizing the number of needle sticks. However, because this is an invasive device, the risk of infection is always present. In addition, the patient needs instructions in care of the needle or catheter and of the insertion site.

Insulin pumps

Insulin pumps are computerized devices that deliver a programmed dose of insulin at a specified rate continuously to the patient. The pump action most closely mimics the body's normal release of insulin.

The pump is a portable, self-contained device that's about the size of a credit card and is worn externally. Typically, the patient wears the pump on his belt or carries it in his pocket. The pump can be worn anywhere as long as the infusion line has a clear path to the injection site.

The pump contains a reservoir in which the insulin is stored. The insulin is delivered from the reservoir to the patient through a small catheter. The catheter can be attached to a needle or soft cannula that's inserted subcuta-

HOW A JET INJECTOR WORKS

A jet injector allows insulin to be administered subcutaneously without a needle. Typically, the device has a spring that, when activated, causes the dose of insulin to be dispersed as a fine pressure stream that penetrates the skin into the subcutaneous tissue.

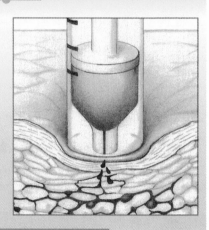

neously and secured in place. The infusion set must be changed to another site every 2 to 3 days for best absorption and to prevent infection at the site. (See *How an insulin pump works.*)

Insulin pumps deliver insulin in small basal doses every few minutes. The pump also can be programmed to release more than one basal rate during the day (based on the patient's needs). The patient can also manually administer additional bolus doses of insulin with the push of a button, such as before mealtime.

Continuous subcutaneous insulin infusion (CSII) delivered by an insulin pump offers the patient relief from multiple injections. Also, its use allows increased flexibility related to mealtimes and exercise. Because the insulin is always available and ready for use, it makes missing mealtime insulin less frequent. Additionally, dosages can be adjusted based on blood glucose values without the patient needing to self-inject.

Other advantages include:
● improvement in glycosylated hemoglobin (HbA$_{1c}$) levels
● less dramatic fluctuations in blood glucose levels
● flexibility and feelings of greater control
● reduction in severe hypoglycemic episodes
● elimination of the unpredictable effects of intermediate-acting and long-acting insulins.

Insulins that can be administered via the pump include insulin lispro, insulin aspart, insulin glulisine, and regular insulin. However, studies have shown that lispro, aspart, and glulisine are more effective in controlling blood glucose levels than regular insulin. Because of their short duration, they're also more effective in managing postprandial blood glucose levels, thus reducing the risk of hypoglycemia.

To determine the amount of insulin to be made available with the pump, these guidelines are used:
● An average of the total number of units of insulin used per day is obtained.
● From that average, about 50% is identified for the basal infusion and the

HOW AN INSULIN PUMP WORKS

The insulin pump delivers a continuous preprogrammed basal rate of insulin to the patient via a catheter that's inserted through the skin into the subcutaneous tissue.

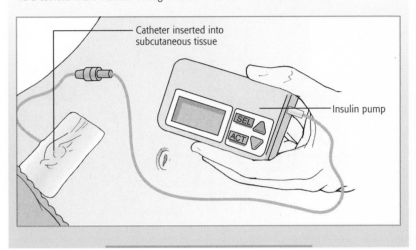

Catheter inserted into subcutaneous tissue

Insulin pump

remaining 50% is identified for bolus administration.

● The basal infusion rate is then divided by 24 hours to determine an hourly basal rate.

● Then the hourly basal rate is adjusted to match the patient's increases or decreases in blood glucose, such as more insulin for early morning hyperglycemia and less for periods of high activity.

The best way to determine the bolus mealtime doses is to calculate the amount of a carbohydrate that the patient plans to eat in that particular meal This amount is divided by the total number of units of insulin per day to ascertain the number of grams of carbohydrate covered by one unit of insulin.

Types of pumps

Insulin pumps work on either an open-loop or closed-loop system. The open-loop system is most commonly used. It infuses insulin but can't respond to changes in blood glucose levels.

With an open-loop system, the pump delivers insulin in basal doses every few minutes as well as bolus doses that the patient sets manually. The system consists of a reservoir, a small pump, an infusion rate selector that allows insulin release adjustments, a battery, and a catheter that's attached to the patient. Usually, the infusion rate selector automatically releases about one-half of the total daily insulin requirement. The patient releases the remainder in bolus doses before meals and snacks.

The closed-loop system is a self-contained system that detects and responds to changes in blood glucose levels. The system commonly includes a glucose sensor, a programmable computer, a power supply, a pump, and an insulin reservoir. The computer triggers

USING AN INSULIN PUMP

To better prepare your patient to use an insulin pump, strongly urge him to review the manufacturer's instructions. In addition, be sure to cover these important topic areas:

- pump function, including significance of the various buttons on the pump, pump alarms, and features
- type of insulin used
- reservoir refill or change
- prescribed insulin infusion rate (basal dose)
- bolus dose amounts
- parameters for administering bolus doses
- blood glucose self-monitoring, including values requiring bolus doses
- dietary plan, including timing of meals with bolus doses and carbohydrate intake
- troubleshooting pump problems
- care of the insertion site
- care of the pump when sleeping, bathing, or showering
- daily inspection of insertion site
- catheter changes, including procedure and frequency
- danger signs and symptoms to report to the health care provider.

the continuous delivery of insulin in appropriate amounts from the reservoir based on circulating blood glucose levels.

Risks of pump therapy

If the pump malfunctions or if the catheter becomes blocked or displaced from the subcutaneous tissue, the patient can experience a rapid escalation of blood glucose, possibly leading to ketoacidosis. This is because only rapid-acting or short-acting insulins are used. Newer devices with a safety alarm indicating a pump problem have helped to minimize this risk.

Another major risk is infection at the site of the subcutaneous catheter. Meticulous skin and catheter care is necessary. In addition, the catheter must be changed every 2 to 3 days. (See *Using an insulin pump.*)

Although the device weighs about 3 oz, some individuals find that wearing the external pump device is uncomfortable and awkward. In addition, they may feel that it brings attention to their disease.

One major disadvantage of insulin pump therapy is the high cost of the equipment and supplies. Most insurance companies and third-party payers cover insulin pump therapy; however, plans vary in the amount of coverage provided. Medicare covers pumps and supplies for diabetes care, but the patient must meet specific eligibility requirements.

Other methods

Several alternative methods for insulin administration are being investigated. The National Diabetes Information Clearinghouse, part of the National Institute of Diabetes and Digestive and Kidney Diseases, a division of the National Institutes of Health, provides a valuable resource on devices being studied. (See *Insulin administration devices under development.*)

One method of insulin delivery receiving attention is inhaled insulin, which is delivered much the same way as medications used for asthma. (See *Insulin inhaler,* page 124.)

Cutting edge

INSULIN ADMINISTRATION DEVICES UNDER DEVELOPMENT

The National Diabetes Information Clearinghouse is researching several promising new methods for insulin administration. These methods include:

- Implantable insulin pump — similar to the external insulin pump, this device is implanted under the abdominal skin to deliver small amounts of insulin continuously. Bolus doses can be administered before meals and snacks by the patient via a remote control device. The pump is refilled every 2 to 3 months.
- Automated glucose feedback control system — this device continually collects minute samples of skin fluid via an external electrode. The information is downloaded at the end of 3 days to provide a tracking of blood glucose values. The device has implications for providing continuous glucose monitoring feedback with insulin pump therapy.
- Insulin patch — similar to other transdermal patches, the insulin patch provides a continuous low dose of insulin via sound waves or electric current to ensure delivery through the skin.
- Insulin pill — this method of insulin therapy is in a tablet form so that it can be absorbed into the bloodstream before it's destroyed by GI secretions.
- Buccal insulin spray — this method of insulin therapy is delivered in liquid form into the mouth, where it's absorbed through the tongue, throat, and buccal membranes.
- Artificial pancreas — a surgically implanted device, the artificial pancreas simulates the action of the normal pancreas. It senses blood glucose levels and secretes insulin. A remote control device also allows the patient to release additional insulin.

In a recent study, researchers attempted to determine whether patients with type 1 diabetes, who were receiving rapid- or short-acting insulin along with intermediate- or long-acting insulin, would find it easier to use inhaled rapid-acting insulin instead of multiple daily injections of the same. The study showed that all members of the study experienced a decrease in their HbA$_{1c}$ levels and similar blood glucose measurements 2 hours after meals. However, the group using inhaled insulin showed lower blood glucose levels at bedtime. This group also experienced fewer episodes of hypoglycemia but had an increase in the number of *severe* hypoglycemic episodes. Researchers determined that inhaled insulin may be a viable alternative for patients who are unable or don't want to take insulin injections before meals. An adverse effect of the inhaled insulin is a mild to mod-

erate cough. Further studies are needed, including the long-term safety implications related to the effects of the inhaled insulin on the lungs.

CARE OF INSULIN AND EQUIPMENT

Insulin and the equipment used for administration, such as syringes and needles, require special care. As with any other medication and supplies, instruct your patients to store them out of the reach of children. Additional safety measures include proper insulin storage, syringe and needle reuse, and syringe disposal.

Insulin

Typically, insulin is stored in a cold place, such as the refrigerator, based on the manufacturer's instructions. However, studies have shown that injecting cold insulin can increase the patient's

INSULIN INHALER

The inhaled form of insulin is delivered in a device similar to the device used for inhaled asthma medications.

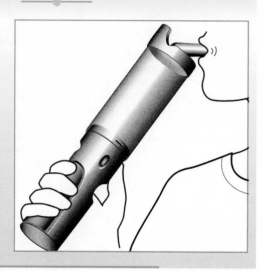

pain on injection. Ideally, the patient should be instructed to remove the insulin from the refrigerator at least ½ hour before use.

⚡ **ALERT** *Insulin shouldn't be stored in extremes of heat or cold. Instruct the patient that it should never be stored in the freezer, in direct sunlight, or in the glove compartment or trunk of a car.*

All insulin vials have an expiration date on the label. Instruct patients to check the expiration date and never to use a vial of insulin beyond that date.

⚡ **ALERT** *When using any insulin that's clear, have the patient check for particles or discoloration. For cloudy insulins, such as NPH, advise the patient to check for a frosty appearance or crystals on the inside of the vial and for small particles in the solution. Warn the patient not to use such insulin vials and to return any unopened vials to the pharmacy if any of these changes are noted.*

Syringes and needle reuse

If a patient reuses a syringe, the needle must be kept clean by ensuring that it remains capped; it also must be completely sterile before injection. Teach the patient how to maintain sterility of the syringe and needle when preparing the injection.

Using alcohol to clean the needle isn't advised. The needles have a protective specialized covering that aids insertion. Using alcohol would remove this covering. Patients should never let anyone else reuse their syringe or reuse another person's syringe.

Repeatedly reusing syringes can increase the risk of infection. Reuse also dulls the needle, placing the patient at risk for injury.

⚡ **ALERT** *Keep in mind that manufacturers don't guarantee the sterility of syringes that are reused. Discourage the reuse of insulin syringes in patients who are ill, have open wounds on their hands, or have an increased risk of infection.*

Syringe and needle disposal

Syringes and needles (also called *sharps*) are considered medical waste and must be disposed of properly according to infection control precautions. In the home, the patient should discard the syringe and needle into an opaque, heavy-duty plastic bottle that has a screw cap or into a plastic or metal box that can be closed securely and firmly. The container should be impervious so that the needles can't break through the plastic. The container shouldn't be recycled.

Local areas may have strict regulations about the discarding of syringes and needles. Advise the patient to check with his local waste management company to determine the specific guidelines. When traveling, advise the patient not to discard the syringes and needles. Rather, the patient should pack the used syringes and needles in a hard plastic container, such as a plastic pencil box, and bring them home to be discarded.

INSULIN INJECTION

Insulin is injected subcutaneously via a syringe with a relatively short needle. Absorption occurs mainly through the capillaries.

Injection preparation

After ensuring that the insulin hasn't expired and doesn't show any discoloration or particles, the patient draws up the insulin into the syringe and takes these steps:

● Roll the insulin between the palms of hands, and gently rotate the vial several times to warm it and mix it.

● Wipe the rubber cap with an alcohol pad or cotton ball moistened with alcohol.

● Pull the syringe plunger back until the volume of air in the syringe equals the volume of insulin to be withdrawn.

● Uncap the syringe, and without inverting the vial, insert the needle into the vial and inject the volume of air.

● Invert the vial and withdraw the prescribed amount of insulin while keeping the needle's bevel tip below the level of the insulin solution.

● Tap the syringe gently to clear any air from the syringe while the needle is still in the solution.

● Withdraw the needle and cover it with the sheath.

If two different types of insulin are to be given, and if the insulins are compatible, the patient should combine them in one syringe.

✷ **ALERT** *Tell the patient never to mix insulin glargine or insulin detemir in the same syringe with other insulins.*

To prepare an insulin injection when combining insulin, the patient should follow these steps:

● Pull the syringe plunger back until the volume of air in the syringe equals the volume of cloudy insulin to be withdrawn, wipe the rubber stopper of the insulin vial with alcohol, and then insert the needle into the vial containing the cloudy insulin and inject the air. Don't let the needle touch the insulin solution. Withdraw the needle.

● Pull the syringe plunger back until the volume of air in the syringe equals the volume of the clear insulin to be withdrawn, wipe the rubber stopper of the insulin vial with alcohol, and then insert the needle into the insulin vial and inject the air. Invert the vial and withdraw the prescribed amount of insulin.

● Remove the needle from the vial and clean the rubber stopper of the cloudy insulin vial with an alcohol pad. Insert the needle and invert the vial; withdraw the cloudy insulin to the prescribed amount. Remove the needle and cover it with its sheath. (See *Mixing insulins,* page 126.)

Site selection

The recommended sites for insulin administration are those containing the most subcutaneous fat. These include

MIXING INSULINS

These illustrations highlight the key steps for combining clear and cloudy insulins in one syringe.

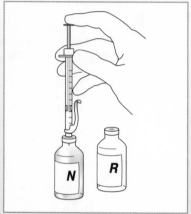

1. Inject air into cloudy insulin.

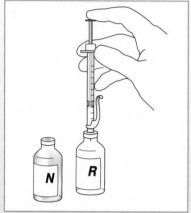

2. Inject air into clear insulin.

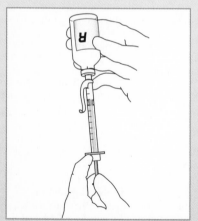

3. Withdraw clear insulin.

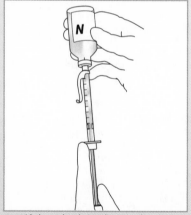

4. Withdraw cloudy insulin into clear in syringe.

the abdomen, anterior and lateral thigh, buttocks, and dorsal area of the arm. (See *Identifying insulin injection sites.*) If the patient chooses to use his abdomen, advise him to avoid a 2″ (5.1 cm) area around the umbilicus.

Also, areas that contain large blood vessels or nerves, such as the inner aspect of the thighs, or areas with scar tissue, broken blood vessels, or varicose veins should be avoided.

IDENTIFYING INSULIN INJECTION SITES

These illustrations identify the appropriate sites for insulin injection.

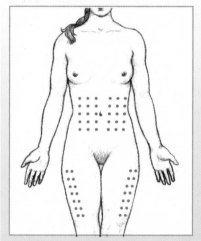

Front view

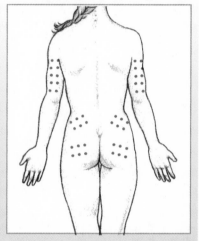

Back view

Site absorption considerations

Not all insulin injection sites promote the same level of drug absorption. Insulin is more rapidly and consistently absorbed when the abdomen is used, followed by the outer aspect of the upper arms, then the outer aspects of the thighs; insulin absorption is slowest from the buttocks. Studies have shown, however, that no significant difference in insulin absorption from sites exists when insulin glargine is given.

Other factors that affect insulin absorption include getting a massage or exercising around the time of injection because of the increase in circulation to the area. So, if the patient were planning to jog or walk briskly, he would be cautioned to avoid using the thighs for injection. Similarly, a patient who would be playing tennis would be cautioned not to use the site of the arm that would be holding the racket.

Temperature can also affect absorption: heat increases absorption, whereas cold decreases it. Caution patients who may be using hot tubs or engaging in cold water swimming.

Site rotation considerations

Repeated injections into the same site can lead to changes in the subcutaneous tissue and increases or decreases in the amount of fat in the area, which in turn can affect absorption of the insulin. Therefore, strongly advise the patient to develop a site rotation plan for his injections. The plan should be based on the patient's insulin regimen, body type, and personal preferences and must be consistent. (See *Site rotation instructions*, page 128.)

Injection administration

When teaching your patients how to administer an insulin injection, follow these steps:

SITE ROTATION INSTRUCTIONS

For the patient requiring insulin therapy with injections, site rotation is crucial to ensuring optimal effectiveness of the therapy and thereby promoting better blood glucose control. Include these tips about site rotation in your teaching plan:

- Rotate injection sites within one area before switching to another area.
- Keep the injections about 1″ (2.5 cm) apart from a previous injection (about the width of two fingers).
- If you inject into more than one area because of more than one injection in a day, try to give the injection in the same area at the same time of day—for example, use the abdomen for morning doses and the thighs for afternoon or evening doses.
- If you use different types of insulin, designate a site for a specific type of insulin—for example, rapid-acting insulin in the arm and long-acting insulin in the thighs.
- Stay away from any areas that are bruised or scarred or that have broken blood vessels or varicose veins.
- When using the abdomen, stay at least 2″ (5.1 cm) away from your belly button.
- Use a written record or locator to keep track of the sites used.

● Clean the injection site with an alcohol pad, starting at the center of the site and moving outward in a circular motion. Let the skin air-dry to avoid stinging.

● If you wish, open a second alcohol pad and place it between the index and middle fingers of your nondominant hand.

● Remove the protective needle sheath.

● With your nondominant hand, grasp the skin around the injection site and firmly elevate the subcutaneous tissue to form a 1″ (2.5-cm) fat fold. If the patient is heavy, you may be able to spread the skin taut rather than forming a fold.

● Position the needle with the bevel up, and tell the patient that he'll feel a prick as you insert it quickly — in one motion — at a 90-degree angle.

ALERT *When administering insulin glargine, inject it at a 45-degree angle.*

● Inject the drug slowly.

● After injection, remove the needle gently but quickly at the same angle used for injection.

● Cover the injection site with an alcohol pad, and apply gentle pressure.

ALERT *Don't massage the site after removing the needle. Massage enhances drug distribution and promotes absorption, which could lead to too-rapid absorption of the insulin dose and, subsequently, to hypoglycemia.*

● Check the injection site for bleeding or bruising. If bleeding continues, apply pressure. If a bruise develops, apply ice. Watch for adverse reactions at the injection site for 30 minutes.

● Dispose of the equipment according to standard precautions. To avoid needle-stick injuries, don't recap the needle, and discard in a sharps disposal.

INSULIN SCHEDULES

The insulin therapy regimen that's prescribed is highly individualized. For patients with type 1 diabetes, insulin replacement is a lifelong treatment. For those with type 2 diabetes, insulin therapy may be used alone or added to the patient's oral regimen to promote better glycemic control.

Compliance with therapy is essential. Therefore, the type of insulin regimen prescribed must take into account the patient's age, lifestyle, general health status (including any comorbidities), self-management skills, motivation, and desired glycemic control.

Schedules for type 1 diabetes

The typical protocol for insulin therapy in patients with type 1 diabetes involves multiple daily injections or CSII. Studies performed by the Diabetes Control and Complications Trial (DCCT) showed that this type of regimen in conjunction with education and self-monitoring of blood glucose levels (SMBG) significantly reduced HbA_{1c} levels and the risk of microvascular complications.

Multiple daily injection regimens typically involve four injections per day, mealtime administration of insulin to simulate normal pancreatic secretion, and basal dose administration to control blood glucose levels throughout the night and between meals. Typically, a rapid-acting insulin, such as lispro, aspart, or glulisine, is used as the mealtime insulin to control postprandial glucose levels. Regular insulin may also be used. NPH, glargine, or detemir may be used as the basal insulin, usually administered at bedtime to control fasting blood glucose levels. Depending on the patient's response and blood glucose levels, an injection of basal insulin may be added to the regimen at breakfast to provide better control of blood glucose levels throughout the day and to reduce blood glucose levels before dinner.

⚡ **ALERT** *Keep in mind that a patient receiving insulin is at greater risk for hypoglycemia. Be sure to teach the patient about the signs and symptoms of hypoglycemia and measures to combat it.*

A formula is typically used to determine the total daily dose of insulin that a patient should receive. For a patient who's just starting insulin therapy, insulin requirements are identified as approximately 0.2 to 0.4 units/kg of body weight. About 50% of the total daily insulin is designated for mealtime administration, with this 50% being divided among the meals. The remaining 50% is designated as the basal insulin to be administered at bedtime or twice daily. Adjustments are individual, based on blood glucose levels. In addition, adjustments in dosage may also be warranted when the patient exercises, because of the increased risk of hypoglycemia.

Schedules for type 2 diabetes

Insulin therapy typically is added to the regimen for a patient with type 2 diabetes when therapy with diet, exercise, and oral antidiabetic agents fails to achieve glycemic control. Research has also suggested that insulin therapy should be introduced earlier in the course of treatment for patients with type 2 diabetes. The DCCT study showed that pancreatic beta cell function progressively deteriorates over time, thus earlier use of insulin may prevent or delay the beta cells from this deterioration. In addition, good glycemic control is associated with a reduction in microvascular complications and some macrovascular complications, and a decreased risk of cardiac disease. Subsequently, morbidity and possibly mortality are decreased.

Typical insulin regimen schedules may include:

● intermediate-acting insulin (NPH) at bedtime with oral antidiabetic agents
● insulin glargine at bedtime with oral antidiabetic agents
● intermediate-acting insulin in the morning and at bedtime in combination with oral antidiabetic agents
● insulin-only therapy such as with: twice-daily dosing using premixed insulins, such as 70/30 NPH regular, Humulog 75/25, Humulog 50/50, or Novolog 70/30; or the patient mixing short or rapid-acting insulin with intermediate-acting insulin (regular and NPH);

thrice-daily dosing using NPH and regular at breakfast, regular at dinner, and NPH at bedtime; or four-times daily dosing using a once-per-day long-acting insulin glargine or detemir, plus premeal rapid-acting insulin lispro, glulisine, or aspart.

EVALUATION OF GLYCEMIC CONTROL

Goals for glycemic control must be highly individualized. Adjustments may be needed for certain populations, including children, pregnant women, and older adults. However, if patients experience frequent or severe hypoglycemic episodes, goals may need to be adjusted.

Key components of monitoring glycemic control include blood glucose levels (fasting and 2-hour postprandial), HbA_{1c} levels, fructosamine levels, and patient SMBG.

Blood glucose levels

Fasting and 2-hour postprandial blood glucose levels are used to monitor glycemic control. According to the American Diabetes Association, glycemic control is indicated by fasting blood glucose levels ranging from 90 to 130 mg/dl (5 to 72 mmol/L) and 2-hour postprandial levels less than 180 mg/dl (10 mmol/L).

HbA_{1c} levels

HbA_{1c}, also called *glycosylated hemoglobin*, provides information about the average blood glucose levels over the past 2 to 3 months. The HbA_{1c} level is considered the primary method for evaluating glycemic control.

According to the American Diabetes Association, target HbA_{1c} levels indicating glycemic control should be less than 7% and as close to normal as possible without hypoglycemia. The American College of Endocrinologists, however, has issued a tighter target level of less than or equal to 6.5%. It's believed that a level of less than 6% may be associated with a greater reduction in risk of complications. However, this restricted

target range must be weighed against the possible increased risk of hypoglycemia.

HbA_{1c} levels typically are performed at least biannually in patients who are achieving their glycemic target ranges and are demonstrating stable glycemic control. Testing frequency is increased to four times per year in patients who aren't achieving their glycemic goals or in those who have undergone changes in their therapy regimen.

Fructosamine levels

Fructosamine is a serum protein that, like hemoglobin, combines to form a glycosylated product. Fructosamine levels are highly correlated with HbA_{1c} levels. Although the cost is variable, measuring fructosamine levels is simpler, and thus is being evaluated as an alternative to measuring HbA_{1c} levels. In addition, fructosamine levels reflect glycemic control over a shorter period of time (2 to 4 weeks), compared with the 6 to 12 weeks for HbA_{1c}.

⚡ **ALERT** *Although fructosamine levels correlate with HbA_{1c} levels, comorbidities involving increased serum proteins or ingestion of large amounts of vitamin C (ascorbic acid) can affect the validity of the results.*

The U.S. Food and Drug Administration has approved a device for self-monitoring of fructosamine levels at home. Studies are currently evaluating the effectiveness of monitoring fructosamine levels.

Self-monitoring of blood glucose levels

SMBG is recommended for all individuals with diabetes, but most importantly for those receiving insulin therapy. General recommendations for SMBG include:

● testing three or more times per day for patients with type 1 diabetes and pregnant women taking insulin
● frequent testing for patients with type 2 diabetes who are taking insulin

(frequency depends on treatment regimen)

- testing once daily for patients with type 2 diabetes not taking insulin.

Self-monitoring blood glucose provides an accurate measurement of glucose values, thus serving as a guide to appropriate food intake. Self-monitoring also empowers the patient to develop (with his health care provider) an exercise regimen and a medication schedule, with adjustments made as appropriate. Patients using SMBG can minimize episodes of hyperglycemia and maintain glucose levels within a normal range.

A common routine for SMBG in patients with type 1 diabetes is testing before each meal, 2 hours after each meal, at bedtime, and during the night. Testing should be done more frequently when medication therapy changes, when the patient becomes ill or is experiencing unusual stress, or when he's experiencing signs and symptoms of hypoglycemia.

A wide range of glucose meters are available for self-monitoring. They vary in the amount of blood needed for testing, time required to obtain results, size, memory to store results, and cost of the meter and testing strips. Newer meters provide such functions as an increased memory for storage of information, smaller size and ease of use, automatic timers, and alarms and safety features. In addition, some meters are available that allow blood glucose level testing and insulin administration all in one device.

Typically, blood for SMBG is obtained from the fingertip. However, new glucose meters allow blood sample collection from other sites, such as the upper arm, forearm, base of the thumb, and thigh. Although desirable, there may be some limitations with the use of alternative site testing. Studies have shown that glucose changes in the blood are more rapidly demonstrated in the fingertips than in other parts of the

body. Blood glucose levels in the alternative sites appear to change more gradually after a meal, administration of insulin, and exercise. (See chapter 12 for patient-teaching information for SMBG.)

Specific routines and target goals of SMBG should be developed in collaboration with all individuals involved in the patient's care. Patients performing SMBG require thorough education about the procedure, frequency of testing and testing sites, acceptable parameters for target levels, and levels that require notifying their health care provider.

Selected references
Alternative Devices for Taking Insulin. "National Diabetes Information Clearinghouse (NDIC)" [Online]. Available at: *www.diabetes.niddk.nih.gov/dm/pubs/insulin/index.htm* [2005 December 7].
American Diabetes Association. "Insulin Delivery. Resource Guide 2004" [Online]. Available at: *www.diabetes.org/utils/printthispage.jsp?PageID=DRFESOURCESGUIDE_241678* [2005 December 6].
American Diabetes Association. "Insulin Storage and Syringe Safety information" [Online]. Available at: *www.diabetes.org/utils/printthispage.jsp?PageI+TYPE1DIABETES3_263609* [2005 December 6].
Cheng, A., and Zinman, B. "Principles of Insulin Therapy," in Kahn, C.R. et al., *Joslin's Diabetes Mellitus*, 14th ed. Philadelphia: Lippincott Williams and Wilkins, 2005.
D'Arrigo, T. "New Device: Remembers Your Last Shot," *Diabetes Forecast* 54(10):53, 54. October 2001.
Diabetes Forecast July 2004. Lumbar, T. "Tips for Site Rotation" [Online]. Available at: *www.diabetes.org/utils/printthispage.jsp?PageID=DIABETESFORECAST3_261841* [2005 December 6].

Edelman, S.V., and Morello, C.M. "Strategies for Insulin Therapy in Type 2 Diabetes," *Southern Medical Journal* 98(3): 363-71, March 2005.

Einhorn, D. "Advanced in Diabetes for the Millennium: Insulin Treatment and Glucose Monitoring," *Medscape General Medicine.* Available at: *www.medscape.com/viewprogram/ 3429_pnt* [2005 November 11].

Fain, J.A. "Unlock the Mysteries of Insulin Therapy," *Nursing* 34(3):41-43, March 2004.

Hill, K. "Insulin Detemir: Evidence, Efficacy, and Application [Online]. Available at: *www.findarticles.com/p/ articles/mi_m)MDR/is_10_8/ai_ n8709119/print* [2005 December 12].

Skyler, J.S., et al. "Use of Inhaled Insulin in a Basal/Bolus Insulin Regimen in Type 1 Diabetic Subjects: A 6-month, Randomized, Comparative Trial," *Diabetes Care* 28(7):1630-635, July 2005.

United States Food and Drug Administration. "Diabetes Information" [Online]. Available at: *www.fda.gov/diabetes/ insulin.html* [2005 December 6].

United States Food and Drug Administration. "Insulin Preparations, FDA Consumer Magazine" [Online]. Available at: *www.fda.gove/fdac/features /2002/chart_insulin.html* [2005 December 6].

Votey, S., et.al. "Diabetes Mellitus, Type 1—A Review" [Online].Available at: *www.emedicine.com/emerg/ topic133.htm* [2005 December 7].

8

Complementary and alternative medicine

For centuries, people have searched for cures for different ailments and for products that help to maintain optimal health; this movement has sometimes extended beyond the scope of traditional medical practice to also include natural healing methods — also known as *complementary and alternative medicine* (CAM). CAM refers to measures that can be used in conjunction with traditional medical therapies, thereby complementing their use.

OVERVIEW OF CAM
IN DIABETES

Studies have examined the use of CAM and nontraditional therapies to help alleviate the complications of diabetes. For example, in October 2002, the *American Journal of Public Health* cited that in a national survey of data collected from 1997 to 1998, up to 57% of people with diabetes were believed to be using CAM. Another study reported by *Diabetes Care* explored the use of CAM in specific populations with diabetes: 39% of Navajos; 33% of Vietnamese; and 49% of the largely Latino and Hispanic population in south Texas.

One reason for this increased use is because CAM takes a whole body (holistic) approach, thus helping to ease the complications associated with diabetes that affect multiple body systems. With a chronic disease such as diabetes, the goal of CAM is to experience symptomatic relief, not to treat the disease itself.

Impact on practice

Despite not being well defined, consumers in the United Sates still seek out CAM to remedy multiple ailments before going to their health care professional. For example, sales of Echinacea increase sharply through the winter months because it's thought to prevent (or alleviate) the common cold. Where problems may arise, however, is when consumers see that a product is labeled "all natural" and assume that this natural status automatically ensures its safety and that it can't cause harm.

Natural ingredients, such as those found in grapefruit juice, can interact with chemical elements found in many prescription medications and can alter the medication's effect or increase the risk of additional adverse effects. For example, in the patient taking oral antidiabetic agents, a natural ingredient can enhance the drug's effect, neutralize it, or significantly reduce its effectiveness, perhaps upsetting the patient's glucose control.

With CAM, there's no gold standard for determining the amount of active ingredient in each naturally grown product because growing conditions vary; this factor alone can alter the strength and potency. Additionally, the dose-for-dose equivalency among brand names may not be equal, and manufacturers

WHAT TO EXPLORE BEFORE USING CAM

The patient with diabetes needs accurate information before deciding to use complementary and alternative medicine (CAM). When assisting your patient with his decision, make sure he's aware that CAM:

- involves using products that usually aren't standardized or officially regulated by the U.S. Food and Drug Administration.
- isn't used or understood by all health care professionals.
- lacks adequate regulation of herbal medicines.
- lacks support through research.
- may increase out-of-pocket expenses because it isn't recognized or reimbursed by many third-party payers.

aren't required to prove efficacy. Therefore, when a consumer decides to use CAM, he must first inform his health care professional so that he understands the mode of action and is aware of the risk versus benefit of the product before trying it. Risks for the patient with diabetes may include changes in blood glucose control, interaction with medications, and exacerbation of adverse effects. (See *What to explore before using CAM.*)

SUPPLEMENTS

According to the National Center for Complementary and Alternative Medicine (NCCAM), supplements are defined as substances that are taken by mouth and contain a dietary ingredient designed for addition to the diet. Available in different forms, the supplement shouldn't be substituted for food. Also, it's important to know that some supplements are contraindicated in the patient with diabetes. (See *Contraindicated supplements.*)

Most supplements are considered natural products. However, some individuals may assume that they're safe for use at any time or in any form or amount. Unfortunately, this assumption may not always be true; therefore, if the patient decides to use a natural dietary

supplement, make sure that he's knowledgeable about the product. (See *Guidelines for dietary supplements,* page 136.)

Herbs

Although herbs may be used to combat common ailments, consideration must be given to the impact they may have on glycemic control in the patient with diabetes. (See *Summary of commonly used herbs,* page 137.)

Herbs and glycemic control

Some studies have shown that certain herbs help to maintain optimal glucose levels in the patient with diabetes. (See *Herbs and glycemic control,* page 138.) Such herbs may also make the body's cells more responsive to insulin, thereby enhancing insulin use and reducing insulin and medication requirements. The herbs' effectiveness should be realized within 1 to 2 months; if the patient's blood glucose levels decrease, his medication dosage should be decreased but not discontinued. If his blood glucose levels don't decrease, the patient should stop taking the herb.

If these herbs don't effectively reduce the patient's blood glucose to the desired level, corosolic acid (also called *Queen's crepe myrtle*) may be given.

CONTRAINDICATED SUPPLEMENTS

Some supplements shouldn't be used in the patient with diabetes, including coltsfoot, ephedra, lobelia, and sassafras, and are discussed here.

Coltsfoot

Coltsfoot (*Tussilago farfara*) is an herbal supplement that may be used for such respiratory problems as coughing, asthma, and bronchitis. However, recent studies indicate that it contains potentially liver-toxic substances called *pyrrolizidine alkaloids*, which has led to recommendations against using the herb. The U.S. Food and Drug Administration (FDA) classifies the herb as having "undefined safety," and several other countries restrict its medicinal use. Because coltsfoot has adverse effects on the liver, patients with a history of liver disease or alcohol abuse should avoid using it. Also, patients taking multiple medications should avoid it to prevent overtaxing the liver. Coltsfoot should never be used in combination with antihypertensive agents. This is especially true for patients with diabetes who have hypertension.

Ephedra

Ephedra, also called *ma huang,* is a plant that contains ephedrine, a substance that's regulated by the FDA as a drug when it's created chemically in the laboratory. The substance acts as a powerful stimulant, affecting the nervous system and heart, and can have potentially lethal effects. Ephedrine, like adrenaline, dilates the bronchial muscles, contracts the nasal mucosa, raises blood pressure, and causes a rapid heart rate. Potential psychological effects include depression, nervousness, and insomnia. When taken in combination with caffeine, ephedrine can overstimulate the nervous system, possibly leading to death.

According to the FDA, products containing ephedrine extracts have caused hundreds of illnesses, including myocardial infarction, seizure, and stroke. As a result, dietary supplements containing ephedra

have been banned in the United States since April 2004. The use of this herb can be especially problematic for the patient with diabetes because of their increased risk of cardiovascular disease, hypertension, and stroke.

Lobelia

Lobelia (*Lobelia inflata*), also known as *Indian tobacco,* contains pyridine-derived alkaloids, primarily lobeline. Its pharmacologic actions are similar to, although less potent than, nicotine. Lobeline can cause autonomic nervous system stimulation or depression. At low doses, it produces bronchial dilation and increases respiratory rate; higher doses result in respiratory depression as well as sweating, rapid heart rate, hypotension, and even coma and death. As little as 50 mg of the dried herb or a single milliliter of lobelia tincture has caused these adverse reactions. Because there's a higher risk of heart disease in people with diabetes, it's strongly recommended that lobelia isn't used in this patient population.

Sassafras

Currently, sassafras bark, sassafras oil, and safrole are prohibited by the FDA as flavorings or food additives. Sassafras extract may be sold as a supplement to make tonics and teas. It may be considered a household cure for many ailments, such as GI complaints, colds, rheumatism, skin eruptions, and eye, liver, and kidney ailments. Its adverse effects depress the central nervous system and irritate mucous membranes. Sassafras is known to cause vomiting, which could impact the patient with diabetes and his ability to ingest an adequate diet. Additionally, central nervous system depression can occur, possibly masking the signs and symptoms of hypoglycemia in the patient with diabetes. Sassafras hasn't been shown to be effective in supporting health.

Patient-teaching tip

GUIDELINES FOR
DIETARY SUPPLEMENTS

Patients may use dietary supplements for several reasons. For patients with diabetes, education is important because of underlying problems with blood glucose regulation. Patients with diabetes must be knowledgeable about the supplements, their intended effect, and their possible effect on blood glucose control. Be sure to stress these guidelines:

■ Look for the United States Pharmacopoeia (USP) symbol on supplements. The USP symbol ensures that certain standards for disintegration, dissolution, purity, strength, packing, labeling, and weight variation have been met.

■ Always look for the drug warning label. This label contains important information concerning dosage recommendations, proper administration, active and other ingredients, usage during pregnancy and other conditions, and possible adverse reactions.

■ Check for lot numbers and expiration dates. Many supplements don't have the rapid turnover as other more commonly used over-the-counter items. Be careful not to purchase an already expired item.

■ Buy from stores with quick turnover. Pharmacies tend to be more conscientious about product safety and adherence to policies more so than a store with other specialties.

■ Keep your health care professionals and others involved in your care informed about your use of supplements.

■ Never stop your current prescribed medications when starting supplements. You could risk compromising your health.

■ Stop taking supplements at least 2 weeks before a scheduled surgery. Many herbs and supplemental remedies may interfere with anesthesia and contrast dyes used in X-rays and nuclear medicine testing procedures.

The typical dose of this herb is 480 to 550 mcg, usually 1 to 2 tablets, three times per day. It usually takes up to 2 weeks to achieve the maximum benefit.

Combination herbs

Many herbal treatments involve combinations of multiple ingredients. For example, combination herb therapy is a major component of traditional Chinese medicine where multiple herbs are used in combination. However, each combination or formulation is different because the Herbalist will adjust the amount based on the individual's diagnosis. Each combination is designed to alleviate the patient's symptoms and the overall goal is to benefit the patient. (See *Commonly used herbs in traditional Chinese medicine*, page 139.) However, for the patient with diabetes, caution

should be used as the dosage of herbs in combination is commonly quite high and potentially dangerous.

Chinese people have fewer problems with consuming higher dosages of herbal supplements. However, in Western culture, high doses typically result in poor compliance due to the unpleasant taste associated with higher doses. Subsequently, many dosage formulations contain a large amount of sugar, which ultimately leads to an increase in the patient's blood glucose levels during the first hour after consumption. Later, the herbs cause a gradual and sustained reduction in blood glucose levels.

Nausea is another problem associated with combination herb therapy, which can interfere with the patient's ability to consume an adequate diet. Additionally, the patient may choose not to

SUMMARY OF COMMONLY USED HERBS

This chart highlights some of the more common herbs, including their uses and important cautions related to their use. The health care professional needs to know about herbs the patient with diabetes is taking for various conditions, such as arthritis, infection, colds, flu, or stress.

HERB	COMMON USES	CAUTIONS
Black cohosh	■ Hot flashes, night sweats	■ None known
Chamaelirium	■ For increased fertility, pregnancy problems	■ Don't use during pregnancy because it contains hormones (safety with severe kidney or liver disease is unknown).
Echinacea angustifolia	■ For stimulation of the immune system ■ Blood cleaning agent ■ For fever, acne, and infection ■ Antiviral, antifungal, antibacterial agent	■ Don't use with immunosuppressive drugs because it may counteract the effect.
Echinacea purpurea	■ For stimulation of the immune system ■ Urinary tract infections, burns ■ Cold and flu prevention	■ Suppresses the immune system after 8 weeks of use; worsens immune disorders (human immunodeficiency virus, AIDS, and lupus)
Ginseng	■ Stress reliever ■ Increased energy ■ Mental and physical performance enhancer ■ For stimulation of the immune system	■ Causes inflamed nerves (sciatica) and muscle spasms with long-term use ■ Increases stimulant effect of caffeine (coffee, tea)
Goldenseal	■ Nasal congestion, digestive disorders, eye and ear infections, acquired immunodeficiency syndrome (AIDS) ■ Liver and blood cleaning agent	■ Use for up to 3 weeks without discontinuing for best results.
Passion flower (*Passiflora incarnata*)	■ Boils, cuts, and inflammation ■ Anxiety and sleep ■ Asthma, pain related to shingles	■ Don't use when driving or operating heavy machinery because it may cause drowsiness. ■ Don't use during pregnancy.
Valerian	■ Relaxation and sleep	■ Combine with passion flower for better results. ■ May cause vivid dreams

take herbs because of the inconvenience of the large dosages and high cost.

Vitamins and minerals

Certain vitamins and minerals have some influence over blood glucose control. (See *Vitamin and mineral supplements with diabetes*, page 140.) In addition, they may play a role in reducing risk factors for developing diabetes and its complications. These vitamins should be taken in the following amounts on a daily basis:

HERBS AND GLYCEMIC CONTROL

This chart highlights some of the herbs that help to control the patient's blood glucose levels, including their actions. Due to their effect on blood glucose levels, frequent monitoring is necessary.

HERB	EFFECTS ON DIABETES
Bilberry extract	■ Helps prevent and reduce the severity of diabetic cataracts
Bitter melon whole fruit extract	■ Helps liver pathways to work more effectively ■ Lowers blood glucose levels
Fenugreek seed extract	■ Helps to lower blood glucose levels ■ Helps the liver and kidneys metabolize blood glucose more efficiently
Gymnema sylvestre leaf	■ Helps keep blood glucose levels low ■ May slow weight gain
Mixed bioflavonoids (citrus)	■ Helps vitamin C and E protect against free radical damage ■ Helps to control blood glucose levels ■ Aids in maintaining vision clarity and sharpness (like bilberry)
Vanadyl sulfate	■ Promotes more effective hepatic and muscle cell use of insulin

● Vitamin C (2,000 mg) lowers heart disease risk.

● Vitamin E (400 international units), when used in combination with vitamin C — both antioxidants — become more beneficial than when either is used alone and slows the progression of atherosclerosis.

● Vitamin B_{12} (100 mcg) is used for heart disease prevention.

● Vitamin B_6 (100 mg) supports immunity, used in heart disease, and supports hemoglobin production.

● Niacin (1,200 to 3,000 mg) increases energy, used for heart attack prevention, and decreases cholesterol.

● Magnesium (700 mg) regulates blood pressure and blood glucose levels and is used to manage diabetes and heart disease.

● Mixed flavonoids (1,000 to 2,000 mg) provide antioxidant action, antibacterial effects, and anti-inflammatory effects; used to treat liver and cardiovascular disease.

● Flaxseed oil (1 T) helps to prevent deposits of fats into arteries; however, if used in high doses, decreases high-density-lipoprotein cholesterol.

● Zinc (30 mg) supports a healthy immune system.

● L-carnitine (300 mg three times daily) increases energy production in heart tissue.

Any patient, but especially the patient with diabetes, needs to use vitamin and mineral supplements cautiously. The absorbability, quality, and effectiveness of vitamins vary greatly. Taking vitamins in split dosages during the day, after or with food to optimize absorption, is more beneficial than taking them once per day. In addition, using vitamins in higher dosages than what's recommended (megadoses) can lead to potential adverse effects and toxicities.

COMMONLY USED HERBS IN TRADITIONAL CHINESE MEDICINE

This chart highlights commonly used herbs in traditional Chinese medicine. Although herbs show some therapeutic benefit, caution must be used to assure that they're used properly in the patient with diabetes, who may be using herbs for other conditions. It's also important for the health care professional to be aware of possible herb-medication interactions and adverse effects.

COMMON NAME	BOTANICAL NAME	CONSIDERATIONS
Astragalus	Astragalus membranaceus	■ Enhances glucose tolerance and elevates serum insulin levels; avoid use in organ transplant patients
Cascara sagrada	Rhamnus purshiana	■ Used in colon detoxification; don't use in dehydrated patients
Garlic	Allium sativum	■ Increases risk of bleeding tendencies in high doses; don't use with anticoagulants (including warfarin [Coumadin])
Ginkgo biloba	Ginkgoaceae	■ Increases memory and blood flow to the brain; use with caution, may cause bleeding tendencies; may decrease effectiveness of monoamine oxidase inhibitors
Ginseng	Panax ginseng	■ Reduces blood glucose levels, aids in digestion, and helps to eliminate fatigue
Glucosamine	None (made from extracting shellfish amino sugars)	■ Treats arthritis and promotes bone health ■ Can increase blood glucose levels and insulin resistance ■ Use with caution and only with health care professional's approval when patient is on anticoagulation therapy
Hoelen	Poriae cocos	■ Lowers blood glucose levels; acts as tonic, sedative, and diuretic (shouldn't be used when urination is excessive)
Lycium bark	Lycium chinense	■ Reduces blood glucose levels (slow and lasting action)
Lycium fruit	Lycium chinense	■ Produces sustained decrease in blood glucose; increases tolerance of carbohydrates; enhances blood circulation
Primrose oil	Oenothera biennis	■ Increases immunity and metabolism; improves thyroid function
Red clover	Trifolium pratense	■ Cleans the liver and blood; used to decrease cardiac risks in postmenopausal women; may be used topically for skin conditions; used for cough in children
Rehmannia	Rehmannia glutinosa	■ Enhances glucose tolerance and elevates serum insulin levels
Scrophularia (Chinese figwort)	Scrophularia ningpoensis	■ Enhances glucose tolerance and elevates serum insulin levels but not as much as Rehmannia
Senna	Cassia senna	■ Cleans the colon (strong and harsh to the intestinal tract) ■ Can be used with ginger to counteract GI disturbances; don't use for prolonged periods, may cause bowel dependency
St. John's wort	Hypericum perforatum	■ Can reduce digoxin (Lanoxin) levels in the blood; interferes with the action of hormonal contraceptives and indinavir (Crixivan) (used to treat acquired immunodeficiency syndrome)
Trichosanthes root	Trichosanthes kirilowii	■ Enhances glucose tolerance and elevates serum insulin levels

VITAMIN AND MINERAL SUPPLEMENTS WITH DIABETES

Various vitamin and mineral supplements can affect diabetes. These supplements and their effects are highlighted here.

Vitamin or mineral	Effects on diabetes
Biotin	■ Helps promote more effective use of insulin, pancreatic function (along with chromium) ■ Lowers blood glucose levels
Chromium	■ Promotes more effective action of insulin ■ Helps maintain healthy pancreatic function ■ Lower blood glucose levels
Copper	■ Aids in keeping insulin-secreting pancreatic cells healthy ■ Helps prevent damage to blood vessels and nerves from diabetes ■ Lowers blood glucose levels
Folic acid	■ Helps prevent stroke and limb loss due to diabetic complications (along with vitamin B_{12})
Magnesium	■ Helps to relieve neuropathic pain ■ Aids in more effective insulin action
Manganese	■ Helps prevent blood vessel and nerve damage
Selenium	■ Aids in moving glucose from the blood into the cells (insulin mimic) ■ Provides protection against blood vessel and nerve damage ■ Helps to lower blood glucose levels
Vitamin B_6 (pyridoxine hydrochloride)	■ Helps to prevent myocardial infarction and nerve damage (along with folic acid and vitamin B_{12}) ■ Helps to prevent blindness and vision loss associated with diabetes
Vitamin B_{12} (cyanocobalamin)	■ Helps to reduce neuropathic pain ■ Works with folic acid and vitamin B_6 (see above)
Vitamin C (ascorbic acid)	■ Promotes movement of glucose out of the blood and into the cells (along with vitamin E) ■ Maintains health of blood vessels and kidneys
Vitamin E (mixed tocopherols)	■ Helps maintain health of pancreas and prevent nerve damage (along with B vitamins) ■ Aids in preventing kidney damage, blindness, and heart disease ■ Maintains health of blood vessels and kidneys (along with vitamin C)
Zinc	■ Helps promote movement of glucose from the blood into the cells ■ Aids in more effective insulin action

Recommendations for use

Dietary supplements have long been used in the United States as complementary to traditional forms of medical treatment. In 1994, Congress passed a law that defined dietary supplements and set criteria that must be adhered to before a product can be labeled as a dietary supplement. This act provides protection to the consumer when purchasing supplements. Products must meet these guidelines:

● The product (other than tobacco) must be intended to supplement the diet and contain one or more vitamins, minerals, herbs or other botanicals, amino acids, or any of the previous ingredients.
● It should be taken in tablet, capsule, powder, softgel, gelcap, or liquid form.
● It isn't represented for use as a conventional food or as a sole item of a meal or the diet.
● It's labeled as being a dietary supplement.

✷ **ALERT** *Dietary supplements are regulated as foods, not drugs, so there could be quality issues in the manufacturing process. Additionally, supplements can interact with prescribed or over-the-counter medicines and other supplements. Moreover, a patient needs to consult his health care professional before starting a supplement, especially if the patient is a child, pregnant, or breast-feeding.*

NCCAM is 1 of 27 institutes and centers that make up the National Institutes of Health (NIH). The NIH is one of eight agencies under the public Health and Human Services. NCCAM is dedicated to exploring CAM healing practices in the context of rigorous science, training CAM researchers, and disseminating authoritative information to the public and professionals. This organization is the most financially solvent institution studying the use of CAM in the United States, and validity in its findings can be trusted. (See *NCCAM research findings for supplements*, page 142.) NCCAM can be accessed at *www.nccam.nih.gov/about/aboutnccam/index.htm.*

Much work remains in the study of CAM. Although some supplements show some efficacy in glycemic control, there may be other factors that outweigh the benefits. (See *Cinnamon and diabetes*, page 143.) People with diabetes must be cautious when researching the best treatment regimen.

OTHER TYPES OF CAM

CAM involves more than just the use of herbs. Traditional Chinese medicine and Ayurveda practices are two examples that encompass a wide range of CAM therapies. In addition, other practices, such as yoga, meditation, and prayer, may be used by patients with diabetes.

The patient with diabetes may use other types of CAM based on his individual beliefs. For example, he may believe that restoration of the body's balance is necessary to help restore glucose control. Or he may use these therapies to help manage symptoms or areas that might be problematic, such as for stress or depression, thereby helping to control glucose levels. Moreover, cultural beliefs, such as Native American or Asian American beliefs, may foster the use of other CAM therapies.

Traditional Chinese medicine treats and views illness quite differently than conventional Western medicine. It views the body as being in a balanced state, where the body and mind are at harmony with the environment. However, various factors, such as stress, injury, and emotion, or environmental factors, such as radiation or pollutants, can disrupt or block this flow of energy. When this imbalance occurs, it can cause disease somewhere within the body. The goal of traditional Chinese medicine is to restore the normal flow, which rebalances the body to restore health and well-being. Examples of traditional Chinese medicine that may be used include:

NCCAM RESEARCH FINDINGS FOR SUPPLEMENTS

This chart lists dietary supplements analyzed by the National Center for Complementary and Alternative Medicine (NCCAM).

SUPPLEMENT	EFFICACY	ADVERSE EFFECTS AND POSSIBLE RISKS
Alpha-lipoic acid	■ An antioxidant found to be beneficial in reducing the oxidative stress caused by high blood glucose levels; may increase glucose uptake in muscles; sensitivity of the body to insulin; and weight loss; more research is needed to determine benefits in diabetes.	■ May cause mild anticoagulation effects with doses over 9 capsules per day ■ May cause a significant lowering of blood glucose levels ■ May lower blood levels of minerals such as iron ■ May interact with other medications such as antacids
Chromium	■ An essential trace mineral element; no rigorous study has been done to prove use in diabetes.	■ Believed to promote more efficient insulin action by lowering blood glucose levels, possibly causing blood glucose levels to drop too low ■ May cause kidney problems in people with diabetes ■ May also cause weight gain
Coenzyme Q 10	■ Several studies demonstrate no effect on glucose control; may have possible use in patients with diabetes and heart disease.	■ May interact with anticoagulants such as warfarin (Coumadin) and antihypertensive agents
Garlic (Allium sativum)	■ Findings mixed related to beneficial use in patients with type 2 diabetes.	■ In high doses, increases bleeding tendencies; not to be used with anticoagulants (including warfarin [Coumadin]) ■ May decrease effectiveness of some antiretroviral drugs ■ Possible interaction with oral contraceptives, cyclosporine, and hepatically metabolized drugs
Magnesium	■ Studies indicate that people with diabetes have a low magnesium level, which makes glucose control worse; therefore, supplementation may be beneficial.	■ May interfere with antibiotics, drugs used for osteoporosis prevention, calcium channel blockers used for high blood pressure, muscle relaxants, and diuretics; megadoses may cause irregular heart rate and extremely low blood pressure ■ May cause loss of appetite, nausea, and diarrhea, which may affect the person's ability to ingest an adequate diet to control blood glucose levels
Omega-3 fatty acids	■ Useful in moving calcium in and out of cells, blood clotting; decreases risk of heart disease, reducing inflammation and lowering triglycerides; slows the progression of atherosclerosis. ■ Possible evidence shows that long-chain omega-3 fatty acids play a role in diabetes prevention and treatment.	■ Safe in adults in low to moderate doses; recent concern that certain species of fish oil may be contaminated with substances from the environment ■ In high doses, may interfere with anticoagulants and agents used for high blood pressure; also may leave a fishy aftertaste

- *Qigong* (pronounced "*chee gong*") — The use of a combination of movement, meditation, and breathing, which stimulates energy flow through the body and promotes better immune function; goal is to balance or rebalance all body functions.
- Acupuncture — The practice of inserting tiny needles into specific points of the body, resulting in removal of obstructions thereby helping to restore energy flow and rebalance the body.
- Moxibustion — A form of heat therapy and a variation of acupuncture; use of sticks or cones from the ground leaves of the plant, *Artemesa vulgaris*, which are burned on ointment or a ginger slice; commonly used to stimulate circulation and treat symptoms of neuropathy.
- Cupping — A variation of acupuncture involving the use of suction cups to withdraw excess toxins from specific acupuncture points, thereby removing obstructions and restoring balance.
- Aromatherapy — The use of essential oils from the plant leaves of the herbal plant that leads to relaxation and stress reduction.
- Chinese massage therapy — The use of hands to stimulate the flow of healing energy to aid in the relief of pain and tension and increase circulation; also aids in decreasing stress hormones for anxiety relief.

Ayurvedic, which means *science of life*, medicine is practiced in India. It emphasizes body, mind, and spirit. Practices are aimed at restoring harmony and balance, similar to the practices used in Chinese medicine. Ayurvedic medicine bases diagnosis on three metabolic body types called *doshas*. Each person has one predominant dosha, but all three are present in varying degrees in every cell, tissue, and organ of the body. Traditional Ayurvedic practice concentrates on keeping the internal organs healthy. Indian cultures also use herbal remedies for diabetes treatment. The roots and stems of *Salacia oblonga* (Saptrangi, Ponkoranti), a woody plant

---

Cutting edge

CINNAMON AND DIABETES

The use of cinnamon in treating diabetes has recently increased in popularity. Research done by Dr. Richard A. Anderson, lead scientist at the Human Nutrition Research Center in Beltsville, Md., a branch of the U.S. Department of Agriculture, shows that cinnamon contains a compound called *methylhydroxy chalcone polymer* (MHCP). It was found that MHCP makes fat cells more responsive to insulin by activating an enzyme that causes insulin to bind to cells and inhibiting the enzyme that blocks this process. However, it's too soon to recommend using this spice as a regular treatment. Additional research is needed before its use can be recommended.

---

found in the forests of India, have been used extensively to treat diabetes. This herb acts in the intestinal tract where glucose absorption is inhibited, thus lowering blood glucose levels. This is the primary herb used for diabetes management in Indian populations.

Native American health practices are driven by an inward spiritual belief, which is the pervasive aspect of the culture. Causes of illness are usually considered to be imbalances among the spiritual, mental, physical, and social interactions of the individual and his family or clan. In many Native American cultures, healing can't be effective without considering the spiritual aspect of the individual.

Meditative exercises, such as yoga and *Tai Chi*, have been shown to provide health benefits. Yoga involves the use of posture in conjunction with specific breathing exercises to help decrease stress and develop, maintain, and promote flexibility. *Tai Chi* is a form of

Chinese martial arts based on *qigong*, which incorporates unity of the mind and body.

Relaxation has been shown to have a significant positive effect on health. It works by opposing or reducing the harmful chemical substances that negative emotions and stress cause. These effects persist long after the relaxation session is finished.

Guided imagery and interactive imagery help to reduce stress, thereby helping to balance the body's chemical substances. Reduction of stress helps in improving overall health and management of the patient's underlying condition.

Prayer and spiritual belief can reduce the adverse effects of other therapy, anxiety, and depression. Whether a person engages in solitary or intercessory prayer or spiritual healing by others, forms of spirituality are thought to reduce stress and to help foster an environment conducive to healing.

EVALUATION OF SUCCESS OF CAM

How's the successfulness of CAM measured? Users may have different opinions regarding treatment outcomes. However, the common view among scientists is that the patient improves because he expects to. The user feels the therapy to be a safe solution. While using CAM, the user feels good. Whether it's a psychological or a real sense of well-being is somewhat debatable. But there's freer reign for the patient's imagination and also a sense of hope. These factors have positive physiological as well as psychological effects. When the patient has some control concerning treatment, there's a peaceable, comfortable feeling. This belief holds true for the patient with diabetes as well. As a result, he may participate more openly in treatment or be more motivated to comply with the treatment. A strong patient-professional relationship must exist to promote better outcomes for all therapeutic interventions.

Selected references

Altshuler, L. *Balanced Healing Combining Modern Medicine with Safe & Effective Alternative Therapies.* Gig Harbor, Wash.: Harbor Press, 2004.

"Ampalaya" [Online]. Available at: *www.tribo.org/vegetables/ampalaya.html.*

Bodeker, G., and Kronenberg, F. "A Public Health Agenda for Traditional, Complementary, and Alternative Medicine," *American Journal of Public Health* 92(10):1582-91, October 2002.

"Coltsfoot" [Online]. Available at: *www.botanical.com/botanical/mgmh/c/coltsf88.html.*

Halat, K.M., and Dennehy, C.E. "Botanicals and Dietary Supplements in Diabetic Peripheral Neuropathy," *Journal of the American Board of Family Practice* 16(1):47-57, January 2003.

Hasegawa, G., et al. "Daily Profile of Plasma % CoQ10 Level, a Biomarker of Oxidative Stress, in Patients with Diabetes Manifesting Postprandial Hyperglycaemia," *Acta Diabetologica* 42(4):179-81, December 2005.

Hess, D.J. "Complementary or Alternative? Stronger vs. Weaker Integration Policies," *American Journal of Public Health* 92(10):1579-81, October 2002.

Hodgson, J.M., et al. "Coenzyme Q10 Improves Blood Pressure and Glycaemic Control: A Controlled Trial in Subjects with Type 2 Diabetes," *European Journal of Clinical Nutrition* 56(11):1137-42, November 2002.

Lewith, G.T., et al. "Do Attitudes Toward and Beliefs About Complementary Medicine Affect Treatment Outcomes?" *American Journal of Public Health* 92(10):1604-06, October 2002.

"Lyceum californicum" [Online]. Available at: *www.sci.sdsu.edu/plants/sdpls/plants/Lycium_californicum.html.*

Nettleton, J.A., and Katz, R. "n-3 Long-Chain Polyunsaturated Fatty Acids in Type 2 Diabetes: A Review," *Journal of the American Dietetic Association* 105(3):428-40, March 2005.

Park, C.M. "Diversity, the Individual, and Proof of Efficacy: Complementary and Alternative Medicine in Medical Education," *American Journal of Public Health* 92(10):1568-72, October 2002.

Silenzio, V.M. "What is the Role of Complementary and Alternative Medicine in Public Health?" *American Journal of Public Health* 92(10):1562-64, October 2002.

Stene, L.C., et al. "Use of Cod Liver Oil during the First Year of Life is Associated with Lower Risk of Childhood-Onset Type 1 Diabetes: A Large, Population-Based, Case-Control Study," *American Journal of Clinical Nutrition* 78(6):1128-34, December 2003.

Treating Type 2 Diabetes with Dietary Supplements. Research Report. National Center for Complementary and Alternative Medicine. Available at: *www.nccam.nih.gov/diabetes*.

Yeh, G.Y., et al. "Use of Complementary and Alternative Medicine Among Persons with Diabetes Mellitus: Results of a National Survey," *American Journal of Public Health* 92(10):1648-52, October 2002.

Management of complications

Because diabetes mellitus is a major risk factor for morbidity and mortality, treating its serious and potentially life-threatening complications, such as blindness, nephropathy, heart disease, and stroke, is essential. The nurse can accomplish this by determining the patient's level of knowledge concerning his illness, educating him (as appropriate), and working with him to ensure positive outcomes.

The patient with diabetes mellitus may have lived with the disease for up to 12 years before ever being diagnosed, during which time many complications may have already developed. Complications associated with diabetes can be categorized as acute or chronic. Acute complications include hypoglycemia, diabetic ketoacidosis, and hyperosmolar hyperglycemic state. Chronic complications include those associated with macrovascular and microvascular changes and include hypertension, dyslipidemia, diabetic neuropathy, diabetic nephropathy, and diabetic retinopathy. Other complications include urinary tract and yeast infections and depression.

HYPOGLYCEMIA

Hypoglycemia, also called *low blood glucose* or *insulin reaction*, occurs when blood serum glucose levels fall below critical levels — less than 50 to 60 mg/dl. It can occur during the day or at night. The signs and symptoms are associated with sympathetic nervous system stimulation, which may include tremors, hunger, sweating, pallor, nausea, tachycardia, palpitations, and shivering. Continued, chronic, or severe hypoglycemia can lead to weakness, dizziness, confusion, blurred vision, behavioral changes, and possibly even seizures and coma due to inadequate glucose transport to the brain.

Causes
Hypoglycemia impacts heavily on people with diabetes and is the result of the interaction of insulin excess and compromised physiologic defenses against declining blood glucose levels.

Severe hypoglycemia occurs when the patient ignores or doesn't recognize the early warning signs and symptoms, such as sweating, tremors, and hunger, or when regulatory glucose hormonal control, such as the action of insulin, glucagon, and amylin, fails to return blood glucose levels to normal.

Drug-induced causes
Drug-induced hypoglycemia accounts for 50% of all hospitalizations and results from insulin excess or an adverse effect of medication. Patients typically experience hypoglycemia because of a dosage error, poor understanding of how the drug works and its possible adverse effects, or deficient medical information. Hypoglycemia is the most common problem associated with insulin

therapy. Other antidiabetic agents, such as sulfonylureas and alcohol, also can cause hypoglycemia. (See *Understanding drug-induced hypoglycemia*.)

Several other pharmacologic agents that can cause hypoglycemia include angiotensin-converting enzyme inhibitors, cytotoxic agents, lithium, pentamidine (Pentam 300), propranolol (Inderal), tricyclic antidepressants, and warfarin (Coumadin).

Although the cause is unknown, salicylates have been found to cause hypoglycemia in children but not in adults. Several theories about salicylate-induced hypoglycemia have been proposed. Researchers believe that they act to increase the use of glucose in the peripheral tissues, inhibit gluconeogenesis in the liver, or enhance insulin release.

Non–drug-induced causes
Non–drug-induced causes of hypoglycemia include fasting hypoglycemia and reactive hypoglycemia. Fasting hypoglycemia is caused by a lack of food intake or exercising without sufficient fuel. As a result, the patient commonly experiences symptoms related to the central nervous system that can range from mild to severe, including slurred speech, blurred vision, headache, difficulty in thinking and concentrating, changes in emotional behavior, decreasing level of consciousness, seizures, and coma.

Reactive hypoglycemia occurs in patients who consume high amounts of refined carbohydrates (simple sugars), which ultimately leads to a sharp drop in the patient's blood glucose level. Subsequently, the patient experiences adrenergic symptoms, such as sweating, shakiness, anxiety, rapid pulse, hunger, nausea, faintness, and seizures. However, reactive hypoglycemia is usually less severe than fasting hypoglycemia.

Risk factors
Factors that put the patient at increased risk for hypoglycemia include:
- poor diabetes self-care practices

UNDERSTANDING DRUG-INDUCED HYPOGLYCEMIA

Hypoglycemia that results from a drug can occur in several ways. The drug can:
- increase the release of insulin by activating insulin secretion mechanisms or by a toxic effect on the islet cells of the pancreas that leads to an uncontrolled release of insulin (Examples include disopyramide [Norpace], pentamidine [Pentam 300], quinidine, and quinine.)
- increase the uptake and use of glucose in the peripheral tissues (Examples include angiotensin-converting enzyme inhibitors, beta-adrenergic blockers such as propranolol (Inderal), and biguanides.)
- decrease glucose production by the liver (Alcohol is an example.)
- potentiate the hypoglycemic effects of insulin and sulfonylureas. (Examples include phenylzine [Nardil] and sulfonamides.)

- prolonged starvation before a surgical procedure or protein-calorie malnutrition
- use of anesthetic agents
- Addison's disease, hepatic disease, pancreatic islet cell tumor, and sepsis.

Diagnosis
Hypoglycemia is diagnosed based on the patient's signs and symptoms, which are typically classified as neurologic or neuroglycopenic. They vary with each patient and in their intensity with each episode. (See *Differentiating symptoms of hypoglycemia*, page 148.) A diagnosis may also be determined through blood glucose testing.

Neurologic symptoms
Neurologic symptoms, also called *autonomic symptoms*, commonly occur in

DIFFERENTIATING SYMPTOMS OF HYPOGLYCEMIA

The major symptoms of hypoglycemia are based on whether the symptom is neurogenic or neuroglycopenic.

NEUROGENIC SYMPTOMS	NEUROGLYCOPENIC SYMPTOMS
Adrenergic	■ Behavioral changes
■ Heart pounding	■ Brain damage
■ Nervousness and anxiety	■ Confusion
■ Shakiness and tremulousness	■ Death
Cholinergic	■ Difficulty thinking
■ Hunger	■ Emotional lability
■ Sweating	■ Fatigue
■ Tingling	■ Loss of consciousness
	■ Seizures
	■ Weakness

early or mild hypoglycemia, usually when blood glucose levels drop rapidly to around 60 mg/dl. These symptoms occur as a response to the increase in epinephrine secretion as the body attempts to compensate for lower blood glucose levels.

Neuroglycopenic symptoms
Neuroglycopenic symptoms most commonly occur at night and result from reduced glucose transport to the brain. The symptoms occur as brain glucose levels drop off slowly, but usually won't appear until blood glucose levels drop below 50 mg/dl.

🔆 **ALERT** *Some of the typical neurologic symptoms of hypoglycemia may be absent in an elderly patient due to age-related changes. Additionally, neuroglycopenic symptoms may be mistaken for other conditions that occur in elderly patients such as stroke.*

In children with type 1 diabetes, there's a significantly higher risk of developing severe hypoglycemia that results in seizures or coma. Because of this risk, it was suggested that these children were at greater risk for gross cognitive and behavioral problems. However, recent research has dispelled this theory revealing that there's no association between severe hypoglycemic episodes and the development of cognitive and behavioral problems among children with type 1 diabetes.

Blood glucose tests
A fingerstick blood glucose test using a glucose meter can be used to determine the patient's blood glucose levels; ve-

nous blood glucose levels may also be obtained. Although exact values may vary and a precise range hasn't been established, a blood glucose range of 45 to 75 mg/dl (2.5 to 4.2 mmol/L) suggests hypoglycemia.

Management
Key to managing hypoglycemia is completing a thorough assessment and obtaining a complete medical history (whenever possible) that includes:
● weight and level of fatigue
● insulin usage or ingestion of an oral hypoglycemic
● use of new prescription or over-the-counter medications, including vitamin supplements and herbal remedies
● history of nausea and vomiting or headaches
● history of renal insufficiency or renal failure
● alcohol intake, including a history of alcoholism
● history of hepatic cirrhosis or liver failure
● nutritional status, including a possible deficiency
● signs of infection.

Mild to moderate hypoglycemia
In mild to moderate hypoglycemia, the patient should be aware of signs and symptoms and be prepared to act quickly with some type of readily available glucose source.

Management strategies for hypoglycemia include:
● taking two or three glucose tablets (available at pharmacy)
● taking one tube of glucose gel (available at pharmacy)
● chewing four to six pieces of hard candy (not sugar-free)
● drinking ½ cup of fruit juice
● drinking 1 cup of skim milk
● drinking ½ cup of a soft drink (not sugar-free)
● eating 1 tbs of honey (placed under the tongue for rapid absorption into the bloodstream)

● eating 1 tbs of table sugar or corn syrup.

After taking one of these measures, the patient should retest his blood in 15 minutes if symptoms persist. In addition to retesting his blood, he should eat a small carbohydrate and protein snack, such as cheese or peanut butter and crackers.

Severe hypoglycemia
If the patient experiences severe hypoglycemia, prompt intervention is necessary. (See *Decision-making process for hypoglycemia*, pages 150 and 151.) If he shows such signs and symptoms as an inability to swallow or a loss of consciousness, an I.V. line should be immediately established. Dextrose 50 to 100 ml of 50% glucose, followed by a continuous infusion of glucose, usually dextrose 10%, should be administered; glucagon may also be administered, but must be reconstituted because it comes in powder form in 1-mg vials. In the event that I.V. access (preferred route) can't be obtained immediately, it may be given subcutaneously or I.M.

In a severe hypoglycemic episode, the patient's blood glucose levels are monitored every 15 minutes until they return to normal. As he responds to treatment, and when blood glucose levels rise above 70 mg/dl, 15 to 20 g of carbohydrates may be given. If the patient is alert and can swallow, carbohydrates may be given orally. After the patient is past the acute phase, blood glucose levels are monitored every 1 to 2 hours.

ALERT *Be careful not to overtreat hypoglycemia. Doing so can lead to rebound hyperglycemia, which, in turn, necessitates insulin administration. The additional insulin can lead to an abrupt decrease in blood glucose levels, resulting in another hypoglycemic episode.*

(*Text continues on page 152.*)

DECISION-MAKING PROCESS FOR HYPOGLYCEMIA

This flowchart shows the decision-making process and subsequent follow-up for managing hypoglycemia based on the patient's condition and capillary blood glucose (CBG) levels.

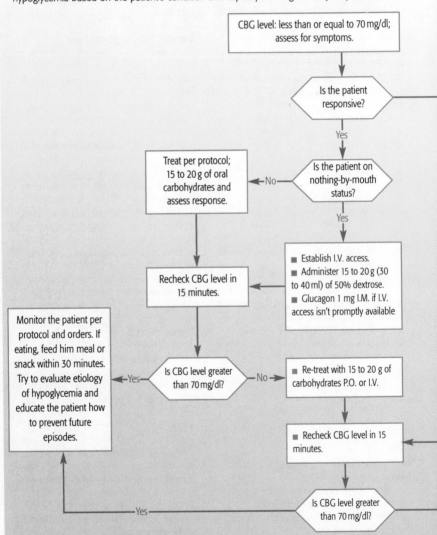

CBG level: less than or equal to 70 mg/dl; assess for symptoms.

Is the patient responsive?

Yes

Is the patient on nothing-by-mouth status?

No → Treat per protocol; 15 to 20 g of oral carbohydrates and assess response.

Yes

- Establish I.V. access.
- Administer 15 to 20 g (30 to 40 ml) of 50% dextrose.
- Glucagon 1 mg I.M. if I.V. access isn't promptly available

Recheck CBG level in 15 minutes.

Is CBG level greater than 70 mg/dl?

Yes → Monitor the patient per protocol and orders. If eating, feed him meal or snack within 30 minutes. Try to evaluate etiology of hypoglycemia and educate the patient how to prevent future episodes.

No → Re-treat with 15 to 20 g of carbohydrates P.O. or I.V.

- Recheck CBG level in 15 minutes.

Is CBG level greater than 70 mg/dl?

Yes

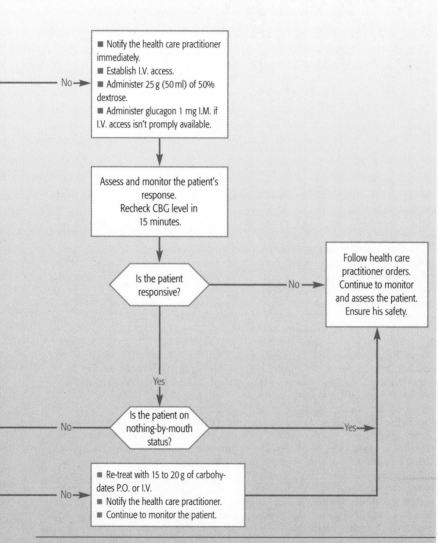

- Notify the health care practitioner immediately.
- Establish I.V. access.
- Administer 25 g (50 ml) of 50% dextrose.
- Administer glucagon 1 mg I.M. if I.V. access isn't promply available.

No →

Assess and monitor the patient's response.
Recheck CBG level in 15 minutes.

Is the patient responsive? — No → Follow health care practitioner orders. Continue to monitor and assess the patient. Ensure his safety.

Yes

Is the patient on nothing-by-mouth status? — No / — Yes →

- Re-treat with 15 to 20 g of carbohydrates P.O. or I.V.
- Notify the health care practitioner.
- Continue to monitor the patient.

No →

Adapted from Tomky, D. "Detection, Prevention, and Treatment of Hypoglycemia in the Hospital," *Diabetes Spectrum* 18(1):39-44, January 2005, with permission of the publisher.

PREVENTING AND MANAGING HYPOGLYCEMIA

For the patient with diabetes, prevention and management of hypoglycemic episodes is important to the overall regimen. Unfortunately, hypoglycemia can occur even when the patient is meticulous in his regimen. Therefore, he needs thorough education on ways to prevent and manage this acute complication. Include these topics in your teaching plan:

■ possible causes
■ signs and symptoms
■ blood glucose level monitoring, including levels suggesting hypoglycemia
■ need for early recognition and prompt treatment of symptoms
■ preparation of simple carbohydrate snacks for immediate use
■ medical alert identification
■ consistent and regular plan for eating and medication
■ exercise and effects on blood glucose levels, including use of snacks
■ signs and symptoms for notifying the health care practitioner.

Prevention

It's essential to educate patients and families on how to prevent the development of hypoglycemia. (See *Preventing and managing hypoglycemia*.)

The patient who uses oral hypoglycemic agents or insulin must understand the signs and symptoms, causes, and treatment of hypoglycemia. He needs to be reminded that insulin absorption can vary even when he injects the correct amount. Inform the patient that weight loss, exercise programs, or the resolution of an infection can cause excess insulin secretion. Instructions should include the importance of regularity in the quantity and timing of food intake, the importance of monitoring blood glucose levels, and the need to consume additional carbohydrates with exercise. Because alcohol interferes with the counter-regulatory response to insulin-induced hypoglycemia and impairs glycogen breakdown, the patient must be cautioned to drink alcohol only with or shortly after a meal that contains enough carbohydrates to prevent hypoglycemia.

The patient also should be instructed to wear a medical alert identification bracelet or necklace and to carry a readily available source of sugar or simple carbohydrates. Keeping blood glucose levels as close to the normal range as possible helps to prevent long-term complications.

DIABETIC KETOACIDOSIS AND HYPEROSMOLAR HYPERGLYCEMIC NONKETOTIC SYNDROME

Diabetic ketoacidosis (DKA) and hyperosmolar hyperglycemic nonketotic syndrome (HHNS) are two metabolic complications associated with diabetes that involve insulin deficiency and severe hyperglycemia. DKA is a severe metabolic disturbance resulting from an absolute or relative insulin deficiency. DKA occurs most commonly in patients with type 1 diabetes, but can also occur in patients with type 2 diabetes. It's considered a medical emergency and is characterized by hyperglycemia, ketosis, dehydration, and electrolyte imbalance. Because a deficiency of circulating insulin occurs, there's an eleva-

UNDERSTANDING DKA

This illustration depicts the various mechanisms involved with diabetic ketoacidosis (DKA).

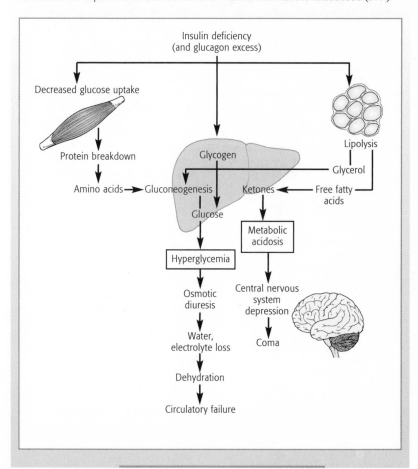

tion of hormones, such as glucagon, catecholamines (epinephrine and norepinephrine), cortisol, and growth hormone, which leads to higher hepatic and renal glucose production and impaired glucose utilization in peripheral tissue. (See *Understanding DKA.*) This impairment leads to hyperglycemia and a change in metabolism causing DKA; severe cases lead to changes in the osmolality of extracellular spaces, causing HHNS.

HHNS is a life-threatening emergency involving a relative insulin deficiency when compared to insulin requirements and commonly affects older patients with type 2 diabetes. HHNS is characterized by severe hyperglycemia, absence of significant ketosis, profound dehydration, and neurologic impairment. Glycosuria results from elevated glucose levels, which spill over into urine, impairing the concentrating capacity of the kidney and exacerbating water loss. Under normal conditions, the kidneys act as a safety valve to eliminate glucose above a certain threshold and prevent further accumulation. However, decreased intravascular volume or underlying renal disease decreases the glomerular filtration rate, causing glucose levels to rise. The loss of more water than sodium leads to hyperosmolarity. Insulin is present, but it isn't enough to reduce blood glucose levels, particularly in the presence of significant insulin resistance.

Causes
DKA and HHNS are most commonly caused by infection, such as respiratory and urinary tract infections. Other causes include taking drugs that affect carbohydrate metabolism, such as dobutamine (Dobutrex), glucocorticoids, phenytoin (Dilantin), terbutaline (Brethine), and thiazide diuretics. Such conditions as alcohol abuse, intestinal obstruction, myocardial infarction, pancreatitis, stroke, and trauma can also cause DKA and HHNS. Additionally, a patient with a new onset of diabetes is at risk for DKA.

Diagnosis
Signs and symptoms usually begin within 24 hours of the insulin deficiency. The patient may have a rapid onset of drowsiness, stupor, and coma. However, if the patient is experiencing extremely mild symptoms, he may wait a day or so before he seeks medical attention.

Signs and symptoms associated with DKA and HHNS include:
- history of polyuria, polydipsia, and polyphagia
- weight loss
- nausea and vomiting (may be coffee ground in appearance and positive for occult blood)

- abdominal pain (only in DKA)
- dehydration
- weakness, poor skin turgor
- Kussmaul's respirations (only in DKA)
- tachycardia, hypotension
- alteration in mental status
- shock
- coma (more common in HHNS).

Laboratory evaluation of patients with suspected DKA and HHNS should include plasma glucose levels, blood urea nitrogen (BUN) and creatinine levels, serum ketones, electrolytes, osmolality, urinalysis, and urine ketones by dipstick as well as initial arterial blood gas analysis, complete blood count with differential, and an electrocardiogram. Blood, urine, and throat cultures should be taken if infection is suspected. (See *Comparing laboratory findings in DKA and HHNS.*)

The diagnostic criteria for DKA include:
- blood glucose level greater than 250 mg/dl
- arterial pH less than 7.3
- bicarbonate level less than 15 mEq/L
- moderate ketonuria or ketonemia.

The diagnostic criteria for HHNS include:
- blood glucose level greater than 600 mg/dl
- arterial pH greater than 7.3
- bicarbonate level greater than 15 mEq/L
- mild ketonuria or ketonemia
- serum osmolality greater than 320 mOsm/kg.

Management
DKA and HHNS require immediate medical attention. Therapy is aimed at correcting fluid and electrolyte imbalances, maintaining normal glucose metabolism, providing adequate insulin to restore and maintain normal glucose metabolism and correct acidosis, preventing complications, and supplying patient education. Identifying comorbidities and frequent patient monitoring are essential. Patients should also be

COMPARING LABORATORY FINDINGS IN DKA AND HHNS

This chart differentiates the findings associated with diabetic ketoacidosis (DKA) and hyperosmolar hyperglycemic nonketotic syndrome (HHNS).

VARIABLES	DKA			HHNS
	Mild	*Moderate*	*Severe*	
Plasma glucose level (mg/dl [mmol/L])	>250 (13.9)	>250	>250	>600 (33.3)
Arterial pH level	7.25 to 7.3	7 to 7.24	<7.0	>7.3
Serum bicarbonate level (mEq/L)	15 to 18	10 to <15	<10	>15
Urine or serum ketones	Positive	Positive	Positive	Small or negative
Effective serum osmolality (mOsm/kg)	Variable	Variable	Variable	>320
Anion gap	>10	>12	>12	Variable
Alternative sensoria in mental obtundation	Alert	Alert, drowsy	Stupor, coma	Stupor, coma

Adapted from Kitabchi A.E., et al. "Hyperglycemic Crises in Diabetes," *Diabetes Care* 27(Suppl 1):S94-102, January 2004, with permission of the publisher.

carefully assessed and treated for underlying causes of HHNS. (See *Decision-making steps for DKA,* pages 156 and 157, and *Decision-making steps for HHNS,* pages 158 and 159.)

Fluid and insulin therapy

In mild DKA and if the patient can drink and tolerate fluids, the focus and first goal of treatment is on rehydration with fluid therapy. In moderate to severe DKA and HHNS and if the patient doesn't have cardiac compromise, I.V. fluid therapy consisting of normal saline solution is infused to restore volume and maintain perfusion to the heart, brain, and kidneys. When renal function is adequate, potassium can be added to correct intracellular-extracellular fluid and electrolyte shifting until the patient is stable and can tolerate fluids by mouth. Successful fluid therapy is based upon an increase in the patient's blood pressure, improved renal function, stabilization of fluid status, and resolution of the patient's clinical manifestations. To avoid fluid overload in the patient with cardiac or renal problems, frequent assessment of those body systems as well as mental status and serum osmolality is necessary.

The second goal of fluid therapy is achieved more slowly and aimed at replacing total body fluid losses. An I.V. infusion of half-normal saline solution is initially administered. When the pa-

(Text continues on page 159.)

DECISION-MAKING STEPS FOR DKA*

Patients with diabetic ketoacidosis (DKA) need prompt intervention. This flowchart highlights the steps in treating adult patients with DKA.

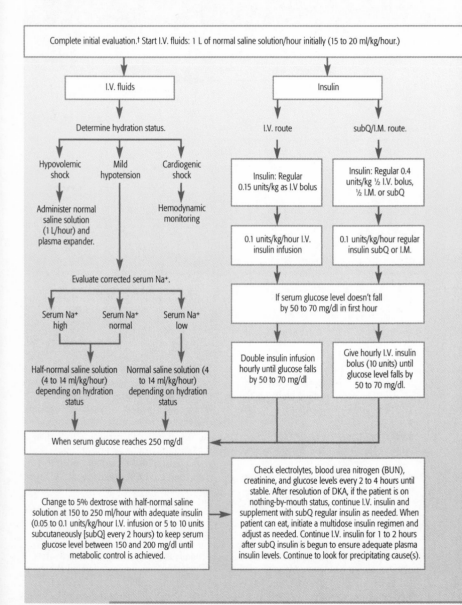

Complete initial evaluation.† Start I.V. fluids: 1 L of normal saline solution/hour initially (15 to 20 ml/kg/hour.)

I.V. fluids

Insulin

Determine hydration status.

I.V. route

subQ/I.M. route.

Hypovolemic shock — **Mild hypotension** — **Cardiogenic shock**

Administer normal saline solution (1 L/hour) and plasma expander.

Hemodynamic monitoring

Insulin: Regular 0.15 units/kg as I.V bolus

Insulin: Regular 0.4 units/kg ½ I.V. bolus, ½ I.M. or subQ

0.1 units/kg/hour I.V. insulin infusion

0.1 units/kg/hour regular insulin subQ or I.M.

Evaluate corrected serum Na+.

Serum Na+ high — **Serum Na+ normal** — **Serum Na+ low**

Half-normal saline solution (4 to 14 ml/kg/hour) depending on hydration status

Normal saline solution (4 to 14 ml/kg/hour) depending on hydration status

If serum glucose level doesn't fall by 50 to 70 mg/dl in first hour

Double insulin infusion hourly until glucose falls by 50 to 70 mg/dl

Give hourly I.V. insulin bolus (10 units) until glucose level falls by 50 to 70 mg/dl.

When serum glucose reaches 250 mg/dl

Change to 5% dextrose with half-normal saline solution at 150 to 250 ml/hour with adequate insulin (0.05 to 0.1 units/kg/hour I.V. infusion or 5 to 10 units subcutaneously [subQ] every 2 hours) to keep serum glucose level between 150 and 200 mg/dl until metabolic control is achieved.

Check electrolytes, blood urea nitrogen (BUN), creatinine, and glucose levels every 2 to 4 hours until stable. After resolution of DKA, if the patient is on nothing-by-mouth status, continue I.V. insulin and supplement with subQ regular insulin as needed. When patient can eat, initiate a multidose insulin regimen and adjust as needed. Continue I.V. insulin for 1 to 2 hours after subQ insulin is begun to ensure adequate plasma insulin levels. Continue to look for precipitating cause(s).

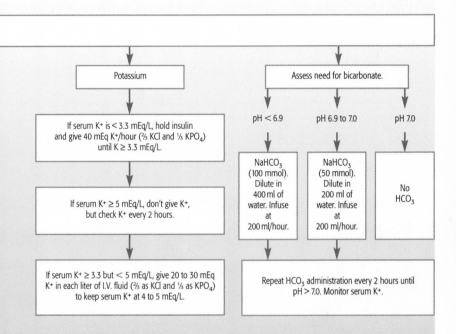

Potassium

If serum K+ is < 3.3 mEq/L, hold insulin and give 40 mEq K+/hour (⅔ KCl and ⅓ KPO₄) until K ≥ 3.3 mEq/L.

If serum K+ ≥ 5 mEq/L, don't give K+, but check K+ every 2 hours.

If serum K+ ≥ 3.3 but < 5 mEq/L, give 20 to 30 mEq K+ in each liter of I.V. fluid (⅔ as KCl and ⅓ as KPO₄) to keep serum K+ at 4 to 5 mEq/L.

Assess need for bicarbonate.

pH < 6.9

pH 6.9 to 7.0

pH 7.0

NaHCO₃ (100 mmol). Dilute in 400 ml of water. Infuse at 200 ml/hour.

NaHCO₃ (50 mmol). Dilute in 200 ml of water. Infuse at 200 ml/hour.

No HCO₃

Repeat HCO₃ administration every 2 hours until pH > 7.0. Monitor serum K+.

*DKA diagnostic criteria: blood glucose > 250 mg/dl, arterial pH < 7.3, bicarbonate < 15 mEq/L, and moderate ketonuria or ketonemia.

†After history and physical examination, obtain arterial blood gas analysis, complete blood count with differential, urinalysis, blood glucose, BUN, electrolytes, chemistry profile, and creatinine levels STAT as well as an electrocardiogram. Obtain chest X-ray and cultures as needed.

Adapted from American Diabetes Association. Position Statement. "Hyperglycemic Crisis in Patients with Diabetes Mellitus," *Diabetes Care* 26(Suppl 1):S111, January 2003, with permission of the publisher.

DECISION-MAKING STEPS FOR HHNS*

Patients with hyperosmolar hyperglycemic nonketotic syndrome (HHNS) need prompt, immediate intervention. This chart highlights the steps in treating adult patients with HHNS.

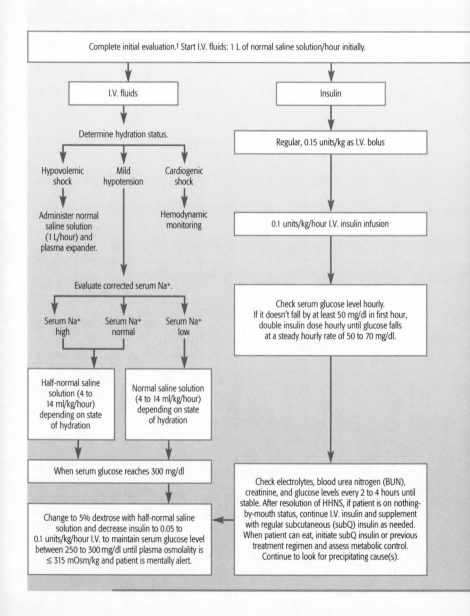

Complete initial evaluation.† Start I.V. fluids: 1 L of normal saline solution/hour initially.

I.V. fluids

Determine hydration status.

- Hypovolemic shock
- Mild hypotension
- Cardiogenic shock

Administer normal saline solution (1 L/hour) and plasma expander.

Hemodynamic monitoring

Evaluate corrected serum Na⁺.

- Serum Na⁺ high
- Serum Na⁺ normal
- Serum Na⁺ low

Half-normal saline solution (4 to 14 ml/kg/hour) depending on state of hydration

Normal saline solution (4 to 14 ml/kg/hour) depending on state of hydration

When serum glucose reaches 300 mg/dl

Change to 5% dextrose with half-normal saline solution and decrease insulin to 0.05 to 0.1 units/kg/hour I.V. to maintain serum glucose level between 250 to 300 mg/dl until plasma osmolality is ≤ 315 mOsm/kg and patient is mentally alert.

Insulin

Regular, 0.15 units/kg as I.V. bolus

0.1 units/kg/hour I.V. insulin infusion

Check serum glucose level hourly. If it doesn't fall by at least 50 mg/dl in first hour, double insulin dose hourly until glucose falls at a steady hourly rate of 50 to 70 mg/dl.

Check electrolytes, blood urea nitrogen (BUN), creatinine, and glucose levels every 2 to 4 hours until stable. After resolution of HHNS, if patient is on nothing-by-mouth status, continue I.V. insulin and supplement with regular subcutaneous (subQ) insulin as needed. When patient can eat, initiate subQ insulin or previous treatment regimen and assess metabolic control. Continue to look for precipitating cause(s).

```
┌──────────────────────────────────────┐
│                                      │
└──────────────────────────────────────┘
                  │
                  ▼
        ┌──────────────────┐
        │    Potassium     │
        └──────────────────┘
                  │
                  ▼
```

If serum K⁺ is < 3.3 mEq/L, hold insulin and give 40 mEq K⁺/hour (⅔ KCl and ⅓ KPO₄) until K⁺ ≥ 3.3 mEq/L

If serum, K⁺ ≥ 5 mEq/L, don't give K⁺, but check potassium every 2 hours.

If serum K⁺ ≥ 3.3 but < 5 mEq/L, give 20 to 30 mEq K⁺ in each liter of I.V. fluid (⅔ as KCl and ⅓ as KPO₄) to keep serum K⁺ at 4 to 5 mEq/L.

*HHNS diagnostic criteria: blood glucose > 600 mg/dl, arterial pH > 7.3, bicarbonate > 15 mEq/l, mild ketonuria or ketonemia, and effective serum osmolality > 320 mOsm/kg of water. This protocol is for patients admitted with mental status change or severe dehydration who require admission to an intensive care unit. For less severe cases, see management guidelines. Effective serum osmolality calculation: 2[measured Na (mEq/L)] + glucose (mg/dl)/18.

†After history and physical examination, obtain arterial blood gas analysis, complete blood count with differential, urinalysis, blood glucose, BUN, electrolytes, chemistry profile, and creatinine levels STAT as well as an electrocardiogram. Obtain chest X-ray and cultures as needed.

Adapted from American Diabetes Association. Position Statement. "Hyperglycemic Crisis in Patients with Diabetes Mellitus," *Diabetes Care* 26(Suppl 1):S111, January 2003, with permission of the publisher.

tient's blood glucose levels reach 250 mg/dl, the I.V. solution is changed to 5% dextrose in half-normal saline solution to prevent hypoglycemia and cerebral edema — complications that may occur when the serum osmolarity rapidly declines.

It's important to remember that adequate fluids must always be given first and should be based on the recommendations in the American Diabetes Association algorithm. If insulin is given before fluids, the fluid will move intracellularly, causing potential worsening of hypotension, collapse of the vasculature, or death.

Insulin should be given as an initial bolus of 0.15 unit/kg of body weight I.V. followed by a continuous infusion of regular insulin at a dose of 0.1 unit/kg (5 to 7 units/hour) in adults, after potassium loss has been excluded. If the patient's plasma glucose doesn't fall by 50 mg/dl from the initial value in the first hour, his hydration status must be checked. If it's acceptable, then the infusion may be doubled every hour until the glucose level steadily declines by 50 to 75 mg/hour.

When the plasma glucose reaches 250 mg/dl in DKA or 300 mg/dl in HHS, it may be possible to decrease the insulin infusion rate to 0.05 to 0.1 unit/kg of body weight (3 to 6 units/hour), and dextrose (5% or 10%) may be added to the I.V. fluids. The rate of insulin administration or the concentration of dextrose may need to be adjusted to maintain the glucose level until acidosis in DKA and hyperosmolarity in HHNS are resolved.

In DKA and HHNS, ketonemia (elevated levels of ketones in the blood) takes longer to resolve than hyperglycemia. During insulin therapy for DKA or HHNS, blood samples should also be obtained every 2 to 4 hours to monitor serum electrolyte, glucose, BUN, and creatinine levels, osmolality, and venous pH (only for DKA). With mild DKA, regular insulin either given subcutaneously or I.M. every hour is as effective as I.V. administration in lowering blood glucose and ketone bodies. Assess effectiveness of glucose therapy on an hourly basis.

Electrolyte replacement therapy

Electrolyte replacement therapy is also critical in the treatment of DKA and HHNS. Initially, potassium levels may be normal or high, even though the total body level of potassium is depleted because insulin therapy, correction of acidosis, and volume expansion decrease serum potassium concentration levels. Throughout the patient's care, he should be monitored for signs of hypokalemia, which includes fatigue, malaise, confusion, muscle weakness, shallow respirations, abdominal distention or paralytic ileus, hypotension, and a weak pulse. After urine output is established, potassium replacement is initiated after serum levels fall below 5.5 mEq/L. Generally, 20 to 30 mEq of potassium should be given in each liter of I.V. fluid to maintain the serum potassium level between 4 and 5 mEq/L.

Bicarbonate therapy is typically used in patients with DKA who have pH values less than 6.9. Because severe acidosis can lead to multiple adverse vascular effects, 100 mmol of sodium bicarbonate is added to 400 ml of sterile water and given at a rate of 200 ml/hour. In patients with a pH of 6.9 to 7.0, 50 mmol of sodium bicarbonate is diluted in 200 ml sterile water and infused at a rate of 200 ml/hour. No bicarbonate is necessary if the patient's pH level is greater than 7.0.

★ **ALERT** *Never rapidly infuse large amounts of sodium bicarbonate because potassium values may decline and result in hypokalemia-induced arrhythmias. Rapid bicarbonate administration is only used in acute cardiorespiratory arrest situations or to treat hyperkalemia-induced cardiac arrhythmias.*

As with potassium, total phosphate concentration increases with insulin therapy (in patients with DKA) even though total body stores of phosphate are depleted. Phosphate replacement may be considered when the patient's serum phosphate level falls below 1 mEq/L and when cardiac and skeletal muscle weakness and respiratory depression (due to hypophosphatemia) is a concern. Because phosphate replacement can cause hypocalcemia with no signs or symptoms of tetany, serum calcium level should be monitored closely.

Hypomagnesemia may manifest as arrhythmias, muscle weakness, seizures, stupor, and agitation. Unless the patient is in renal failure, magnesium administration is warranted.

Documentation of clinical parameters, fluid and electrolytes, laboratory values, insulin therapy, and urinary output should be maintained.

Treatment-related problems

The most common treatment-related problems associated with DKA and HHNS include hypoglycemia, from aggressive treatment with insulin; and hypokalemia, from treatment with insulin and bicarbonate. Patients may also become hyperglycemic when insulin therapy is discontinued and no subcutaneous insulin is given. Patients recovering from DKA may also become hyperchloremic as a result of the excessive use of saline fluid and electrolyte replacement.

Although rare, cerebral edema may also result from treatment and is the primary cause of death in children who have been treated for DKA. Fatal cases of cerebral edema have also been reported with HHNS in children and adults. One factor contributing to its development is the rapid decline in blood glucose levels. I.V. osmotic diuretics, such as mannitol, may be used in the treatment. Cerebral edema may be prevented by gradually replacing sodium and water deficits in patients with hyperosmolality and adding dextrose to the hydrating solution after the blood glucose level reaches 250 mg/dl.

Prevention

Strategic planning and self-management guidelines should be a priority in educating the patient and his family about preventing DKA and HHNS. Sick-day management instructions must cover how to maintain blood glucose control when ill and should be reviewed periodically. Teach the patient about:

● when to contact the health care practitioner

● what blood glucose goals should be and how to use supplemental short-acting insulin when ill or if an infection is present

● ways to suppress fever and treat infection

● how to initiate an easily digestible liquid diet containing carbohydrates and salt.

Also teach the patient never to omit insulin and to seek medical advice when he first feels sick. Either the patient or his family must monitor glucose levels frequently and test urine for ketones. It's important that family members or staff recognize the early symptoms of dehydration in elderly patients, who are commonly hospitalized due to this complication.

When the patient's blood glucose level is greater than 300 mg/dl, insulin should be administered, and his temperature, respiratory and pulse rate, and body weight should be recorded and communicated to the health care practitioner.

HYPERTENSION

About 73% of adults with diabetes have elevated blood pressure (greater than or equal to 130 mm Hg systolic and 80 mm Hg diastolic) or use prescription medications for hypertension. Hypertension affects 20% to 60% of all patients with diabetes and increases the risk of microvascular complications, including retinopathy, nephropathy, and neuropathy. An effective mnemonic for teaching blood pressure control to patients with diabetes is ABC:

● A = A_{1C} (hemoglobin)
● B = blood pressure
● C = cholesterol.

Blacks, overall, have a higher incidence of hypertension than Whites or Asians. It's also more common among lower socioeconomic groups and patients with a genetic predisposition.

Causes

The exact cause of primary hypertension is unknown; however, certain risk factors have been identified, including family history, advancing age, sleep apnea, and race. Secondary hypertension is caused by several problems, including coarctation of the aorta, renal artery stenosis, brain tumor, endocrine dysfunction, and numerous medications, such as hormonal contraceptives, cocaine, and sympathetic stimulants.

Diagnosis

Patients with hypertension may exhibit such signs and symptoms as headache, epistaxis, dizziness, and blurred vision. Diagnosis of hypertension is based on blood pressure readings that are greater than 130 mm Hg systolic and 80 mm Hg diastolic on two or more successive occasions. Patients with diabetes who have hypertension show signs and symptoms of extracellular fluid volume problems, microalbuminuria, elevated systolic hypertension, and orthostatic hypertension.

Management

The American Diabetes Association recommends that blood pressure for patients with diabetes should be reduced to less than 130 mm Hg systolic and 80 mm Hg diastolic. In patients with proteinuria (greater than 1 g/day) and renal insufficiency, the target blood pressure should be 125 mm Hg systolic and 75 mm Hg diastolic.

General guidelines

● Because obesity is closely related to hypertension, weight reduction should

BLOOD PRESSURE AND A HIGH-CARBOHYDRATE DIET

A recent study at the University of Texas Southwestern Medical Center, Division of Nutrition and Metabolic Diseases, showed that a long-term high-carbohydrate diet can impact the blood pressure of patients with type 2 diabetes. In the study, patients ate a high-carbohydrate diet for 6 weeks and then a diet high in monounsaturated fats for 6 weeks, with 1 week off between the two diets. The diet sequence was randomly assigned so that one patient ate the high-carbohydrate diet while another ate the high monounsaturated fat diet. The calorie content of each diet was the same. Then, the patients were given the option to continue the diet for an additional 8 weeks. After 8 weeks, systolic blood pressure readings in patients eating the high-carbohydrate diet were found be approximately 6 points higher. Their heart rates also were elevated by 7 to 8 beats/minute. In patients who consumed the high monounsaturated fat diet, systolic and diastolic blood pressure readings were 3 to 4 points lower than initial readings, and there was a statistically significant lowering of the heart rate. The researchers proposed that a long-term high-carbohydrate diet may lead to an increase in blood pressure in patients with type 2 diabetes.

be encouraged to reduce blood glucose and lipid levels.

● Reducing sodium intake and monitoring carbohydrate intake can help lower blood pressure in patients with primary or essential hypertension (elevated blood pressure without an identifiable cause). (See *Blood pressure and a high-carbohydrate diet.*)

● Daily exercise, such as brisk walking, is effective in lowering blood pressure and improving cardiovascular function; thus, it's an important part of the treatment plan in the patient with diabetes.

● Smoking cessation helps to reduce the risk of developing stroke, heart disease, and peripheral arterial disease.

● Alcohol is acceptable in moderation. Men should limit alcohol to no more than two drinks per day, whereas women should limit alcohol to no more than one drink per day.

Medication therapy

Patients with diabetes who have hypertension are usually on more than one antihypertensive drug to control elevated blood pressure. Drug therapy has been shown to reduce cardiovascular and microvascular complications, including diabetic retinopathy, and slow down the progression of diabetic nephropathy. Such medications include angiotensin-converting enzyme (ACE) inhibitors, beta-adrenergic blockers, calcium channel blockers, and diuretics.

ACE inhibitors and calcium channel blockers are usually the drugs of choice because beta-adrenergic blockers can mask signs of hypoglycemia. ACE inhibitors, such as enalapril (Vasotec), provide greater protection against coronary artery disease, heart disease, and myocardial infarction and are shown to have beneficial effects on renal function; they also reduce microalbuminuria.

Thiazide diuretics may also be used as initial therapy. However, they can contribute to hyperglycemia and hypokalemia; therefore, close monitoring of serum potassium levels is warranted.

Antihypertensive drugs may be taken alone or in combination. Although they may cause adverse effects, the ultimate focus for the patient with diabetes is blood pressure control. In addition, laboratory test results should be obtained before antihypertensive therapy begins to evaluate for organ or tissue damage or other risk factors. These tests include complete blood count; blood chemistry, including potassium, sodium, and creatinine levels; fasting blood glucose; and total cholesterol and lipoprotein levels (high-density, low-density, and very-low-density lipoprotein). Moreover, an electrocardiogram is performed as a baseline.

Prevention

The patient with diabetes should have his blood pressure obtained at every routine visit to his health care practitioner. In addition, he should be encouraged to institute lifestyle changes, including diet and exercise, to enhance glucose control and help in controlling his blood pressure.

DYSLIPIDEMIA

Dyslipidemia refers to abnormal lipid levels in the blood, which contribute to the risk of cardiovascular disease in the patient with diabetes.

Lipids serve three major functions in the body. They:
● store nutrients (triglycerides)
● form the precursors for adrenal and gonadal steroids and bile acids (cholesterol)
● transport complex lipids throughout the body (lipoproteins).

Lipids are important to body tissue, but high cholesterol and triglyceride levels cause cardiovascular complications in patients with diabetes.

Causes

There are four major components involved in dyslipidemia: decreased high-density lipoprotein (HDL) cholesterol level, increased low-density lipoprotein (LDL) cholesterol level, increased triglyceride level, and increased lipoprotein level.

HDL (good) cholesterol protects against heart disease. An HDL level of less than 40 mg/dl increases the risk of developing heart disease. An HDL level

of 60 mg/dl or more helps to lower the patient's risk of heart disease.

High levels of triglycerides can also raise the risk of heart disease. For example, levels that are borderline high (150 to 199 mg/dl) or high (200 mg/dl or more) may need dietary or pharmacologic treatment in some people.

Patients with diabetes have an increased risk of hyperlipidemia (high lipid levels) due to prolonged hyperglycemia — the fats circulating in the blood bind to sugars. High lipid levels lead to atherosclerosis (another cause of dyslipidemia in patients with diabetes) through increased plasma cholesterol, particularly LDL cholesterol levels. Obese or overweight patients are at greater risk for atherosclerosis.

Primary hyperlipidemia is commonly hereditary and caused by mechanisms involved in lipid metabolism. Secondary hyperlipidemia occurs in relation to a diet that's high in cholesterol, total fat, saturated fat, and excess calories as well as associated with diabetes mellitus, renal disease, and excessive alcohol intake. Medications, such as beta-adrenergic blockers, thiazide diuretics, glucocorticoids, and estrogen therapy, can contribute to hyperlipidemia.

Diagnosis

Because patients with dyslipidemia are usually asymptomatic, the National Cholesterol Education Program recommends that those older than age 20 have their cholesterol level tested every 5 years. (For specific blood levels, see *Cardiovascular risk based on lipoprotein levels in diabetes*, page 164.)

Management

Although treatment usually depends on the patient's lipid levels and cardiovascular status, initial therapeutic steps typically include changes in diet and exercise and adherence to a medication regimen.

CARDIOVASCULAR RISK BASED ON LIPOPROTEIN LEVELS IN DIABETES

The patient's risk of cardiovascular disease is determined by his total cholesterol level as well has his low-density lipoprotein (LDL) level. This chart shows that the greater the total cholesterol and LDL levels, the higher the patient's risk of heart disease.

	RISK CATEGORY
Total cholesterol level	
Less than 200 mg/dl	Desirable
200 to 239 mg/dl	Borderline high
240 mg/dl and above	High
LDL cholesterol level	
Less than 100 mg/dl	Optimal
100 to 129 mg/dl	Near or above optimal
130 to 159 mg/dl	Borderline high
160 to 189 mg/dl	High
190 mg/dl and above	Very high

Dietary measures

The goal of diet, also called *medical nutrition therapy*, is for the patient to attain and maintain optimal blood glucose and A_{1C} levels, LDL and HDL cholesterol levels, triglyceride levels, blood pressure, and body weight. These goals can be accomplished by educating the patient about healthy food choices and various types of physical activity, which help to prevent and treat obesity, dyslipidemia, cardiovascular disease, hypertension, and nephropathy.

A nutritional assessment should include determining the patient's food intake and underlying issues, including renal and metabolic functioning, and financial and cultural considerations. These areas are important in determining the most optimal nutrition plan for the patient to ensure glycemic control as well as one that the patient will adhere to consistently.

Because carbohydrates are an important source of energy and glucose for the brain and central nervous system, the patient with diabetes should follow a diet that includes healthy amounts of carbohydrates. (See chapter 5, Nutritional therapy, for more information.) Indeed, the recommended range is that carbohydrates should account for about 45% to 65% of total calories consumed. However, the patient should monitor the amount and type of carbohydrates he consumes during a meal to help predict his glycemic response and to avoid hyperglycemia after a meal. The patient with diabetes who has lipid abnormalities must also reduce his intake of total

CRITERIA FOR METABOLIC SYNDROME

This chart identifies the key areas that are used to determine if a patient has metabolic syndrome.

RISK FACTORS	DEFINING LEVEL
Abdominal obesity (given as waist circumference)	
Males	> 40" (> 102 cm)
Females	> 35" (> 88 cm)
Triglycerides	≥ 150 mg/dl (≥ 1.7 mmol/L)
High-density lipoprotein cholesterol	
Males	< 40 mg/dl (< 1 mmol/L)
Females	< 50 mg/dl (< 1.3 mmol/L)
Blood pressure	≥ 130/85 mm Hg
Fasting glucose	≥ 110 mg/dl (≥ 6.1 mmol/L)

Adapted from Grundy, S.M., et al. "NHLBI/AHA Conference Proceedings Definition of Metabolic Syndrome," *Circulation* 109:433-38, January 2004, with permission of the publisher. Available at: *http://www.//circ.ahajournals.org/cgi/content/full/109/3/433.*

saturated fats and cholesterol. A triglyceride level of 150 mg/dl or more is an indication of metabolic syndrome (a group of conditions occurring as a cluster in one individual — obesity, hypertension, hyperglycemia, and abnormal cholesterol levels) and increases the risk of heart disease. (See *Criteria for metabolic syndrome*.)

Sodium should also be reduced in patients with dyslipidemia and hypertension. Dietary fiber provides a sensation of being full, and large amounts of soluble fiber (oats, barley, peas, corn, apples, and bananas) may be beneficial to serum lipid level. Refined sugars and alcohol should also be restricted.

Exercise
Regular exercise plays an important role in managing diabetes. Moreover, it decreases the risk of cardiovascular disease, such as hypertension and hyperlipidemia; improves glycemic control;

and has beneficial effects on insulin sensitivity. Initially, physical activity should be limited and then gradually increased in duration and frequency. For example, the patient can start off at 10 to 20 minutes 2 to 3 days per week and gradually increase to 30 to 45 minutes 3 to 5 days per week. He should never start an exercise program without first consulting with his health care practitioner and devising an appropriate routine.

The patient also needs to be instructed about testing his glucose levels before beginning exercise. If the blood glucose level exceeds 250 mg/dl, the patient should then test his urine for ketones and avoid exercise if there's ketonuria. His feet should be inspected daily and proper footwear must be worn. Exercising in extremely cold or hot weather should be avoided. The patient's progress should always be monitored and positive feedback should be given to encourage him to continue with the exercise plan.

Medication therapy

Medication therapy is an important component in the overall management plan for the patient with diabetes and dyslipidemia. Treatment goals include lowering total serum cholesterol and LDL levels and raising the HDL level. Statins are prescribed for the patient with diabetes older than age 40 with a total cholesterol of 135 mg/dl, without cardiovascular disease (but may also be prescribed for the patient with diabetes who also has cardiovascular disease). Statin therapy also aims to achieve a reduced LDL level of 30% to 40%, regardless of the baseline LDL level. The primary goal is an LDL level of less than 100 mg/dl. Routine antilipid drugs aren't prescribed to the patient with diabetes unless he has lipid abnormalities.

Statins, such as pravastatin (Pravachol), lovastatin (Mevacor), simvastatin (Zocor), and atorvastatin (Lipitor), are first-line medications in the treatment of hyperlipidemia.

ALERT *Because statins reduce cholesterol synthesis in the liver, the patient's liver enzyme levels may be increased. Therefore, liver function tests must be monitored. Keep in mind that statins are contraindicated in the patient with active liver disease or one who's pregnant.*

An adverse effect of statins is muscle myopathies; therefore, the patient should be instructed to call the physician if he experiences muscle weakness and pain or if his urine is brown. If combination therapy is needed, other cholesterol-lowering drugs may be added such as nicotinic acid (niacin [Nicobid]), fibric acid derivatives (gemfibrozil [Lopid]), and bile acid sequestrants (cholestyramine [Questran]).

Prevention

Prevention of lipid abnormalities is directly related to following a healthy lifestyle that includes a nutritious heart healthy diet and daily exercise.

DIABETIC NEUROPATHY

The longer a patient has diabetes, the greater his risk of developing diabetic neuropathy — a debilitating disorder that occurs in nearly 50% of patients with diabetes. Some patients with neuropathies are asymptomatic and thus don't immediately seek medical attention. Therefore, the American Diabetes Association makes the following screening recommendations: for patients with type 2 diabetes, immediate screening because diabetic neuropathy is usually present at diagnosis; for patients with type 1 diabetes, 5-year interval, because diabetic neuropathy is commonly diagnosed late. For both types, follow-up screening should take place every year thereafter.

Diabetic neuropathy can cause motor deficits, silent cardiac ischemia, orthostatic hypotension, vasomotor instability, gastroparesis, bladder dysfunction, and sexual dysfunction. It's also common in patients who have poor blood glucose level control, elevated blood pressure, and hyperlipidemia, in those who are overweight, and in those who smoke or abuse alcohol.

Because of thickened wall muscles and slow and impaired nerve conduction, nutrients can't reach the nerves they supply, resulting in diabetic neuropathy. It's slow and progressive in onset, results in loss of function, and is usually irreversible. These factors lead to decreased sensations in the feet with decreased sensitivity to pain. Therefore, the patient can't even feel a small cut, puncture, or blister. In these patients, foot trauma is a common occurrence and foot ulcers and amputations are a major cause of morbidity and disability.

Types

Diabetic neuropathy may be categorized as sensorimotor or autonomic neuropathy.

Diabetic sensorimotor neuropathy

Diabetic sensorimotor neuropathy, also known as *peripheral neuropathy*, commonly affects the nerves of the lower extremities. Muscular symptoms include balance problems, muscle weakness, ataxic gait, and atrophy. Sensory symptoms include pain, paresthesia, numbness, paralysis, cramping, and nighttime falls.

Diabetic autonomic neuropathy

Diabetic autonomic neuropathy affects the cardiovascular, GI, genitourinary, sudomotor (sweat glands), and endocrine systems. It causes fatigue, exercise intolerance, syncope, dizziness, changes in digestion, loss of bowel and bladder control, pruritus, limb hair loss, changes in perspiration, and changes in sexual response.

Diabetic autonomic neuropathy can cause many complications. It may lead to hypoglycemia unawareness, including skin flaking and cracks, increasing the patient's risk for ulcerations; damage to the digestive system, causing constipation; and gastroparesis, a condition in which the stomach empties too slowly, causing blood glucose level to fluctuate. In addition, the patient may not be able to sense a full bladder, resulting in urinary retention and incomplete voiding, which could cause urinary tract infections and overflow incontinence. Further, if there's damage to the sweat glands in the patient with diabetic autonomic neuropathy, body temperature can't be properly regulated. Lastly, the patient's pupils may become affected, causing them to become less responsive to changes in light.

Causes

A combination of metabolic and vascular mechanisms may cause diabetic neuropathy. Metabolic causes include having diabetes for an extended period, elevated blood glucose level, low insulin level, and hyperlipidemia. Vascular causes include damage to the blood vessels and nutrient supply to the nerves, inherited traits that increase susceptibility, autoimmune factors, and heavy smoking or alcohol abuse.

Risk factors

Risk factors associated with the development of diabetic neuropathy must be identified for effective preventive management. Patients who have had diabetes for over 10 years, who have poor control of their diabetes, or who have cardiovascular, retinal, or renal complications are at increased risk for diabetic neuropathy. In addition, patients with decreased sensation in the feet and those with peripheral vascular disease are also at risk. Elderly people have an increased risk of falling.

Diagnosis

Assessment of diabetic neuropathy involves screening for peripheral vascular disease. The initial screening should include taking a thorough history for intermittent claudication, decreased or absent pedal pulses, foot ulceration, muscle pain, and burning or cramping that's relieved by rest. Absent peripheral pulses due to occlusive peripheral arterial disease is more common in the patient with type 2 diabetes. As the disease progresses, he may report awakening at night because of throbbing pain that's only relieved by placing the leg in a dependent position.

On physical examination, foot structure and skin integrity should be observed for skin breaks, especially between the toes and under the metatarsal heels; reddened or calloused areas; decreased or absent pedal pulse; delayed capillary refill; and protective sensation. Signs of peripheral neuropathy include loss of vibratory and position sense, loss of deep tendon reflexes (especially loss of the ankle jerk), trophic ulceration, footdrop, muscle atrophy, and excessive callus formation, especially overlying pressure points such as the heel.

Protective sensation is assessed using the Semmes-Weinstein 5.07 (10-g) monofilament test. Bony deformities, such as hammer toe, Charcot's foot deformity, bunions, and problems with gait and balance, should also be recorded. The American Diabetes Association recommends a thorough foot examination for all patients with diabetes once per year, but one should be given by the physician at every visit to identify those at risk. Patients should also be asked about daily foot inspections at home.

Another diagnostic tool is the ankle-brachial index (ABI); it's a noninvasive test where the physician uses a hand-held Doppler device to evaluate for vascular disease. The cuff is slowly deflated until a Doppler-detected pulse returns. It's then repeated on the leg, with the cuff wrapped around the distal calf and the Doppler placed over the dorsalis pedis or posterior tibial artery. The ankle systolic pressure divided by the brachial systolic pressure gives the patient's ABI. (An ABI of less than 1 suggests vascular disease.)

Management

In the patient with diabetes who has diabetic neuropathy, appropriate wound care is necessary for ulcers to prevent infection, wound progression, and possible amputation. In addition, medication is available to treat neuropathic pain associated with diabetic neuropathy. Teaching the patient about appropriate foot care is also a key component of the treatment plan.

Wound care

Debridement and infection control are two of the most important components in the care of foot ulcers in patients with diabetes. Debridement removes necrotic and infected tissue, calluses, and foreign bodies from the ulceration to promote wound healing and decrease the risk of infection. The ulcer should be surgically debrided down to viable bleeding tissue. Immediately after the procedure, the wound should be flushed thoroughly with sterile normal saline solution. (Clean, granulating

wounds shouldn't be debrided.) If debridement isn't an option as a result of significant vascular compromise, enzymatic debridement may be considered.

After debridement, apply a moist sodium chloride dressing or isotonic sodium chloride gel (Normlgel, Intra-Site gel) or a hydroactive paste (Duoderm). Optimal wound coverage requires wet-to-damp dressings, which support debridement, absorb exudate, and protect surrounding healthy skin. A polyvinyl film dressing (OpSite, Tegaderm) that's semipermeable to oxygen and moisture and impermeable to bacteria is a good choice for wounds that are neither very dry nor highly exudative. Bandaging an anatomical area, such as a heel ulcer, requires a highly conformable dressing such as an extra-thin hydrocolloid dressing. (See *Wound coverage recommendations*.)

Medication therapy

Duloxetine (Cymbalta), a selective serotonin norepinephrine reuptake inhibitor that's used to treat major depressive disorder, is also approved for use in managing the pain associated with diabetic peripheral neuropathy. The usual dosage is 60 mg per day, and studies have shown that doses above this level don't provide additional relief. For patients with renal disease, a lower starting dose may be necessary. The most common adverse effects associated with the drug include nausea, dizziness, sleepiness, and fatigue. In addition, constipation, dry mouth, decreased appetite, and weakness as well as increased liver enzyme levels may occur. In clinical trials, patients taking duloxetine showed an average weight loss of just over 2.2 lb (1 kg) over a 13-week period.

Foot care

Foot care is essential in the patient with diabetic neuropathy due to decreased sensation in the feet and sensitivity to pain. The patient with diabetes must also closely monitor the skin of his feet because a constant state of elevated

WOUND COVERAGE RECOMMENDATIONS

Wound coverage recommendations include:

■ dry wounds — Hydrocolloid dressings, such as Duoderm or IntraSite Hydrocolloid, are impermeable to oxygen, moisture, and bacteria, and maintain a moist environment.

■ exudative wounds — Absorptive dressings — for example, calcium alginates (Kaltostat, Curasorb) — are highly absorptive and appropriate for exudative wounds.

■ infected superficial wounds — Silvadene (silver sulfadiazine) may be used if the patient isn't allergic to sulfa drugs. If a sulfa allergy exists, either bacitracin-zinc or Neosporin ointment is a good alternative.

■ dry eschar wounds — Protection by covering should be applied until the eschar dries and separates. Occasionally, painting the eschar with povidone-iodine (Betadine) is beneficial to maintain sterility while eschar separation occurs.

In addition, platelet-derived growth factors (PDGF) can be topically applied and have a modestly beneficial effect in promoting wound healing. Becaplermin gel 0.01% (Regranex), a recombinant human PDGF that's produced through genetic engineering, is approved by the U.S. Food and Drug Administration to promote healing of foot ulcers in patients with diabetes. Regranex is meant for a healthy, granulating wound, not one with a necrotic wound base.

Last, collagen comprises a significant fraction of the necrotic soft tissues in chronic wounds. In such cases, enzymatic debridement may be used. The enzyme collagenase, derived from fermentation of *Clostridium histolyticum*, helps remove nonviable tissue from the surface of wounds. However, it isn't a substitute for an initial surgical excision of a grossly necrotic wound.

---

blood glucose levels can dehydrate the skin. Because of the neuropathy, the nerves can't control the moisture and the oil and the feet can become externally dry, leading to peeling, cracking, and fissures. As a result, the patient's feet are at greater risk for becoming infected. Patient education is extremely important in maintaining the integrity of the feet and preventing ulcers. (See *Guidelines for foot care*, page 170.)

Prevention

The patient with diabetes should receive an annual foot examination to identify problem areas, with scheduled follow-up evaluations (as appropriate). He should be instructed to visually inspect his feet every day and institute appropriate skin care measures.

DIABETIC NEPHROPATHY

Diabetic nephropathy occurs in just under one-half of all patients with diabetes, with increased prevalence in Native Americans, Hispanics, and Blacks. About 20% to 30% of patients with type 1 or type 2 diabetes develop diabetic nephropathy, the leading cause of end-stage renal disease (ESRD) in the United States and Europe. Diabetic nephropathy accounts for approximately 40% of new cases of ESRD. According to the National Institute of Diabetes & Digestive & Kidney Diseases, approximately 36% of patients who have diabetes mellitus require dialysis or kidney transplantation. Microalbuminuria has been identified as the earliest stage of diabetic nephropathy in patients with type 1 diabetes; it's also used as a marker for the development of nephropathy in patients with type 2 diabetes. Progression

Patient-teaching tip

GUIDELINES FOR FOOT CARE

The patient with diabetic neuropathy is at risk for problems involving his feet. Therefore, he needs education and instruction about daily foot care, including these guidelines:

- Maintain management of diabetes — Monitor blood glucose levels daily and keep them in the target range.
- Inspect the feet daily — Check for red spots, cuts, and blisters or puncture wounds. If you can't see the bottom of the foot, use a mirror to inspect them or have a family member do it.
- Wash the feet every day — Use lukewarm water (optimal temperature is 95°F [35°C]), and dry them thoroughly, especially between the toes.
- Use moisturizing lotion — After bathing, apply a moisturizing lotion to the feet. Avoid putting lotion between the toes.
- Wear socks at all times — Never go barefoot, and wear clean socks to avoid blisters and keep your feet warm. Don't wear socks or knee-high stockings that are too tight below your knee; they should be soft and able to absorb moisture and not have thick seams, creases, or holes that can irritate the skin. Don't allow your feet to get sunburned.
- Wear shoes at all times — Leather or canvas shoes are preferable; don't wear sandals, open-toed shoes, or straps between the toes. Always inspect the inside of the shoes for tears or cracks in the lining before inserting your feet. Check the shoes for nails or pebbles. Break in new shoes gradually. Make sure that there's plenty of room for your toes. Buy shoes in the middle of the day when your feet are normally larger.
- Trim your toenails — If you can clearly see your toenails, trim them straight across with a nail clipper. Smooth the edges with an emery board or a nail file. Never use a razor blade. See your physician or podiatrist if you can't reach your feet, if the toenails are very thick or ingrown, if the toes overlap, or if you have poor circulation.
- Watch water temperature — Always check your bath water with an elbow before stepping in. Never use hot water bottles, heating pads, or electric blankets to warm your feet. Because of decreased sensation, you may not feel your feet burning.
- Keep the blood flowing — Don't cross your legs at the knees or ankles. When sitting down, put your feet up whenever possible. Move your ankles up and down and wiggle your toes two to three times per day for 5 minutes. If you smoke, stop; if you don't smoke, don't start.

of microalbuminuria to macroalbuminuria suggests ultimate progression to ESRD. (See *Progression of end-stage renal disease in diabetes.*)

Causes
The severity of the nephropathy depends upon the comorbidities of the patient, such as atherosclerosis, hypertension, and neuropathy. Hyperglycemia is an important risk factor for persistent proteinuria.

Diagnosis
Patients with type 2 diabetes may have microalbuminuria or proteinuria upon diagnosis because they may have had the disease for years but it went unrecognized. Screening for patients with type 1 diabetes should begin 5 years after diagnosis.

Early in diabetic nephropathy, before other symptoms are present, the kidneys are still able to filter waste and function normally. The only sign of kidney disease may be a slight increase in protein and albumin (which is responsi-

PROGRESSION OF END-STAGE RENAL DISEASE IN DIABETES

This chart depicts the number of patients with type 1 and type 2 diabetes who develop end-stage renal disease.

PREVALENCE OF TYPE 1 AND TYPE 2 DIABETES IN THE UNITED STATES AND PROGRESSION OF MICROALBUMINURIA AND DIABETIC NEPHROPATHY

	TYPE 1 DIABETES	TYPE 2 DIABETES
Prevalence of disease*	0.85 to 1.7 million	15.3 to 16.2 million (estimated 5.9 million undiagnosed)
Prevalence of microalbuminuria at 15 years†	21%	28%
Prevalence of macroalbuminuria at 15 years†	21%	14%‡
Progression to end-stage renal disease 10 years after onset of macroalbuminuria†	50%	10%‡

*Data from www.diabetes.org/main/info/facts/facts.jsp (Accessed June 2003.)
†Data from www.niddk.nih.gov/health/diabetes/diq/ (Accessed June 2003.)
‡Higher prevalence and progression in certain racial subgroups, such as African Americans and Pima Indians.

ble for controlling fluid balance in the body) in urine. However, as diabetic nephropathy progresses, the kidney becomes hypertrophied, the glomerular basement membrane thickens, and glomerulosclerosis, known as *Kimmelstiel-Wilson syndrome*, takes place. As the kidney becomes less adept at filtering wastes, more protein from the blood spills into the urine.

Screening for microalbuminuria may be performed using a random urine collection, in the practitioner's office, to measure albumin-to-creatinine ratio; a 24-hour creatinine clearance urine collection; or a timed urine collection, such as for 4 hours or overnight. Microalbuminuria is present if urinary albumin excretion is greater than or equal to 30 mg in 24 hours.

Urinary albumin excretion is highly variable. For example, exercise within 24 hours, infection, fever, heart failure, marked hyperglycemia, marked hyper-

tension, pyuria, and hematuria may elevate urinary albumin excretion over baseline values. Therefore, the patient must provide 3 specimens over a 3- to 6-month period; of those three specimens, two would need to be abnormal before establishing a diagnosis.

The assessment findings provide clues to the stage of the patient's renal disease:

● Stage I — At the time diabetes is diagnosed. Kidney size and the glomerular filtration rate (GFR) are increased. Blood glucose control can reverse the changes.

● Stage II — Two to 3 years after diagnosis. Glomerular basement membrane thickens and the decline in renal function is initiated. The GFR is elevated and scar formation occurs, known as *glomerulosclerosis.*

● Stage III — Seven to 15 years after diagnosis. Microalbuminuria first appears. Glomerular damage has pro-

gressed and hypertension may be present. Patients are asymptomatic.
- Stage IV — Overt, or dipstick-positive, diabetes. The GFR is decreased. Almost all patients have hypertension. There's suboptimal glucose control.
- Stage V — ESRD; the GFR has fallen to 10 ml/minute. Renal replacement therapy is needed.

In addition, serum creatinine level may be obtained, which is an indirect measurement of the GFR. The normal value is 0.8 to 1.3 mg/dl, and a change in this value may indicate major functional loss.

Management
Strict glycemic control, through intensive diabetes therapy, is essential in the treatment of diabetic nephropathy. The Diabetes Control and Complications Trial and the United Kingdom Prospective Diabetes Study demonstrated that maintaining strict blood glucose control with intensive insulin and nutritional therapy as well as implementing lifestyle changes (smoking cessation) reduces the onset of microalbuminuria and overt nephropathy in patients with type 1 and type 2 diabetes.

Medication therapy
Aggressive antihypertensive medication should be initiated because it may slow the decline of the GFR. ACE inhibitors, such as enalapril (Vasotec) or captopril (Capoten), are the first-line drugs of choice for all patients with diabetic nephropathy, unless contraindicated. If the adverse effects aren't tolerated, an angiotensin II receptor blocker, such as losartan (Cozaar) or valsartan (Diovan), may offer comparable protection. The primary goal of antihypertensive drugs is to decrease the blood pressure to and maintain it at less than 130 mm Hg systolic and 80 mm Hg diastolic. A patient with diabetes who's in the later stages of diabetic nephropathy may require insulin adjustment because the kidneys lose their insulin-degradative function.

Dietary measures
Nutritional therapy and exercise, limitations in total saturated fats, reduced cholesterol levels along with statin therapy, and good glycemic control are important components in educating the patient with diabetes about diabetic nephropathy. In addition, studies have shown that a protein-restricted diet (0.6 g/kg body weight/day) modestly slows down the GFR.

ESRD treatment options
The patient with diabetic nephropathy who progresses to stage V, ESRD, has the following options:
- hemodialysis — removes the blood's waste products through filtration outside of the body
- peritoneal dialysis — filters through the membrane lining the abdominal cavity; fluid is instilled into the peritoneal space and then drained
- kidney transplantation.

Prevention
Prevention of diabetic nephropathy focuses on optimizing glucose levels and blood pressure control. Annual screening for microalbuminuria is recommended for patients with type 1 diabetes who have had the disease for 5 years or more; patients with type 2 diabetes, beginning at the time of diagnosis; and patients with pregnancy-induced diabetes.

DIABETIC RETINOPATHY
Diabetic retinopathy is the major cause of blindness in the United States among adults ages 20 to 74, and it's directly linked with how *long* the patient has had diabetes, with severity strongly associated with poor glycemic control.

The primary problems associated with diabetic retinopathy are microvascular damage and occlusion of the small blood vessels of the retina — the light-sensitive tissue at the back of the eye. Diabetic retinopathy commonly accompanies diabetic nephropathy, and

PROGRESSION OF DIABETIC RETINOPATHY

This flowchart shows the pathophysiologic events associated with diabetes that cause changes in the eye, ultimately leading to proliferative diabetic retinopathy.

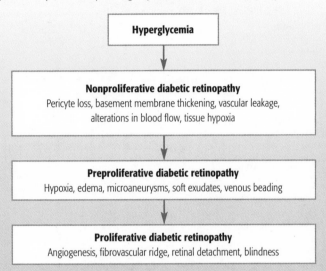

Hyperglycemia

↓

Nonproliferative diabetic retinopathy
Pericyte loss, basement membrane thickening, vascular leakage, alterations in blood flow, tissue hypoxia

↓

Preproliferative diabetic retinopathy
Hypoxia, edema, microaneurysms, soft exudates, venous beading

↓

Proliferative diabetic retinopathy
Angiogenesis, fibrovascular ridge, retinal detachment, blindness

patients with type 1 and type 2 diabetes are at equal risk.

Diabetic retinopathy usually progresses from nonproliferative or background retinopathy to proliferative retinopathy. (See *Progression of diabetic retinopathy.*)

Nonproliferative retinopathy is characterized by increased vascular permeability. Blood vessels within the retina develop microaneurysms that leak fluid, causing macular edema and the formation of exudates. Proliferative diabetic retinopathy is characterized by abnormal growth of new blood vessels on the retina. These new vessels rupture and bleed into the vitreous humor, which prevents light from reaching the retina. These blood vessels form scar tissue, which can exert a pull on and detach the retina.

Risk factors

Risk factors for developing diabetic retinopathy include fluctuating glucose levels, nephropathy, and high blood pressure. Some research also suggests that pregnancy in patients with type 1 diabetes may aggravate retinopathy for a short period.

Diagnosis

Patients with type 1 diabetes should have a comprehensive eye examination with dilation within 3 to 5 years of the diagnosis of diabetes. Patients with type 2 diabetes should have the same type of examination shortly after being diagnosed. A comprehensive eye examination by an ophthalmologist or optometrist, including a dilated eye examination, reveals exudates and macular edema. The patient might complain of blurred vision. If proliferative retinopa-

VISUALIZING LASER THERAPY

With laser therapy, the laser beam is directed to the affected area. Here, the beam helps to seal microaneurysms and decrease bleeding, thereby reducing edema.

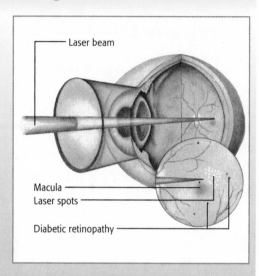

Laser beam

Macula
Laser spots

Diabetic retinopathy

thy is present, the eye examination reveals new blood vessels on the retina that bleed. The patient also might complain of seeing black or red spots or lines.

Management

For the patient with diabetic retinopathy, management focuses on glycemic control, blood pressure regulation with medication therapy, and possible laser therapy.

The Diabetes Control and Complication Trial and the United Kingdom Prospective Diabetes Study demonstrated that improved blood glucose control reduced or delayed the risk of developing diabetic retinopathy.

Medication therapy

Data suggest that ACE inhibitors lower blood pressure and may be effective in slowing the progression of the retinopathy.

Laser therapy

Laser therapy can seal microaneurysms and decrease bleeding. (See *Visualizing laser therapy*.) Scattering of laser burns across the retina (called *panretinal photocoagulation*) significantly reduces (not restores) vision loss and also reduces the risk for *further* vision loss. Laser burns appear to be more effective in patients' whose eyes demonstrate high-risk characteristics such as vitreous hemorrhage.

Prevention

Patients with diabetes should be identified early and routinely to detect diabetic retinopathy. Patients with type 1 diabetes should have a comprehensive eye examination within 5 years of diagnosis. Those with type 2 diabetes should have similar eye examinations soon after they're diagnosed. Follow-up examinations should be done annually. In addition, measures to optimize glucose control and blood pressure can reduce the risk and progression of diabetic retinopathy.

URINARY TRACT INFECTIONS

Patients with diabetes are at increased risk for chronic infections, specifically frequent urinary tract infections (UTIs), which are the most common type of infection in patients with diabetes. Most UTIs in patients with diabetes are asymptomatic and are caused by bacteria that can also live in the digestive tract, in the vagina, or around the urethra. One factor that predisposes patients to reinfection is incomplete urinary voiding. It's more common in women because of the short urethra, which is easily accessible to organisms from the vagina and rectum. UTIs can lead to severe kidney disease, thus causing renal failure.

Causes

Causes of UTI in patients with diabetes are the same as those for any patient and include bacteria, such as *Escherichia coli*, *Proteus vulgaris*, and streptococcus, and fungal infection caused by *Candida albicans*. In addition, high glucose concentrations in urine provide an optimal medium for bacterial growth.

Diagnosis

A urine culture and sensitivity reveals the offending organism. In addition, the patient may report frequency, urgency, burning or pain, lower abdominal discomfort, nocturia, low-grade fever, and flank or suprapubic tenderness. The patient's urine may appear dark and have a strong odor.

Management

Management focuses on antimicrobial therapy specific to the causative organism. In addition, strict glucose control must be maintained. Urinary antiseptics such as phenazopyridine (Pyridium), and nonopioid analgesics may be helpful.

Prevention

Optimal glucose control is essential in preventing UTIs. Patients must be educated about the signs and symptoms of UTIs and to seek treatment immediately if urgency, burning, dysuria, or other signs of cystitis or UTI occur. Female patients should be taught the importance of voiding after sexual intercourse and the need to consume water throughout the day. Cranberry juice may also be recommended because it acidifies urine; it's also been shown to reduce the incidence of UTIs in older women. Patients with diabetes who get UTIs should also be instructed to avoid taking nephrotoxic drugs, including aminoglycosides such as gentamicin (Garamycin).

YEAST INFECTIONS

Women with diabetes tend to develop recurring yeast infections when they have poor control of the disease. When blood glucose levels aren't under control, the resulting high glucose environment allows yeast to proliferate in vaginal secretions.

Susceptibility to yeast infections and vaginitis may also increase when women with type 2 diabetes enter menopause. Menopause slows estrogen production, decreasing the amount of nourishment supporting the vaginal lining. This makes it easier for yeast and bacteria to grow.

The American Diabetes Association's *Complete Guide to Diabetes* provides the following precautions for menopausal women to help prevent yeast infections:
- keep blood glucose levels under control
- bathe regularly to keep fecal bacteria from entering the vagina
- consider hormone replacement therapy.

Some health care practitioners also recommend eating low-fat yogurt with active cultures on a daily basis to help battle yeast in the digestive tract.

Causes

Yeast infections are typically caused by *Candida albicans*.

Diagnosis

Culture or gram stain of vaginal secretions reveals evidence of the offending organism and infection. In addition, the patient may report itching, burning, and a vaginal discharge with a curdlike cheesy consistency.

Management

Treatment focuses on antifungal therapy to eradicate the causative organism. Treatment may be topical or systemic. In addition, comfort measures are used to relieve itching and burning. Perineal care is essential.

Prevention

Optimal glucose control is essential in preventing yeast infections. Patients must be educated about the signs and symptoms of yeast infections and to seek treatment immediately if itching, burning, or discharge occur. Female patients should be taught proper perineal care measures.

DEPRESSION

Although depression isn't considered prevalent in people with diabetes, studies show that they have a higher *risk* of developing depression than those who don't have diabetes. Treatment of depression helps the patient manage the symptoms of both diseases. If the patient with diabetes develops complications, such as neuropathy, or can't maintain good glycemic control, he may become depressed, possibly feeling a lack of control over the disorder. Studies suggest that people with diabetes who have a history of depression are more likely to develop diabetic complications than those without depression.

Depression can interfere with good diabetes self-care. For example, the patient may not monitor his blood glucose levels as required. Also, he may not follow the diet regimen that the practitioner and the nutritionist prescribed. Sometimes the patient, family, and friends don't recognize the symptoms of depression and the patient goes untreated for a long period. Episodes of depression can be triggered by stress, difficult life events, adverse effects of medications, or other factors.

Causes

The cause of depression in the patient with diabetes can be due to several factors. He may feel helpless or hopeless about dealing with a chronic disease. In addition, he may be experiencing difficulty in achieving optimal glucose control despite compliance with therapy. In addition, even with tight glucose control, there's no guarantee that the patient won't develop complications. Physiologically, metabolic changes, such as severe hypoglycemic episodes, can affect brain chemistry (including neurohormonal levels), possibly leading to depression.

Diagnosis

The patient with diabetes exhibits signs and symptoms of depression just as another patient would. He may report feelings of sadness, difficulty sleeping, changes in appetite, or difficulty concentrating or making decisions. The patient may exhibit low self-esteem, easy distractibility, and poor coping. Typically, psychological testing is done to determine if the patient is experiencing major depression.

Management

Psychotherapy, or "talk" therapy, and antidepressants are two types of treatment. Short- or long-term psychotherapy with a well-trained therapist can help the patient find ways to relieve and cope with depression.

Medication therapy

Prescription antidepressants are generally well tolerated and safe for the patient with diabetes. Antidepressants can take several weeks to work and can be combined with psychotherapy. It's important for the patient to know that antidepressants can take time to become effective. In addition, he needs to know the adverse effects of the drugs and how blood glucose levels may be affected. Scientists report that psychotherapy and antidepressants have positive effects on mood and glycemic control. Ideally, the mental health professional will be part of the management team and will be in close communication with the health care practitioner providing the care for the patient with diabetes.

Selective serotonin reuptake inhibitors, such as fluoxetine (Prozac) and sertraline (Zoloft), have fewer adverse effects and are used as first-line drug therapy. In 2004, duloxetine (Cymbalta) was approved for depression and diabetic peripheral neuropathy. When prescribed, the patient needs close follow-up for diabetes and depression.

Prevention

Prevention of depression focuses on close monitoring of the patient, his glucose control, and his ability to adjust to this chronic condition. Ensuring optimum support in all areas may help to promote positive coping skills.

Selected references

"Adherence to Statin Therapy and LDL Cholesterol Goal Attainment by Patients With Diabetes and Dyslipidemia." Available at: *http://care.diabetes journals.org/cgi/content/full/28/3/595? maxtoshow=&HITS=10&hits=10&RE-SULTFORMAT=&fulltext=dyslipi-demia&searchid=1131045237012_802 4&stored_search=&FIRSTINDEX= 0&sortspec=relevance&journalcode=di-acare.* Accessed December 22, 2005.

"The Aetiology of Diabetic Neuropathy: The Combined Roles of Metabolic and Vascular Defects" [Online]. Available at: *www.ncbi.nlm.nih.gov/entrez/ query.fcgi?cmd=Retrieve&db=PubMed &list_uids=7554777&dopt=Abstract.*

"The ALLHAT Study" [Online]. Available at: *www.clinical.diabetesjournals.org/ cgi/content/full/21/3/102.*

American Diabetes Association Position Statement. "Hyperglycemic Crisis in Patients with Diabetes Mellitus," *Diabetes Care* 26(Suppl 1):S112, January

2003. Available at: *www.care.diabetes journals.org/cgi/content/full/26/suppl_ 1/s109.*

American Diabetes Association Reviews Diabetic Neuropathies. *www.medscape. com/viewarticle/502295.*

Clinical Management of Diabetic Retinopathy (DR). *www.medscape. com/viewarticle/506671_6.*

"Controlling Hypertension in Patients with Diabetes" [Online]. Available at: *www.aafp.org/afp/20021001/1209.html.*

"Defining and Reporting Hypoglycemia in Diabetes" [Online]. Available at: *www.care.diabetesjournals.org/cgi/con-tent/full/28/5/1245?maxtoshow=&HIT S=10&hits=10&RESULTFORMAT= &fulltext=hypoglycemia&andorexact-fulltext=and&searchid=113070850668 9_5880&stored_search=&FIRSTIN-DEX=0&sortspec=relevance&resource-type=1&journalcode=diacare.*

"Depression" [Online]. Available at: *www.diabetes.org/type-2-diabetes/ depression.jsp.*

"Detection, Prevention, and Treatment of Hypoglycemia in the Hospital" [Online]. Available at: *www.spectrum. diabetesjournals.org/cgi/content/full/18/ 1/39#FIG1.*

"Diabetes, Depression and Stress" [Online]. Available at: *www.ncpamd.com/ dmdepression.htm.*

"Diabetic Dyslipidemia" [Online]. Available at: *www.diabetes.org/uedocuments/ ADACardioReview3.pdf.*

"Diabetic Foot Ulcerations" [Online]. Available at: *www.medscape.com/ viewarticle/456305_7.*

"Diabetic Foot Ulcers: Prevention, Diagnosis and Classification" [Online]. Available at: *www.aafp.org/afp/ 980315ap/armstron.html.*

"Diabetic Ketoacidosis" [Online]. Available at: *www.healthopedia.com/diabet-ic-ketoacidosis/.*

"Diabetic Nephropathy" [Online]. Available at: *www.care.diabetesjournals.org/ cgi/content/full/25/suppl_1/s85 www.care.diabetesjournals.org/cgi/con-tent/full/26/suppl_1/s94.*

"Diabetic Neuropathies" [Online]. Available at: *www.care.diabetesjournals.org/ cgi/content/full/28/4/956.*

"Diabetic Neuropathies: Current Treatment Strategies" [Online]. Available at: *www.medscape.com/viewarticle/496605_8*.

"Diabetic Neuropathies: The Nerve Damage of Diabetes" [Online]. Available at: *www.diabetes.niddk.nih.gov/dm/pubs/neuropathies*.

"Diabetic Retinopathy" [Online]. Available at: *www.ncbi.nlm.nih.gov/entrez/query.fcgi?cmd=Retrieve&db=pubmed &dopt=Abstract&list_uids=16184249 &itool=iconfft&query_hl=12*; *www.care.diabetesjournals.org/cgi/content/full/25/suppl_1/s90*; *www.care.diabetesjournals.org/cgi/content/full/26/suppl_1/s99*.

"Diabetic Retinopathy: What You Should Know" [Online]. Available at: *www.nei.nih.gov/health/diabetic/retinopathy.asp*.

"Diabetic Ulcers" [Online]. Available at: *www.emedicine.com/med/topic551.htm*.

"Don't Forget the Five C's of Foot Care" [Online]. Available at: *www.amlab.com/education/foot_care.asp*.

Grundy, S.M, et. al. "NHLBI/AHA Conference Proceedings Definition of Metabolic Syndrome," *Circulation* 109:433-438, January 2004. Available at: *www.circ.ahajournals.org/cgi/content/full/109/3/433*.

"High Blood Cholesterol: What You Need To Know" [Online]. Available at: *www.nhlbi.nih.gov/health/public/heart/chol/wyntk.htm*.

"High Blood Pressure" [Online]. Available at: *www.emedicinehealth.com/articles/11073-1.asp*.

"Hyperglycemic Crises in Diabetes" [Online]. Available at: *www.care.diabetes journals.org/cgi/content/full/27/suppl_1/s94*.

"Hyperglycemic Crises in Patients With Diabetes Mellitus" [Online]. Available at: *www.care.diabetesjournals.org/cgi/content/full/26/suppl_1/s109*.

"Hyperosmolar Hyperglycemic State" [Online]. Available at: *www.aafp.org/afp/20050501/1723.html*.

"Hypertension in Diabetes" [Online]. Available at: *www.diabetes.org/uedocuments/ADACardioReview_2.pdf*.

"Hypoglycemia" [Online]. Available at: *www.diabetes.niddk.nih.gov/dm/pubs/hypoglycemia/index.htm*.

Kahn, C.R., et. al. *Joslin's Diabetes Mellitus*, 14th ed. Philadelphia: Lippincott Williams and Wilkins, 2005.

Ignatavicius, D.D., and Workman, M.L. *Medical-Surgical Nursing, Critical Thinking for Collaborative Care*, 5th ed. Philadelphia: W.B. Saunders Co., 2006.

"Lipids and Lipoproteins in Patients with Type 2 Diabetes" [Online]. Available at: *www.care.diabetesjournals.org/cgi/content/full/27/6/1496?maxtoshow= &HITS=10&hits=10&RESULTFOR-MAT=&fulltext=dyslipidemia&searchi d=1131045379275_8060&stored_searc h=&FIRSTINDEX=0&sortspec=rele-vance&journalcode=diacare*.

"Management of Diabetes in the Elderly" [Online]. Available at: *www.journal.diabetes.org/clinicaldiabetes/v17n11999/Pg19.htm*.

"Management of Hyperglycemic Crises in Patients with Diabetes" [Online]. Available at: *www.medscape.com/viewarticle/421556*.

"Management of the Diabetic Foot: Preventing Amputation" [Online]. Available at: *www.medscape.com/viewarticle/426899*.

"Management of Type 2 Diabetes Mellitus" [Online]. Available at: *www.guide-line.gov/summary/summary.aspx?doc_i d=6147&nbr=003975&string=man-agement+AND+diabetes+AND+com-plications*.

"National Diabetes Statistics" [Online]. Available at: *www.diabetes.niddk.nih gov/dm/pubs/statistics/index.htm#7*.

"National Diabetes Surveillance System" [Online]. Available at: *www.cdc.gov/diabetes/statistics/index.htm*.

"Nephropathy in Diabetes" [Online]. Available at: *www.care.diabetesjournals.org/cgi/content/full/27/suppl_1/s79*.

"Nutrition Principles and Recommendations in Diabetes" [Online]. Available at: *www.care.diabetesjournals.org/cgi/content/full/27/suppl_1/s36*.

"Prevent Diabetes Problems: Keep Your Heart and Blood Vessels Healthy" [Online]. Available at: *www.diabetes.niddk.nih.gov/dm/pubs/complications_heart/index.htm*.

"The Prevention and Treatment of Complications of Diabetes Mellitus: A Guide for Primary Care Practitioners" [Online]. Available at: *www.aepo-xdv-www.epo.cdc.gov/wonder/prevguid/p000 0063/p0000063.asp#head0040010050 00000.*

"Preventive Foot Care in Diabetes" [Online]. Available at: *www.care.diabetes journals.org/cgi/content/full/27/suppl_1/s63.*

"Retinopathy in Diabetes" [Online]. Available at: *www.care.diabetesjournals. org/cgi/content/full/27/suppl_1/s84.*

Shah, M., et al. "Effect of a High Carbohydrate versus a High cis-Monosaturaed Fat Diet on Blood Pressue in Patients with Type 2 Diabetes" *Diabetes Care* 28(111):2607-12, November 28, 2005.

"Standards of Medical Care in Diabetes" [Online]. Available at: *http://care.diabetesjournals.org/cgi/content/full/28/su ppl_1/s4?maxtoshow=&HITS=10&hits =10&RESULTFORMAT=&fulltext=d yslipidemia&searchid=1131045521435 _8091&stored_search=&FIRSTIN- DEX=0&sortspec=relevance&journal-code=diacare.*

"Summary of Implications of Recent Clinical Trials for ATP III Treatment Algorithm" [Online]. Available at: *www.guideline.gov/summary/summa- ry.aspx?doc_id=5503&nbr=003746&st ring=hyperlipidemia+AND+guide- lines.*

"Treatment of Depression in Patients with Diabetes Mellitus" [Online]. Available at: *www.ncbi.nlm.nih.gov/entrez/query. fcgi?cmd=Retrieve&db=PubMed&list_ uids=7713850&dopt=Citation.*

"The Treatment of Hypertension in Adult Patients With Diabetes" [Online]. Available at: *www.medscape.com/ viewarticle/424458.*

"Treatment of Hypertension in Adults with Diabetes" [Online]. Available at: *www.care.diabetesjournals.org/cgi/ content/full/26/suppl_1/s80.*

"Type 2 Diabetes Mellitus Complications" [Online]. Available at: *www.medscape.com/viewarticle/ 442883_7.*

"Vascular Complications of Diabetes" [Online]. Available at: *www.bmj.bmj journals.com/cgi/content/full/320/7241/ 1062.*

"WOCN's Evidence-Based Pressure Ulcer Guideline" [Online]. Available at: *www.nursingcenter.com/prodev/ce_arti- cle.asp?tid=587527.*

"You're Not Alone — Women, Diabetes and Sexual Health" [Online]. Available at: *www.diabeteshealth.com/ read,3,1064.htm.*

"Your Guide to Lowering High Blood Pressure" [Online]. Available at: *www.nhlbi.nih.gov/hbp/treat/bpd_type. htm.*

Management of special populations and situations

Even under ideal conditions, maintaining blood glucose levels is challenging. However, for certain populations, such as pregnant women, children, and elderly patients, managing diabetes presents some additional challenges. Moreover, certain situations, such as labor and delivery and hospitalization, further impact diabetes control.

PREGNANCY AND DIABETES

When type 1 diabetes is identified for the first time during pregnancy, it's called *gestational diabetes mellitus* (GDM). It's defined as a carbohydrate intolerance of varying degrees of severity with the onset or first recognition during pregnancy.

Type 1 diabetes and GDM can lead to pregnancy complications for the woman and her fetus, especially if glucose levels aren't well controlled. These patients are at greater risk for cesarean deliveries and chronic hypertension. The fetus or neonate is at risk for macrosomia, hypoglycemia, hypocalcemia, and hyperbilirubinemia.

Incidence and risk

GDM affects approximately 4% of all pregnancies in the United States, but this rate may range from 1% to 14% based on the population and the diagnostic measures used. The general consensus is that GDM is increasing world-

wide. However, specific statistics are unavailable because of the lack of uniform standards for detection and diagnosis.

These incidence rates include women who may have previously undiagnosed type 2 diabetes. Type 1 diabetes occurs in 5% to 10% of the general population and is commonly identified by the presence of anti-insulin antibodies, islet cell antibodies, or the presence of the antigen glutamic acid decarboxylase. The same percentage can be found among women with GDM. It's believed that these women have evolving type 1 diabetes, but haven't yet experienced overt signs or symptoms, and are diagnosed through prenatal screening for GDM. In a study done between 1994 and 2002, a 12% increase in GDM was reported in a multiethnic population of women connected with Kaiser Permanente of Colorado. It's estimated that by 2025, the total number of pregnancies complicated by GDM will increase by 120%.

Similar to type 2 diabetes, GDM is a result of the body's increased resistance to insulin. As such, many of the risk factors for GDM are the same as for type 2 diabetes. However, as many as 35% to 50% of all women who develop GDM have no risk factors. (See *Risk factors for GDM*.)

RISK FACTORS FOR GDM

Risk factors for gestational diabetes mellitus (GDM), which are similar to those for type 2 diabetes, include:

- age 25 or older
- body mass index (BMI) greater than 27
- ethnicity (Hispanic, Native American, African American, South or East Asian, and Pacific Island populations)
- family history of diabetes, primarily a first-degree relative
- glycosuria
- history of a previous delivery birth weight of greater than 4,000 g (9 lb)
- multiparity
- previous child born with birth defects
- previous history of GDM
- previous polyhydramnios
- previous stillbirth.

Physiologic effects on blood glucose control

To understand the role of insulin resistance in pregnancy, it's necessary to grasp the normal physiologic changes associated with gestation in the nondiabetic patient. The fetus relies completely on an uninterrupted fuel supply from the mother to grow and develop properly. (See *Fuel metabolism during pregnancy*, page 182.) Therefore, the glycemic state of the mother directly impacts the growth of the fetus.

As pregnancy progresses, the woman begins to experience increased storage of glycogen in the tissues, increased peripheral glucose utilization, and an increase in hepatoneogenesis (new glucose production by the liver). The increased glucose circulation produces an increased insulin response, causing the beta cells of the pancreas to hypertrophy.

Glucose is transported to the fetus across the placenta and provides a steady influx of fuel. Conversely, the woman experiences a decrease in the gluconeogenic amino acid alanine, which leads to a lower fasting blood glucose level. In a pregnancy uncomplicated by diabetes, the fasting glucose level

may decrease as much as 20%, with a mean fasting blood glucose level as low as 56 mg/dl during 28 to 38 weeks' gestation.

In combination, the increased glycogen storage, the increased usage of glucose peripherally, the increased insulin production, and the decreased maternal alanine levels all lead to an increased hypoglycemic state. The American Association of Diabetes Educators reports, "The early months of a nondiabetic pregnancy can be described as a period of maternal anabolism during which maternal fat storage takes place."

In the second trimester, the need for insulin further increases due to the production of hormones that work against its ability to lower blood glucose levels. Human placental lactogen, prolactin, estrogen, and free and bound cortisol block insulin receptors, leading to an increased insulin-resistant state. An increased metabolism of fat (whenever a fasting state occurs) leads to increased concentrations of free fatty acids and plasma and urinary ketones. An extended fast, such as more than 4 hours, can lead to severe hypoglycemia.

In contrast, the postprandial blood glucose level is higher and remains

FUEL METABOLISM DURING PREGNANCY

The fetus relies completely on the mother for its fuel supply to ensure adequate growth and development. This chart summarizes the changes occurring in the mother during the first and second trimesters to provide adequate fuel to the fetus.

EARLY GESTATIONAL FUEL METABOLISM	LATE GESTATIONAL FUEL METABOLISM
■ ↑ Tissue glycogen storage	■ ↑ Diabetogenic hormones (human placental lactogen, estrogen, progesterone, free and bound cortisol)
■ ↑ Peripheral glucose utilization	■ Impaired peripheral insulin sensitivity
■ ↑ Insulin response to glucose secondary to pancreatic cell hypertrophy	■ ↑ Need for insulin levels (two- to threefold increase)
■ ↑ Production of free fatty acids (FFAs) and ketones	■ ↑ Fat metabolism → fasting ketosis ■ ↑ FFAs and ketones
■ ↓ Maternal alanine → lower fasting blood glucose (FBG), ↑ hypoglycemia	■ ↓ FBG and mean glucose levels ■ ↑ Postprandial levels
■ ↑ Hepatic glucose production	

higher longer to promote further fuel delivery to the fetus. It isn't unusual for the maternal basilar insulin requirement to double or even triple by the end of the pregnancy, even in a nondiabetic patient.

As insulin is released in response to glucose level, hunger results from the increased circulating insulin level. When an increased level (an anabolic steroid) is present, the body increases its fuel intake. Coupled with an increased blood glucose level resulting from insulin resistance, the body is further stimulated to feel hunger. While there's more than an adequate supply of glucose in the blood, the use of that supply is limited by the inability of the cells to access it for energy. Glucose toxicity leads to further hepatoneogenesis, further complicating hyperglycemia.

Screening for gestational diabetes

All pregnant women should be screened for glucose intolerance based on the recommendation of the Second and Third International Workshop-Conferences on GDM. The American Diabetes Association (ADA), in a position statement on the detection and diagnosis of gestational diabetes, recommends that a risk assessment be done at the first prenatal visit, and those at high risk for GDM should be screened as soon as possible. (See *Risk assessment for GDM.*)

As mentioned earlier, a percentage of women may have preexisting diabetes that's been undiagnosed and — with the additional insulin resistance brought on by pregnancy — may exhibit hyperglycemia early.

RISK ASSESSMENT FOR GDM

This chart identifies possible factors and their associated risk for developing gestational diabetes mellitus (GDM).

FACTOR	LOW RISK	AVERAGE RISK	HIGH RISK
Age	< 25	≥ 25	≥ 25
Ethnicity	Caucasian	Hispanic, African American, Native American, Asian, Pacific Islander	Hispanic, African American, Native American, Asian, Pacific Islander
Body mass index	< 25	25 to 27	> 27
Family history of diabetes	Negative	Negative	First-degree relative
History of impaired glucose tolerance	Negative	Negative	Previous GDM, impaired fasting glucose, impaired glucose tolerance, glycosuria, or diabetic symptoms
History of poor obstetric outcomes	Negative	Negative	Previous stillbirth, macrosomia, birth defect, or polyhydramnios

ALERT *The first trimester is the most critical time for the fetus because all of its organs are developing. As such, the earlier diabetes is detected, the healthier the environment for the fetus.*

General screening recommendations
In the initial risk assessment, if the woman is considered to be at low risk, routine screening isn't necessary. Women considered at low risk for GDM:
● are younger than age 25
● have a normal body mass index (BMI) before pregnancy (before age 25)
● have no first-degree relative with diabetes
● are a member of an ethnic group with a low prevalence of GDM
● have no history of impaired glucose tolerance

● have no history of poor obstetric outcomes.

An average-risk patient should be tested for hyperglycemia at 24 to 28 weeks' gestation. If a woman is considered to be at high risk, an initial glucose screening should be done as soon as possible. If not diagnosed with GDM, additional screening should occur at 24 to 28 weeks' gestation.

Initial screening
Initial screening for GDM includes obtaining a fasting plasma glucose level or a casual plasma glucose level on two separate occasions. A fasting plasma glucose level greater than 126 mg/dl or a casual plasma glucose level greater than 200 mg/dl indicates GDM. According to the ADA, women meeting this criteria don't require additional testing or a glucose challenge. If the pregnant woman doesn't meet the guidelines for diagnosis of GDM based on

DIAGNOSIS OF GDM WITH 100-G OGTT

This chart indicates the plasma glucose levels that meet the criteria for diagnosing gestational diabetes mellitus (GDM) with the 100-g oral glucose tolerance test (OGTT). Keep in mind that the patient must have levels that meet or exceed the values listed for at least two of the time intervals to confirm the diagnosis of GDM.

TIME INTERVAL	PLASMA GLUCOSE LEVELS	
	mg/dl	mmol/L
Fasting	95	5.3
1 hour	180	10.0
2 hours	155	8.6
3 hours	140	7.8

the initial screening level, follow-up testing is necessary.

Follow-up testing

The ADA identifies two methods for follow-up testing. These methods are defined as a one-step and two-step approach.

The one-step approach involves performing a 100-g oral glucose tolerance test (OGTT) without previous plasma or serum glucose screening. This method may be less cost prohibitive in high-risk ethnic populations or high-risk patients, as defined earlier.

The two-step approach most commonly used in the United States involves a 50-g, 1-hour glucose challenge test (GCT). This is followed by a 100-g OGTT if the GCT value exceeds the threshold. The cut-off of greater than

140 mg/dl identifies 80% of women with GDM, while a level of 130 mg/dl identifies approximately 90%. Two or more readings obtained with the OGTT must meet or exceed the set values to diagnose GDM. (See *Diagnosis of GDM with 100-g OGTT.*)

In some cases, a 75-g OGTT may be used. However, this test isn't considered as reliable and valid in detecting at-risk mothers when compared to the 100-g OGTT.

Patient preparation. When preparing the patient for the OGTT, encourage her to fast for at least 8 hours but no longer than 14 hours because this could potentially lead to increased ketonuria. Also instruct her to consume at least 150 g of carbohydrates per day for 3 days before the test. In addition, advise her to continue her normal level of activity. Inform the patient that she will need to remain seated during testing and not be allowed to smoke.

Risks associated with gestational diabetes

Screening for and detection of GDM identifies pregnancies at increased risk for complications, perinatal morbidity, and mortality for the fetus and mother. Complications can be identified at any time in the pregnancy, but with GDM in particular, the most common problems occur during the last month of pregnancy, during delivery, or soon after.

Maternal risks

While much information centers around the effects of hyperglycemia on the fetus, concern should be raised for the mother as well. Because GDM is an insulin-resistant state, regular monitoring of the woman's blood pressure, weight, and urinary protein excretion is essential. Due to the pathogenesis of insulin resistance, the mother is more likely to retain fluid, thereby leading to an increased risk of hypertension.

Preeclampsia is a significant cause of maternal morbidity and may indicate the need to schedule an early delivery. In a recent study, it was found that women with GDM were more likely to experience medical complications, specifically preeclampsia, compared with nondiabetic pregnant women. Another study revealed that women with GDM were specifically 2.5 times more likely to have preeclampsia.

GDM also increases maternal risk for urinary tract infections (UTIs). Elevated glucose levels commonly increase the severity of UTIs making them more difficult to treat. UTIs can also cause premature labor.

Long-term maternal risks include developing type 2 diabetes after pregnancy and later in life. Consequently, educating the patient on how to prevent diabetes through risk modification, such as reducing weight and increasing activity, must be a primary focus of care after delivery. Recommendations include:
● OGTT repeated at 6 to 12 weeks postpartum to identify type 2 diabetes
● reassessment of glucose levels at least every 3 years if postpartum glucose levels are normal.

Studies about the development of type 2 diabetes after a previous diagnosis of GDM reveal that the incidence of developing type 2 diabetes ranges from 2.6% to 70%. The greatest risk occurs in the first 5 years after pregnancy, and plateaus after 10 years. Recent data show that an increased duration of lactation may help prevent the development of type 2 diabetes in young and middle-age women.

Fetal and neonatal risks
The most common fetal complication of GDM or preexisting diabetes is macrosomia — birth weight of more than 4,000 g (9 lb) or above the 90th percentile for gestational age on a standard growth chart. In the general population, only 10% of pregnancies are complicated by macrosomia, while 20%

to 32% of pregnancies among women with diabetes involve neonates with the disorder.

Macrosomia develops when an increased glucose level leads to an earlier development of the fetus' pancreatic cells. As the fetal glucose level increases, insulin is produced in excessive amounts, which causes growth of the fetal tissues, particularly the liver, cardiac tissue, muscle, and subcutaneous fat. The fetus not only receives larger amounts of glucose, but also amino acids and fatty acid fuels. This excess of nutrients stimulates fetal growth at an accelerated rate. As the chest-to-head and shoulder-to-head ratios increase, the risk of prolonged labor, shoulder dystocia, and birth trauma also increase. Subsequently, women with GDM are more likely to require a cesarean delivery.

Neonates with macrosomia and those who are large for gestational age (LGA) also experience an increased demand for oxygen. If demand exceeds supply, asphyxia may result. While it isn't known for sure, intrauterine hypoxia is a likely explanation for stillbirths in pregnancies affected by diabetes. However, stillbirth has decreased dramatically due to increased detection of GDM and monitoring throughout gestation. Respiratory distress syndrome, once commonly associated with diabetes during pregnancy, also is an infrequent complication because of increased monitoring and advances in obstetric care.

Hypoglycemia, however, remains common among neonates delivered by women with diabetes. With delivery, the direct, continuous glucose supply from the woman ceases, requiring the neonate to readjust. Subsequently, the first few hours of a neonate's life may be compromised by severe hypoglycemia.

A normal blood glucose level for the neonate ranges from 40 to 60 mg/dl, but a level of less than 40 mg/dl may be considered critical. If euglycemia is maintained throughout pregnancy, the risk of hypoglycemia following delivery is the same as that for the neonate of a nondiabetic woman. According to the ADA, although uncomplicated GDM with less severe fasting hyperglycemia hasn't been associated with increased perinatal mortality, GDM of any severity increases the risk of fetal macrosomia. Neonatal hypoglycemia, jaundice, polycythemia, and hypocalcemia may complicate GDM as well.

Antepartum management of diabetes

Regardless of the type of diabetes, prevention of the risks associated with diabetes is key. This is best achieved through the maintenance of near-normal glycemia throughout the pregnancy.

In gestational diabetes

Extensive education, glucose monitoring, medical nutrition therapy and, if necessary, insulin are key components in the care of a woman with GDM. Therefore, a team approach is vital to the delivery of a healthy neonate. The woman should be identified as the center of the team, with a certified diabetes educator (CDE), registered dietitian (RD), and primary health care practitioner listed as other key members. Additional team members to help meet the medical, physical, and emotional needs of the patient might include an exercise physiologist, social worker, or spiritual care provider.

The woman with GDM requires extensive teaching so that she understands the full ramifications of hyperglycemia to herself and her fetus. Usually the woman experiences shock, fear, or denial after being diagnosed with GDM. She may not feel different physically, and as such, may not realize the importance of her role in ensuring a healthy neonate. Having reached 24 to 28 weeks' gestation (normal screening timeline for GDM) without difficulty, she may feel as if she's past a point

where harm can come to the fetus. Stress the importance of early diagnosis and treatment as well as the primary role she must play to reinforce positive outcomes for her and the neonate.

The patient also may experience a sense of guilt, as if she has done something wrong throughout her pregnancy, or as if she's being punished for choices she made, such as food selections or the amount of weight she has gained. Explanations of the underlying insulin resistance, the increased need for insulin, and the effects of hormones related to pregnancy can help to alleviate these feelings.

Provide written guidelines about what's required of the patient so that she can review them at a later time. This helps to reinforce what she's been told initially but may not have absorbed. Instructions typically include following up with the RD, CDE, or other team members to achieve tight glycemic control, measures to improve pregnancy outcomes, and sources of emotional and psychological support for her and her partner, if present.

Medical nutrition therapy

Medical nutritional therapy (MNT) is commonly considered the primary treatment for GDM, and as such, all affected women should be referred to an RD. Diet recommendations include a carbohydrate-controlled diet, with small, frequent meals to ensure adequate nutrition for the mother and fetus, as well as appropriate weight gain, while preventing ketosis. The initial appointment should occur within 1 week of diagnosis, with subsequent visits scheduled 1 to 3 weeks thereafter, including a 6-week postpartum visit.

The goals for MNT include achieving and maintaining euglycemia and adequate nutrition for appropriate gestational weight gain. It's important to cover several topics during the initial nutritional assessment. (See *Initial nutritional assessment*.)

Height, current and prepregnancy weight, BMI, and pregnancy history are some of the more obvious items to be obtained. Of special concern is the obese pregnant woman. Recent research on the impact of obesity on GDM and pregnancy outcomes revealed that obese women have a two- to three-fold higher risk of adverse pregnancy outcomes than those who were overweight or normal weight when treated with diet alone, regardless of glucose levels achieved.

Laboratory results of the patient's GCT, OGTT, hemoglobin, hematocrit, ketones, and glycosylated hemoglobin (HbA$_{1c}$) levels can help individualize the meal plan and determine the energy level needed for the patient.

Address existing issues that may impact the patient's food plan — for example, GI issues that could include eating disorders; discomforts such as heartburn, nausea, vomiting, and constipation; allergies; food intolerances; cravings; aversions; current appetite level; and pica. A dietary recall of meal and snack food choices, portions, preparation methods, and preferences are an ideal way to gather data. Lifestyle factors also may affect how and when the patient eats. Type of work and schedule, educational level, cultural influences, religious matters, financial concerns, substance abuse, exercise patterns, and limitations should all be assessed at the initial visit.

Encourage the patient to keep a detailed food record to provide information for review at future visits. When viewed in correlation with self-monitoring of blood glucose (SMBG) results, appropriate recommendations can then be made. The blood glucose level is the guiding factor in MNT.

Nutrient recommendations. Carbohydrates are the primary nutrient affecting postprandial glucose levels. Therefore, they should be spread evenly throughout the day, divided into three meals and two to four snacks. Calories from

INITIAL NUTRITIONAL ASSESSMENT

When the patient with gestational diabetes mellitus undergoes an initial nutritional assessment, these areas must be addressed:

- height and weight (body mass index)
- pregnancy history
- review of laboratory data (oral glucose challenge, oral glucose tolerance test, hemoglobin, hematocrit, glycosylated hemoglobin)
- GI history
- typical daily intake recall
- exercise patterns and limitations
- lifestyle factors (work schedule; education level; family, ethnic, cultural, and religious influences; financial concerns; possible substance or physical abuse)
- pregnancy-related discomforts (nausea and vomiting, heartburn, constipation, cravings, bloating).

carbohydrates are typically distributed as:

- 10% of calories at breakfast
- 30% of calories for lunch and dinner
- 30% divided between snacks.

Adequate levels of carbohydrates are essential to provide the fetal brain with sufficient levels of glucose. When inadequate levels of carbohydrates are available, the body resorts to ketosis to provide adequate amounts. The recommended daily allowance (RDA) for carbohydrate intake during pregnancy is 175 g per day. Increased maternal levels of cortisol and growth hormone early in the morning can lead to increased levels of insulin resistance, limiting carbohydrates at breakfast to 30 g to 45 g. An evening snack is usually needed to help prevent starvation ketosis during the night. Periods of fasting lasting for longer than 10 hours should be avoided for the same reason.

RECOMMENDED GLUCOSE LEVELS

This chart shows the targeted goals for blood glucose levels developed by the American Diabetes Association (ADA) and the American College of Obstetrics and Gynecology (ACOG). Although the values differ somewhat, they're used as a basis for determining the need for additional therapy.

TIME	ADA RECOMMENDATIONS	ACOG RECOMMENDATIONS
Fasting	< 105 mg/dl	< 95 mg/dl
1 hour postprandial	< 155 mg/dl	< 140 mg/dl
2 hour postprandial	< 130 mg/dl	< 120 mg/dl

Protein intake doesn't directly increase glucose levels after meals, and can be included in meals and snacks to promote satiety. The RDA for protein in pregnancy is an additional 25g per day, added to the recommended 56 g per day.

In addition, fat should be included in the pregnant patient's diet to ensure appropriate fetal brain development. However, fats are limited to 20% to 40% of total calorie intake, with one-third or less coming from saturated fats. Eating high-fat foods can delay the absorption of glucose from the bloodstream into the body's cells, thereby contributing to an extended period of hyperglycemia.

Self-monitoring of blood glucose

SMBG provides direct feedback to the patient and health care team. The optimal testing times remain controversial. General consensus includes a fasting blood glucose level and a measure of the glucose level either at 1 hour or 2 hours postprandially. Together these values will provide an overview of the pregnant woman's glycemic state. Postprandial monitoring reveals improved glycemic control, decreased incidence of LGA infants, and direct feedback of the effects of food on the glucose level.

(See chapter 12, Daily care regimens, for more information on SMBG.)

The ADA and the American College of Obstetrics and Gynecology provide guidelines and recommendations for targeted glucose levels for women with GDM. (See *Recommended glucose levels.*)

Insulin therapy

When glucose levels exceed the identified range, insulin therapy is recommended. It's used in 20% to 60% of all women with GDM. The use of oral agents in pregnancy remains controversial due to fetal safety issues and, according to the ADA, insulin has most consistently shown a reduction in fetal morbidity when added to MNT. Studies and research continue about the use of oral agents during pregnancy. Currently, they aren't approved by the U.S. Food and Drug Administration for use in GDM. Although currently used in Europe, glargine insulin isn't approved in the United States due to its similarity to the insulin-like growth factor receptor, found in abundant supply in the placenta.

Human insulin is the insulin of choice in treating GDM with dosages based on the results of SMBG. Insulin analogs aren't officially recommended by the ADA to treat GDM. However, studies have demonstrated reduced hyperglycemia with a decreased amount of hypoglycemia at no additional risk to the mother or fetus. It's also been shown that women report an increased ease of use with analogs and the timing of the injections in relation to oral intake. Further testing and research are needed to determine the safety of insulin analogs during pregnancy.

⋙ **ALERT** *Keep in mind that if average blood glucose levels run lower than normal, studies have shown an increased risk of small for gestational age (SGA) infants. While there's been concern for the potential of SGA infants to have an increased risk of developing type 2 diabetes later in life, one study reported that there wasn't an increased risk unless the SGA infant became overweight later in life.*

Women need to be instructed on the potential dangers of undereating in an attempt to avoid insulin therapy. Telling the patient that insulin is made chemically identical to the natural hormone insulin in her body may serve to allay some of her fears regarding medication use in pregnancy.

Although insulin therapy commonly increases fear and trepidation on the part of the patient, it shouldn't hinder therapy when needed. One study suggests that obese women with a BMI of 30 or more who develop GDM have a higher risk of adverse perinatal outcomes than do normal-weight women with GDM. Therefore, achieving glycemic control with insulin therapy may enhance the outcome for these patients.

Urine monitoring

According to the ADA, monitoring urine glucose levels isn't helpful in managing GDM; however, urine ketone testing can be. A first-voided specimen can identify starvation ketosis as well as inadequate carbohydrate consumption throughout the day. Women who participate in regular exercise over 30 minutes may also need to check for

ketones due to increased energy requirements. In the pregnant state, the body quickly moves to use fat storage for additional energy to spare glucose and amino acids for the fetus. Some research has demonstrated increased ketonemia may lead to decreased intelligence test scores and decreased psychomotor skills for the neonate later in life.

Activity

Regular physical activity can improve glucose control and decrease insulin resistance, even in pregnancy. Exercise and physical activity in moderation have been shown to be safe during pregnancy, unless a medical or obstetric contraindication exists. Physical activity can commonly be used in combination with MNT to decrease insulin resistance, thereby avoiding the need for insulin therapy.

Women with GDM should be encouraged to start or continue a pattern of moderate activity and exercise as part of their treatment, if approved by her health care practitioner. Walking, swimming, and arm ergometry can be helpful. However, the heart rate should be kept below 140 beats/minute to avoid overstressing the cardiovascular system. Walking 15 to 30 minutes each day can lower the blood glucose level by 20 to 40 mg/dl and, if done postprandially, can have an additional beneficial effect. Exercise can improve cardiovascular health, helping to reduce the risk of complications. When counseling about exercise and activity, advise the pregnant patient to avoid vigorous activity. The increase in maternal blood volume and carbon dioxide level with pregnancy may result in a shunting of oxygen, fuel, and nutrients from the fetus to the woman. Brief episodes of fetal bradycardia may also occur. Also instruct her to avoid exercises involving mechanical stress on the trunk of the body or exercises requiring her to lie in a supine position. Encourage the patient to assess for uterine contractions during periods of increased activity. In addition, advise her to have a quick source of glucose or carbohydrate readily available during exercise or physical activity to prevent hypoglycemia.

In preexisting type 1 or type 2 diabetes

The basic management guidelines for GDM also apply to pregnant women with preexisting type 1 or type 2 diabetes. However, additional considerations also must be addressed. For example, it's important that women with type 1 or type 2 diabetes have preconception counseling. Some experts suggest that the ideal time for initiating this counseling is at puberty.

Diabetes mellitus is the most common medical complication of pregnancy worldwide, depending on the population described and the criteria used for diagnosis. According to the World Health Organization Department of Reproductive Health and Research (2004), diabetes in pregnancy is the 7th most common condition associated with maternal morbidity and mortality. Only hypertensive disorders, stillbirth, abortion, hemorrhage, preterm delivery, and anemia in pregnancy were ranked higher than diabetes. However, the risk of these conditions increased in pregnancies complicated by diabetes. Before the development of insulin, the mortality rate for mothers with diabetes was 20% with an infant mortality of 60%.

While many advances in health care have helped to decrease the overall rate of maternal and fetal complications, almost one-half of perinatal deaths of neonates born to mothers with preexisting diabetes result from congenital malformations. (See *Potential complications with preexisting diabetes and pregnancy*.)

So, achieving and maintaining blood glucose levels within the normal range throughout the entire pregnancy are essential. Therefore, if a woman isn't planning to have a child in the immediate future and isn't achieving normal glucose levels, close attention must be paid to the form of birth control she's

using, with emphasis on using the most effective method.

Preconception counseling

According to the ADA, diabetes care and education should begin before conception to help prevent spontaneous abortions and congenital malformations in infants of patients with diabetes. This includes care by a multidisciplinary team, such as a diabetologist, internist, or family practice physician skilled in diabetes management; an obstetrician familiar with the management of high-risk pregnancies; diabetes educators, including a nurse, RD, and social worker; and other specialists as necessary. Ideally, the woman with diabetes should be the most active member of the team, asking team members for specific guidance and expertise to help her achieve her goal of a healthy pregnancy and neonate.

Because organogenesis begins in the first few weeks of pregnancy, a normal glucose level is vital to prevent congenital anomalies. Therefore, it's recommended that preconception counseling begin 3 to 6 months before conception. Baseline examinations should include a dilated retinal eye examination by an ophthalmologist; assessment of orthostatic blood pressure changes; 24-hour urine collection for creatinine, creatinine clearance, and microalbumin; thyroid function tests (because of the correlation between type 1 diabetes and thyroid abnormalities); neurologic examinations for autonomic neuropathy; and cardiovascular screening, including a baseline electrocardiogram (ECG), for evidence of cardiac or peripheral vascular disease.

Prevention of complications. Pregnancy has been shown to be an independent risk factor for retinopathy acceleration due to the elevation in the placental lactogen level and other hormones that cause vascular changes. When background retinopathy is present at the start of the pregnancy, there's

POTENTIAL COMPLICATIONS WITH PREEXISTING DIABETES AND PREGNANCY

The woman who enters pregnancy with preexisting diabetes is at risk for many complications as is her fetus. This chart highlights some of the potential complications that can occur.

RISK FACTORS	POTENTIAL COMPLICATIONS
Type 1 diabetes	■ Maternal diabetic ketoacidosis

Hyperglycemia in early pregnancy (especially the first 6 to 8 weeks)	■ Congenital abnormalities:
	  – Sacral agenesis
	  – Central nervous system defects (spina bifida, hydrocephalus)
	  – Anencephalus
	  – Cardiac anomalies (transposition of the greater vessels, ventricular septal defect, atrial septal defect, coarctation of the aorta)
	  – Renal anomalies (agenesis, cystic kidneys, ureter duplex)
	  – Anal and rectal atresia
	  – Situs inversus
	■ Spontaneous abortion

Hyperglycemia later in pregnancy	■ Polyhydramnios ■ Macrosomia ■ Preterm delivery and increased rate of cesarean deliveries ■ Hypoglycemia at birth ■ Blood alterations (hyperbilirubinemia, polycythemia, hypocalcemia) ■ Respiratory distress syndrome ■ Shoulder dystocia ■ Neuropsychological defects ■ Intrauterine death
Preexisting maternal complications: ■ Retinopathy	■ Acceleration of disease, may lead to blindness without treatment
■ Cardiovascular	■ Maternal death
■ Nephropathy	■ Preeclampsia → intrauterine growth retardation, small for gestational age, preterm delivery, stillbirth
■ Neuropathy	■ Peripheral neuropathy, may lead to increased carpal tunnel syndrome symptoms ■ Gastroparesis ↑ leading to nausea, vomiting, hypoglycemia, hyperglycemia ■ Urine retention ■ Orthostatic hypotension ■ Hypoglycemic unawareness

a 16% to 50% risk of progression during the pregnancy. Additionally, women who had no baseline retinopathy present had a 10% increased risk of developing retinopathy.

Preeclampsia is the most common and serious complication associated with diabetes during pregnancy. If the pregnant patient has proteinuria level greater than 190 mg/dl, she has a 31% increased chance of having preeclampsia. Studies indicate that deterioration in renal status isn't that different for women who are pregnant versus those who aren't. Renal disease is progressive and worsens over time, but doesn't seem to be increasingly worse secondary to pregnancy. However, if overt nephropathy is present, women are two to four times more likely to have coronary artery disease (CAD).

Women with untreated CAD have a higher mortality rate during pregnancy, with rates of maternal death being as high as 25% to 50%. As a result, exercise tolerance testing should be included in preconception counseling when appropriate. Women with treated CAD, even following coronary revascularization, can have successful pregnancy outcomes. In addition, statin therapy should be discontinued before conception.

Gestational hypertension (previously called *pregnancy-induced hypertension*), preeclampsia, and chronic, preexisting hypertension rates are all increased in women with diabetes during pregnancy. It's estimated that the rate of preeclampsia and gestational hypertension among this group is twice as high as in the general, nondiabetic population. The use of angiotensin-converting enzyme inhibitors and diuretics are contraindicated in pregnancy. Methyldopa (Aldomet) is commonly recommended as a first-line agent. In addition, beta-adrenergic blockers remain controversial because of their masking of hypoglycemic signs. Prazosin (Minipress) or clonidine (Catapres) can be added as needed for additional control in early pregnancy, and diltiazem (Cardizem) may be prescribed after the end of the first trimester. Throughout pregnancy, the goal is to maintain blood pressure within the range of 110 to 129 mm Hg/ 65 to 79 mm Hg. As the pregnancy continues, blood pressure control commonly becomes more difficult.

The presence of atherosclerotic lesions in the uterine arteries compromise oxygenation of the fetus and — in combination with diabetes, hypertension, and chronic proteinuria — may lead to preterm delivery and stillbirth. There's a tenfold risk of stillbirth in pregnant women with preexisting diabetes and nephropathy when compared to nondiabetic pregnant women without nephropathy.

Self-management skills. An assessment of diabetes self-management skills should be done to determine accurate SMBG levels, insulin dose, and administration techniques. Nutritional assessments and counseling by an RD should be done to assess for adequate calcium, iron, and folic acid intake. The HbA_{1c} level should be within the normal range to help prevent congenital abnormalities. All contraception should be continued until blood glucose levels are normal.

Anticipatory guidance. During preconception counseling, the woman needs information about the possible increased financial burden associated with pregnancy and diabetes, such as the need for additional supplies for monitoring or testing of the fetus throughout pregnancy. The cost-to-benefit ratio should be explored with the patient in relation to preconception care, the time needed to achieve normal blood glucose goals, and the prevention of malformations. Teaching also should address the risks of congenital anomalies, obstetric complications, maternal complications, and exacerbations of preexisting conditions, and how these risks can be prevented or decreased through achieving near-normal blood glucose levels. In addition, for the patient with type 2 diabetes currently being treated with oral agents or diet alone, it's necessary to discuss the use of insulin therapy throughout pregnancy.

If oral agents are being used, the patient should be switched to insulin as soon as possible.

Blood glucose levels. Goals for blood glucose levels should be established at the first preconception visit or at the initial appointment, if there was no counseling before contraception. The ADA reports unplanned pregnancies in two-thirds of women with diabetes.

⚡ ALERT *It's important to note that a woman with polycystic ovarian syndrome (PCOS) may be treated with metformin (Glucophage) to help decrease insulin resistance and help her conceive. If a woman had difficulty conceiving and is now being treated with metformin, she should be counseled about the risk of increased fertility associated with taking the drug to help prevent unplanned pregnancy.*

The ADA recommends these blood glucose level targets with SMBG:
- before meals — 80 to 110 mg/dl (4.4 to 6.1 mmol/l)
- 2 hours after meals — less than 155 mg/dl (less than 8.6 mmol/l).

Due to hypoglycemic unawareness or the risk of severe neuroglycopenia, glycemic goals may need to be modified. When levels are attained that are the safest for the patient and provide the lowest risk of complications for the woman and fetus, contraception can be discontinued. If pregnancy doesn't result within 1 year, fertility testing should be considered. The patient should be tested at the earliest possible time after conception and definitely if menses don't occur within 15 to 18 days following ovulation.

The HbA_{1c} level should be monitored every 1 to 2 months until a stable and identified goal is achieved. Even mild elevations of the HbA_{1c} level may have some impact on the incidence of malformations. As organogenesis occurs during the first 8 weeks of gestation, malformations can occur. Pregnant women should aim for an HbA_{1c} level

of approximately 5% because studies show that levels at the end of the first trimester may result in a 2% to 5% risk of congenital malformations with normal to moderate elevations and a 20% to 40% risk with marked elevations.

Congenital heart defects are the most common malformation, affecting as many as 4% of all pregnancies in women with preexisting diabetes. In addition, spontaneous abortion rates increase dramatically with increases in the HbA_{1c} level.

In pregnancy, the lifespan of the red blood cell is shortened, and as a result, the HbA_{1c} level measures the glycemic control of the preceding 6 to 8 weeks. Consequently, this can be a valuable tool in assessing the overall glycemic control of the pregnant patient.

Insulin adjustments. Insulin therapy may need to be adjusted with the onset of pregnancy. Women with type 1 diabetes can receive two or three injections to help maintain good glycemic control. Attention must be given to the potential nocturnal hypoglycemia if a two-injection therapy is chosen. In pregnancy, women with diabetes will experience an even more pronounced rebound effect from nocturnal hypoglycemia, resulting in an elevated fasting glucose level.

Care during pregnancy
The focus of care and education during pregnancy for the woman with preexisting diabetes should focus on keeping the blood glucose level near normoglycemic and maximizing the patient's health during pregnancy. Treatment will involve the same key elements as GDM: MNT, SMBG, physical activity, and a team approach. Again, the pregnant patient must be the core element in the team, because only she can determine how diligently she'll pursue a healthy outcome for her pregnancy, given proper guidance and information. While normal and near-normal glucose levels can radically reduce the risk of

Patient-teaching tip

DEALING WITH MORNING SICKNESS

The pregnant woman with type 1 diabetes may experience morning sickness. To help her cope and prevent possible hypoglycemia from not eating, instruct her to:
- eat dry crackers or toast before getting out of bed
- eat smaller, more frequent meals
- avoid caffeine, and foods containing caffeine
- avoid foods that are spicy or high in fat
- drink fluids between meals, not during meals
- take prenatal vitamins later in the day
- eat a bedtime snack to prevent hypoglycemia in the morning.

In addition, be sure to instruct the patient to check her glucose level because hypoglycemia can exacerbate nausea.

---

birth defects, it can't totally eliminate risk; the general population has a rate of 2% to 3% risk of congenital birth defects. This percentage dramatically increases, however, with increased hyperglycemia. As a result, the woman needs to fully understand the ramifications of poor glycemic control throughout pregnancy and the vital role she plays in reducing her risk.

Medical nutrition therapy. During the first trimester, the energy required to maintain the fetus is the same as before pregnancy. However, because of variations in blood glucose levels, adjustments may need to be made to the meal plan. Similar to the diet plan for GDM, the recommendation is three meals and two to four snacks per day. If the woman experiences morning sickness, additional precautions and measures can be used. (See *Dealing with morning sickness.*)

Because hypoglycemia can exacerbate morning sickness, inform the patient to check her blood glucose level whenever she's nauseated. Also advise her to carry a quick-acting glucose source at all times. If she vomits after injecting her insulin before food is absorbed, 0.15 mg of glucagon may be given subcutaneously to increase the blood glucose level 30 to 40 mg/dl. This

effect will last for approximately 1 to 2 hours.

Calorie intake should be adjusted at the beginning of the second trimester to allow for increased energy requirements. Additional protein is required only in the second half of pregnancy due to increased protein deposits. A recommended 175 g per day of carbohydrates should provide adequate glucose to the fetus's and the woman's brain without relying on gluconeogenesis or glycogenolysis. Enough glucose is required to fuel the central nervous system (CNS) without having to rely on a further increase, which might possibly lead to ketoacidosis or starvation ketosis. When using carbohydrate counting with an insulin-to-carbohydrate ratio for coverage, insulin doses can be tailored to match food intake. As in GDM, carbohydrate intake should be somewhat restricted first thing in the morning due to increased insulin resistance. Alternatively, separate insulin-to-carbohydrate ratios may be necessary to allow for this difference.

During pregnancy, the patient needs to be aware that scheduled mealtimes and snack times are essential to prevent hypoglycemia. This scheduled eating plan also helps to prevent overeating at a later meal or reduce intake at a regular meal, which could contribute to hyperglycemia. Dietitians should continue to meet regularly with the patient and review blood glucose and urine ketone levels, appetite, and weight gain throughout pregnancy.

The pregnant diabetic patient should be cautioned against drinking alcohol. In addition, she should avoid such foods as shark, swordfish, mackerel, and tilefish. These foods contain high levels of methylmercury, a potent neurotoxin that can cross the placenta, possibly causing damage to the fetal nervous system.

Activity. Physical activity helps women with GDM and also can benefit women with type 1 or type 2 diabetes in pregnancy. The same limitations exist for safe exercise. However, as a result of tighter management of glucose levels, hypoglycemic episodes may be triggered more easily. Activities done before pregnancy without hypoglycemia occurring won't be perceived as being a potential cause of hypoglycemia during pregnancy. Thus, careful monitoring for hypoglycemia and implementing measures to prevent it must be stressed.

Self-monitoring of blood glucose. SMBG is one of the most important tools the pregnant woman has for assisting in the healthy development of her fetus. In addition, urine monitoring for ketones is needed daily on the first urine specimen, and again any time the glucose level exceeds 200 mg/dl. Ketones spill into urine at a lower level than in a nonpregnant woman. In addition, screening for ketones is strongly recommended whenever nausea or vomiting is present or if the patient is ill.

Ketosis can be harmful to the fetus. Near-normal blood glucose level with positive ketones usually suggests starvation ketosis, indicating inadequate calorie intake. If the blood glucose level is mildly elevated, the pregnant patient should be evaluated for incipient ketoacidosis in which infection is the main cause. Ketoacidosis in pregnancy is commonly associated with high perinatal mortality.

Insulin therapy. Women with type 2 diabetes being managed with oral agents should be switched to insulin before conception if possible. If no preconception counseling was given, the switch should be made as soon as possible.

Although various studies have been done to establish the safety of using oral antidiabetic agents during pregnancy, the ADA maintains that insufficient data are available to establish their safety; therefore, insulin should be prescribed for all patients with type 1 or type 2 diabetes during pregnancy. The use of continuous subcutaneous insulin infusion via pump therapy may appeal to some pregnant women and can be especially beneficial in controlling and preventing hypoglycemia.

Fetal surveillance. Monitoring the mother and fetus throughout the gestational period helps identify complications early and determine treatment options. (See *Monitoring to assess fetal health,* page 196.) Ultrasound should be done early in pregnancy to accurately date fetal growth and development. In most cases, it's repeated again in the third trimester.

Women who have markedly high HbA_{1c} levels are at a much higher risk for delivering infants with congenital malformations, typically as high as 20% to 40%. A maternal serum alpha-fetoprotein (AFP) level can be done to help identify neural tube defects, and ultrasonography can be used to screen for CNS, heart, renal, and skeletal anomalies. While these tests aren't 100% sensitive, they're helpful in detecting fetal malformations.

The maternal serum AFP is only a screening test and should be done at 15 to 18 weeks' gestation. It can result in false positives, thereby necessitating further investigation by ultrasound or am-

MONITORING TO ASSESS FETAL HEALTH

When a woman with diabetes is pregnant, threats to herself as well as to her fetus are possible. These tests may be used to assess fetal well-being during pregnancy.

TEST	MEASURES
Fetal movements	■ Overall fetal health
Nonstress test	■ Overall fetal health ■ Response of fetal heart rate (FHR) if uterine contractions are present
Contraction stress test	■ Response of FHR to mild uterine contractions
Biophysical profile	■ Fetal breathing, body movement, muscle tone, and heart rate ■ Amniotic fluid volume
Amniocentesis	■ Fetal lung maturity

niocentesis. Fetal echocardiography can be done at 18 to 22 weeks' gestation to assess for congenital heart defects.

The nonstress test (NST) can be done to assess the overall health of the fetus. It's safe and noninvasive, involving the use of transducers — one to measure the fetal heart rate (FHR) and the other to track uterine contractions. It's normal for the FHR to increase during a contraction and decrease following the contraction. Performed on a regular basis, some practitioners will begin the NST at 32 to 34 weeks' gestation and continue until delivery. If the woman has a history of vascular disease, it may be beneficial to begin earlier and perform more frequent testing.

Recording fetal movements is another noninvasive, safe method to assess overall fetal health. In this method, the patient herself assesses fetal movement. Various methods can be used, including counting how long it takes for the fetus to move 10 times. Another method determines how many times the fetus moves in a 30- or 60-minute period.

Weekly contraction stress tests (CSTs) may be used starting at 32 to 34 weeks' gestation. It's similar to the NST, except the uterus is induced to mild contractions by I.V. oxytocin (Pitocin) or nipple stimulation. A positive CST, evidenced by late deceleration in the FHR after more than 50% of the contractions, can indicate fetal distress and the need for immediate delivery.

To measure the intrauterine environment and the danger of mortality, a biophysical profile can be done. This test measures fetal breathing, body movement, muscle tone, heart-rate activity, and amniotic fluid level. A numeric score of 0, 1, or 2 is given to each parameter, with a possible score of 10. A score of less than 6 indicates the need for further evaluation. It helps to detect fetal compromise early, thereby allowing interventions to prevent fetal demise.

Amniocentesis can be used to assess fetal lung maturity if delivery before 39 weeks' gestation is being considered. Many women who reach 38 weeks' gestation and have good glycemic control may not need to have amniocentesis.

Preparation for delivery. If there's no maternal complication identified and the fetal health doesn't appear to be compromised, many pregnancies can go full term, and the woman may be able to deliver vaginally. Cesarean deliveries are considered whenever there's a risk to the woman or fetus due to complications of preexisting diabetes and pregnancy.

Some health care practitioners feel labor should be induced if the patient doesn't go into spontaneous labor by week 40. As long as the fetus isn't LGA and the cervix is favorable, an induction can be attempted. Should the woman go into preterm labor, the use of β-sympathomimetic therapy such as terbutaline (Brethine) to stop labor, can lead to deterioration in blood glucose control and development of ketosis. Therefore, magnesium sulfate or nifedipine (Procardia) is recommended as the first-line treatment of preterm labor in a woman with type 1 or type 2 diabetes.

Intrapartum management of diabetes

During labor and delivery, insulin resistance that's common in pregnancy is reduced dramatically, leading to a reduction in the amount of insulin required to maintain a near-normal blood glucose level. In addition, most women with GDM return to normal glucose levels shortly after delivery.

For the pregnant woman with type 1 or 2 diabetes, adequate carbohydrate intake is important. I.V. glucose, administered at 2 to 2.5 mg/kg/minute, helps to provide appropriate energy requirements and prevent ketosis. Blood glucose levels need to be measured every 1 to 2 hours and controlled with short-acting insulin either by multiple injections or continuous I.V. infusion. Regardless of how insulin is administered, the key is to maintain euglycemia — glucose levels of 70 to 90 mg/dl — during labor and delivery to help prevent fetal hyperinsulinemia leading to hypoglycemia after delivery.

Various opinions exist as to insulin guidelines if a cesarean delivery is necessary. The morning basal insulin could be withheld and short-acting insulin given based on the blood glucose level. Alternatively, the bedtime basal insulin dose could be given in the morning and every 8 hours thereafter if surgery is delayed.

In addition to frequent glucose measurements, the serum potassium level needs to be assessed. Potassium will follow insulin and glucose into the cells, thereby affecting serum level. ECG monitoring should also be done to identify a problem with the patient.

Postpartum management of diabetes

As with GDM, insulin requirements of the woman with preexisting diabetes mellitus decrease significantly during labor and typically return to normal immediately after delivery. Just as pregnancy doubles or triples insulin requirements throughout the gestational period, the hormones responsible for this dramatic increase now return to normal or near-normal levels after delivery. It isn't unusual for a woman with diabetes to require little or no insulin during the first 24 to 48 hours after delivery.

⭐ **ALERT** *If no reduction in insulin is needed, assess the patient for an underlying infection, such as a UTI or endometritis.*

This propensity for lower-than-normal blood glucose levels can continue through the first few weeks after delivery and is further increased if the woman breast-feeds. Women have reported a drop in blood glucose levels of 50 to 100 mg/dl over a 30-minute breast-feeding session. Despite this additional challenge in managing glucose levels, all women with preexisting diabetes are encouraged to breast-feed. Eating a snack before or during breast-feeding can help offset the drop in blood glucose levels, and a calorie intake similar to that of the third trimester may be warranted. Women with type 2

SIGNS AND SYMPTOMS OF HYPOGLYCEMIA IN THE NEONATE

Unlike an adult or older child, the neonate can't say how he feels. Therefore, the keen observation for these signs and symptoms would lead you to suspect hypoglycemia:

- cardiovascular collapse
- coma or stupor
- episodes of apnea and cyanosis
- episodes of sweating
- irritability
- jitteriness

- seizures
- sudden hypotonia
- tachypnea
- tremors
- weak or high-pitched crying.

diabetes may need to remain on insulin throughout the period of lactation because oral agents are contraindicated.

For the woman with GDM, glucose tolerance should be reevaluated at 6 to 12 weeks postpartum, and if normal, the ADA recommends reassessment at a minimum of every 3 years. However, if impaired fasting glucose or impaired glucose tolerance, known as *prediabetes*, is noted, annual testing is urged. The woman should also receive intensive nutritional counseling and education on the prevention of diabetes, including lifestyle modifications that can serve to lower insulin resistance. In addition, instruct the woman to get annual screening for diabetes and preconception counseling with future pregnancies. After delivery, it's important to discuss contraception and family planning. The use of contraception in all women with diabetes or a previous history of GDM must be emphasized to ensure that preconception care can be provided.

In addition, the children from the pregnancy affected by GDM need to be followed closely for the development of obesity and glucose intolerance.

Management of the neonate

Management of the neonate after delivery includes blood glucose monitoring, assessment for congenital anomalies

and signs of respiratory distress, and measurement of calcium, magnesium, and bilirubin levels.

Peak incidence of hypoglycemia for the infant occurs 6 to 12 hours after delivery and is defined as a blood glucose level less than 35 mg/dl. Because prolonged or severe hypoglycemia may be associated with neurologic complications, treatment should be initiated at 40 mg/dl or more. Early oral feeding is the most efficient and safest treatment and can help prevent hypoglycemia in the neonate. (See *Signs and symptoms of hypoglycemia in the neonate*.)

In the event of a hypoglycemic event in the neonate, oral feedings may be given if the respiratory status is stable. A repeat blood glucose level in 30 minutes is used to assess effectiveness. If the level remains low, I.V. dextrose 10% in water with a possible bolus of 2 ml/kg may be initiated. Typically, blood glucose levels are monitored every 30 minutes until stable, every hour for 2 hours, and then every 4 to 8 hours.

Neonatal hypoglycemia, hyperbilirubinemia, hypocalcemia, and hypomagnesemia can result from maternal hyperglycemia. Hypoglycemia seems to be more prevalent in LGA and macrosomic infants compared to normal-weight infants. Hyperbilirubinemia, present in 11% to 29% of infants of women with diabetes, may be due to chronic fetal hypoxemia, which is a result of an accumulation of glycogen in the fetal liver, an increased lipid synthesis causing increased hepatic enzyme activity, and accumulation of fat in adipose tissue. This increased pathogenesis leads to an increased metabolic rate requiring an increased level of oxygenation, thereby stimulating an increased synthesis of erythropoietin leading to polycythemia. In turn, the polycythemia contributes to hyperbilirubinemia. Macrosomia also leads to an increased risk of hyperbilirubinemia.

Hypocalcemia doesn't usually appear until 24 to 72 hours after birth, and is related to lower parathyroid hormone levels in infants of women with diabetes compared to infants of nondiabetic women. It's also related to the extent and severity of the woman's diabetes. Hypomagnesemia is thought to be related to maternal polyuria and occurs within 3 days after birth in 40% of infants born to women who have diabetes. Prematurity can also lead to lower levels of magnesium. Generally, hypocalcemia and hypomagnesemia don't require treatment.

DIABETES IN CHILDREN

Historically, children with diabetes were diagnosed with type 1 diabetes — hence the name juvenile-onset diabetes. However, this is no longer the case. Normally considered a disease common in adults, type 2 diabetes is being diagnosed more frequently in children. According to the American Association of Diabetes Educators, approximately one-third to one-half of childhood-onset diabetes is type 2 diabetes. The increase in children with type 2 diabetes is a direct reflection of lifestyle choices being made in the United States. Because children are less active physically and are eating less-nutritious foods, their weight is increasing. With the additional weight gain and loss of activity, insulin resistance increases. Subsequently, these changes are directly linked to

an increase in the number of children being diagnosed with type 2 diabetes.

Diabetes can be a challenging disease to manage and is even more so in the pediatric population. Compounded by the rapid growth and development associated with childhood as well as the various stages each child goes through, the health care practitioner is vital to helping young individuals achieve a healthy and optimal life.

Prevention

Prevention is key in dealing with type 2 diabetes in children. The International Diabetes Foundation emphasizes prevention as a major priority, urging government and communities to provide an environment that promotes individual lifestyle changes that help to prevent and reverse obesity.

Prevention efforts should target the entire family — not just the individual child. The behaviors a child learns are from the environment in which he lives.

Nutritional strategies

Overall nutritional strategies should include:
- setting mealtimes and snack times, with healthier food options
- limiting fast food to a maximum of three times per week
- limiting regular soda (For example, 20 oz of soda can contain 65 g of carbohydrates, which is more than what's needed for a regular meal; additionally it's full of empty calories.)
- maintaining portion control (Portions sizes have grown considerably over the past decade and are reinforced by the fast-food industry with larger meals available for only cents more).

Eating a healthy breakfast always should be encouraged. Reinforce the concept there are no "good" or "bad" foods; what's important is the amount eaten at one time. A child needs to be taught how to recognize healthier foods in an environment where they're in charge of their food choices such as in

DIFFERENTIATING TYPE 1 AND TYPE 2 DIABETES IN CHILDREN

Confirming the diagnosis of type 2 diabetes in children can be difficult because children also may exhibit ketoacidosis, which is typically associated with type 1 diabetes. However, additional signs and symptoms may be noted to help differentiate the diagnosis.

	TYPE 1 DIABETES	TYPE 2 DIABETES
Onset	■ Acute (symptomatic)	■ Slow (commonly asymptomatic)
Clinical picture	■ Weight loss ■ Polyuria ■ Polydipsia	■ Obese ■ Strong family history of type 2 diabetes ■ Ethnicity (high-prevalence populations) ■ Acanthosis nigricans ■ Polycystic ovary syndrome
Ketosis	■ Almost always present	■ Usually absent
Insulin	■ C-peptide negative	■ C-peptide positive
Antibodies	■ Islet cell antibodies (ICA) positive ■ Anti-glutamic acid decarboxylase (GAD) positive ■ ICA 512 positive	■ ICA negative ■ Anti-GAD negative ■ ICA 512 negative
Therapy	■ Insulin invariably	■ Oral antidiabetic agents
Associated autoimmune diseases	■ Yes	■ No

Adapted from Alberti, G., et al. "Type 2 Diabetes in the Young. The Evolving Epidemic," *Diabetes Care* 27(7):1801, July 2004, with permission of the publisher.

school. Low-calorie dairy items should be included with a goal of three servings per day. Fruits and vegetables are recommended at five to eight servings per day with an emphasis on those that are high in fiber, which have been associated with a decreased risk of type 2 diabetes in children and adolescents.

Weight control
Specific weight goals need to be individualized. Weight loss should occur only through modest calorie restriction, ensuring a balance between micronutrients and macronutrients. Children need to meet the physical energy requirements for normal growth and development. A primary goal related to weight is to prevent further weight gain while encouraging and promoting the child to maintain his current weight until his age matches that weight. Increased physical activity is helpful in meeting this goal. The emotional connection between food and weight status must be addressed. At times, people eat because of boredom, fear, isolation, and other stressors.

ADA CRITERIA FOR TYPE 2 DIABETES SCREENING

Currently, the American Diabetes Association (ADA) recommends screening children for type 2 diabetes if they meet the following criteria:
- overweight (body mass index of 85th percentile for age and sex, weight for height at 85th percentile, or weight 120% of ideal for height).
Plus any two of the following:
- family history of type 2 diabetes in first- or second-degree relative
- race or ethnicity (American Indian, African American, Hispanic, Asian, and Pacific Islander)
- signs of insulin resistance or conditions associated with insulin resistance (acanthosis nigricans, hypertension, dyslipidemia, polycystic ovarian syndrome).

Adapted from Alberti, G., et al. "Type 2 Diabetes in the Young. The Evolving Epidemic," *Diabetes Care* 27(7):1804, July 2004, with permission of the publisher.

Activity

Physical activity levels have decreased for people of all ages in the United States and should be reviewed with family members. Everyone should be encouraged to remain as physically active as possible. Family physical activities can be helpful for all involved and encourage sharing. Family involvement is vital to the success of lifestyle changes. A helpful suggestion is to encourage the child to take a 5-minute activity break for every 30 minutes of sedentary activity, such as watching TV or working or playing on the computer.

Screening and diagnosis

Diagnosing type 2 diabetes in children can be difficult because ketosis may be present. Evidence of ketosis may suggest type 1 diabetes. Symptoms can assist in differentiating type 1 from type 2 diabetes. (See *Differentiating type 1 and type 2 diabetes in children*.)

Ideally, some experts feel that the diagnosis of type 1 diabetes should be confirmed with antibody testing, and typical cases of type 2 diabetes with fasting C-peptide levels.

Due to more children being diagnosed with type 2 diabetes, the ADA has recommended screening at-risk children based on certain criteria. (See *ADA criteria for type 2 diabetes screening*.)

If the child meets the criteria, then screening is recommended beginning at age 10 or at the onset of puberty (if puberty has occurred before this age). Then screening is repeated every 2 years. A fasting glucose level is the preferred method of screening. The belief is that the child has longer periods in which he may need to live with the comorbidities and long-term effects of diabetes, so the sooner diabetes is identified, the sooner treatment can begin to help achieve a normal blood glucose level.

Treatment

Treatment of diabetes in children, whether type 1 or type 2, should focus on physical and psychological well-being and the prevention of long-term complications. Healthy lifestyle behaviors need to be the central theme in maintaining good health in this population.

Children with diabetes differ from adults in many respects, including insulin sensitivity related to sexual maturity, physical growth, ability to provide self-care, and unique neurologic vulnerabilities to hypoglycemia. Attention to such issues as family dynamics, develop-

DEVELOPMENTAL CONSIDERATIONS AND DIABETES MANAGEMENT

This chart summarizes the developmental tasks of the major stages of type 1 diabetes and how they can impact management of the child and his parents.

DEVELOPMENTAL STAGE (APPROXIMATE AGES)	NORMAL DEVELOPMENTAL TASKS
Infancy (0 to 12 months)	■ Developing a trusting relationship; bonding with primary caregiver(s)
Toddler (13 to 36 months)	■ Developing a sense of mastery and autonomy
Preschooler and early elementary school-age (3 to 7 years)	■ Developing initiative in activities and confidence in self
Older elementary school-age (8 to 11 years)	■ Developing skills in athletic, cognitive, artistic, and social areas ■ Consolidating self-esteem with respect to the peer group
Early adolescence (12 to 15 years)	■ Managing body changes ■ Developing a strong sense of self-identity
Later adolescence (16 to 19 years)	■ Establishing a sense of identity after high school (decisions about location, social issues, work, and education)

Adapted from Silverstein, J., et al. "Care of Children and Adolescents with Type 1 Diabetes," *Diabetes Care* 28(1):186-212, January 2005, with permission of the publisher.

mental stages, and physiologic differences related to sexual maturity all are essential in developing and implementing an optimal diabetes regimen. (See *Developmental considerations and diabetes management*.)

TYPE 1 DIABETES MANAGEMENT PRIORITIES	POSSIBLE FAMILY ISSUES IN TYPE 1 DIABETES MANAGEMENT
■ Preventing and treating hypoglycemia ■ Avoiding extreme fluctuations in blood glucose levels	■ Coping with stress ■ Sharing the "burden of care" to avoid parent burnout
■ Preventing and treating hypoglycemia ■ Avoiding extreme fluctuations in blood glucose levels due to irregular food intake	■ Establishing a schedule ■ Managing the "picky" eater; setting limits and coping with toddler's lack of cooperation with regimen ■ Sharing the burden of care
■ Preventing and treating hypoglycemia ■ Dealing with unpredictable appetite and activity ■ Using positive reinforcement to cooperate with regimen ■ Trusting other caregivers with diabetes management	■ Reassuring child that diabetes is no one's fault ■ Educating other caregivers about diabetes management
■ Making diabetes regimen flexible to allow for participation in school and peer activities ■ Learning short- and long-term benefits of optimal control	■ Maintaining parental involvement in insulin and blood glucose monitoring tasks while allowing for independent self-care for "special occasions" ■ Continuing to educate school and other caregivers
■ Managing increased insulin requirements during puberty ■ Overcoming difficulty with diabetes management and blood glucose control ■ Dealing with weight and body image concerns	■ Renegotiating parents' and teen's roles in diabetes management to be acceptable to both ■ Learning coping skills to enhance ability to self-manage ■ Preventing and intervening with diabetes-related family conflict ■ Monitoring for signs of depression, eating disorders, and risky behaviors
■ Beginning a discussion of transition to a new diabetes team ■ Integrating diabetes into new lifestyle	■ Supporting the transition to independence ■ Learning coping skills to enhance ability to self-manage ■ Preventing and intervening with diabetes-related family conflict ■ Monitoring for signs of depression, eating disorders, and risky behaviors

Because about 70% of new cases of type 1 diabetes in children don't require hospitalization upon diagnosis due to a lack of significant ketosis, outpatient care and education are the priority. These measures can be adequately provided if the health care team has experience with diabetes in the pediatric patient. The ADA recommends that for the care of children and adolescents with type 1 diabetes, each child be evaluated by a diabetes team that includes a pediatric endocrinologist, nurse educator, dietitian, and mental health professional. In addition, a complete history and physical must be completed at the time of diagnosis.

Developmental considerations
Each age-group is unique and presents challenges for maintaining healthy blood glucose levels without an increased risk of hypoglycemia. The child as well as his parents can be affected.

Infants and toddlers
Caring for an infant younger than age 1 can be particularly challenging. The parents experience a great deal of fear and stress upon hearing their child's diagnosis. In addition, the fear of hypoglycemia can be paralyzing and is justified because the infant's ability to react to hypoglycemia with the classic catecholamine response isn't yet developed. Additionally, the infant can't verbalize the complaints related to a low blood glucose level. This increases the risk of seizures and coma leading to developmental issues in the brain.

In addition, parents of children ages 1 to 3 may experience similar fears related to their child developing hypoglycemia. Temper tantrums may be due to normal growth and developmental issues, but also may be related to hypoglycemia. Children in this age-group tend to react negatively to blood glucose monitoring or insulin administration. Parents need to be aware of this, and follow through on all treatment options and assessments of hypoglycemia. A reward system for the child, such as a hug or telling the child what a good job he's done, can lead to more positive behaviors during these procedures.

Treatment of hypoglycemia in the infant or toddler can be impaired by the child's unwillingness to eat or drink the recommended 15 g of carbohydrates per day. Therefore, teach parents how to give glucagon, urging them to have the prescription filled as soon as possible so that it's readily available should the child need it. Also instruct parents in how to prepare glucagon. It's supplied in 1-mg vials of powder, which need reconstitution. Typically, the child weighing less than 44 lb (20 kg) would receive 20 to 30 mcg/kg subcutaneously or I.M. to a maximum of 1 mg. This can be expected to raise the blood glucose level within 5 to 15 minutes.

Preschool and early school-age children
The desire to be independent characterizes children in the preschool and early school ages (3 to 7). Thus, parents may find difficulty in providing and sharing care for the child. Encourage parents to allow the child to assume some role in self-management, such as testing the blood glucose level, relating feelings of hypoglycemia, or choosing foods at snack time from two or three predetermined items. The majority of care, however, remains the responsibility of the parent or caregiver. Due to wide variations in activity levels as well as willingness to eat when scheduled, hypoglycemia may remain undetected, leading to adverse effects on brain development.

School-age children
School-age children may spend as much as 8 to 12 hours away from home and their primary caregiver. They should be expected to begin to assume a much more active role in managing their diabetes. However, shared care among parents and children in the area of management decisions is vital. Children may begin to feel isolated and different in comparison to classmates, and may actually be teased and ostracized by peers. School can present additional challenges. (See "Special settings," page 210.)

Adolescents

Adolescence is a time of dramatic changes, including biological changes in conjunction with increasing physical, cognitive, and emotional maturity. Caring appropriately for diabetes can interfere with many teenagers' desire to fit in or to be like everyone else. Adolescence is an age characterized by experimentation, commonly involving drugs, alcohol, and sex, all of which can impact diabetes. In addition, this age-group reflects increased conflict with their parents. Parental supervision is still required for overall management decisions such as insulin dosages. Studies have shown poorer outcomes with adolescents left to manage their diabetes completely on their own.

Target blood glucose values

Just as children vary in their developmental level, so too, do they vary in their individual blood glucose levels. Children younger than age 6 are more prone to hypoglycemia due to their inability to communicate symptoms and their varied eating habits and activity patterns. In correlation, the ADA recommends special consideration be given to this population, identifying that target blood glucose values may need to be slightly higher to balance the increased risk of hypoglycemia and neurophysiological impairment. In addition, the child needs regular assessment for nocturnal hypoglycemia because reports show that this is a more frequent occurrence than what was previously thought. Therefore, frequent self-monitoring of blood glucose is recommended along with a target HbA$_{1c}$ level of 7.5% to 8.5% for this age-group.

Children ages 6 to 12 are the most willing age-group related to blood glucose management and intensive control. They're able to relate feelings and symptoms associated with hypoglycemia, still require adult supervision, and haven't yet experienced the increased insulin resistance associated with adolescence and puberty. Blood glucose levels need to be monitored during the school day, with the child having immediate access to treatment if needed. HbA$_{1c}$ targets for this age-group are less than or equal to 8%, with a lower goal of less than or equal to 7% if it can be achieved with minimal hypoglycemia.

In adolescence, many factors confound the ability to achieve near-normal glycemia. It's been documented that metabolic control indicated by an HbA$_{1c}$ level of less than or equal to 7% isn't achievable in most adolescents. Studies also show that near-normal blood glucose levels are seldom attainable in children and adolescents after the remission period.

Physically, puberty and the resultant hormone changes lead to increased insulin resistance in teenagers. Emotionally, they're experimenting to determine their own identity separate from their parents. They spend increasingly more time away from parents and thus parental supervision of their diabetes. Additionally, they may be engaging in risky behaviors such as unprotected sexual activity. Unprotected sex can lead to sexually transmitted diseases or unplanned pregnancies. For teen girls, this can present additional problems. (See "Pregnancy and diabetes," page 180.) Alcohol and drug abuse can lead to severe hypoglycemia if not accompanied by adequate food intake. Increased fast food consumption, erratic timing of meals, and time differences regarding school days and off days can interfere with the adolescent's diabetes management.

Nonadherence is a common problem with diabetes management in the adolescent. Girls tend to experiment with mismanagement while boys tend to try more risky behaviors. Girls are more likely to reduce the amount of their insulin in an attempt to stay thin. Teenagers experience feelings of invulnerability as well as a desire to be normal. Thus they may not take the time to check their blood glucose levels before activities such as driving. The ADA recommends that all adolescents be required to test their blood glucose levels and take appropriate action before driving.

The current recommendation for blood glucose values in adolescents and young adults is 90 to 130 mg/dl preprandially and 90 to 150 mg/dl if checked at bedtime or during the night. An HbA_{1c} level of less than or equal to 7.5% is the targeted value, with the ultimate goal of attaining a level of less than or equal to 7%.

Nutritional management

To achieve targeted blood glucose levels, care must be taken with nutritional intake and energy expenditure. Nutrition recommendations must consider the developmental stage and age of each child as well as the need to maintain blood glucose levels without excessive hypoglycemia.

Age-related considerations

Healthy eating habits are the same for children with type 1 or type 2 diabetes. Meal plans need to be individualized, taking into consideration food preferences, cultural and ethnic influences, and family eating habits and patterns as well as patterns of activity.

To determine if the child is receiving adequate nutrition, height and weight gain is documented at every visit or at least four times per year on a growth chart. If these measurements fall below the child's normal growth percentile, the child should be assessed for glycemic control, insulin insufficiency, nutritional adequacy, celiac disease, or other endocrine disorders. Mauriac syndrome is a diabetes-related growth disorder characterized by delayed sexual maturation, delayed linear growth, hepatomegaly, and joint contractures. If weight percentile is elevated, additional encouragement is necessary for healthier food choices and increased physical activity.

Children younger than age 6 usually require three meals plus three snacks

per day. The amount of sleep required based on age will influence the timing of meals and snacks and must be taken into consideration. Nighttime feedings also need to be scheduled for infants and the very young. A flexible schedule, such as every 3 to 4 hours, can help maintain blood glucose in this young population. However, feedings can become a problem when young children decide they don't want to eat. Carbohydrate counting and the use of an insulin analog after eating can assure parents of decreased episodes of hypoglycemia.

Children older than age 6 typically need three meals plus snacks in the mid-afternoon and at bedtime. This may be problematic for adolescents who may not like having to eat snacks while at school because they don't want to bring unwanted attention to themselves. Consequently, insulin requirements and types may need to be adjusted. Frequent follow-up, but at least yearly appointments, with a dietitian are important because energy requirements can change radically in children of all ages secondary to growth and development.

When participating in a scheduled activity, additional carbohydrates can be taken before the activity. Sandwiches or cheese and crackers can be good choices for younger children, while older children may choose to have a sports drink or fruit juice. If an insulin pump is being used, the pump should be removed for the activity, and can be left off for up to 2 hours. The need for additional carbohydrate intake is neutralized and the risk of hypoglycemia is decreased by this practice.

Adjustments for physical activity

It's important to note that with activity, children may develop changes in their blood glucose levels. Ten percent to 20% of hypoglycemic episodes in children occur during periods of exercise in which the frequency, duration, or intensity is greater than expected. In response, there may be an increased gluconeogenic surge causing a hyper-glycemic excursion after exercise. This can then be followed by post-activity, late-onset hypoglycemia 1 to 6 hours after completing the activity. Coaches and school personnel need to be aware of guidelines individualized for each child.

Adjustments with insulin therapy

The insulin therapy regimen for the child will also determine consistency of carbohydrate intake. When a long-acting insulin analog with rapid-acting insulin analog in a basal and bolus manner is used, the scheduling of meal-times is more flexible. In addition, this type of dosing allows for decreased concerns over hypoglycemia. However, because of the increased number of injections required, some children and their families may not choose this method of glycemic control. Intermediate-acting insulins also can be used, but will require scheduled, regular mealtimes and snack times. Moreover, a honeymoon phase is common in newly diagnosed diabetes. As the initial hyperglycemia is relieved, glucose toxicity abates, and there's some functionality of beta-cells, leading to secretion of small amounts of insulin. The beta-cells continue to deteriorate, and the need for additional exogenous insulin returns.

Insulin requirements

Determining what a child's insulin requirements are isn't based on a set formula. Typically, requirements are based on body weight, age, and pubertal status. Infants and toddlers may require small doses of insulin, which may need to be diluted. Diluents are available for specific types of insulin and can be mixed at the pharmacy or at home.

Studies have shown that a regimen of 6 to 7 insulin injections per day using a basal bolus approach is ideal. This regimen involves a long-acting insulin analog, such as insulin glargine, in conjunction with a rapid-acting insulin analog before meals and snacks. Unfor-

tunately, the required number of injections makes it an undesirable choice for many children and their families. An alternative regimen involves the administration of a rapid-acting insulin with small doses of an intermediate-acting insulin to provide coverage for meals and snacks. Thus, the insulin regimen prescribed for most children involves two to three doses of a rapid- or short-acting insulin along with intermediate-acting insulin.

Use of an insulin pump is an alternative method of administration. However, a specific age for starting pump therapy hasn't been determined.

Typically, a child newly diagnosed with type 1 diabetes receives 0.5 to 1 units/kg if the child's body weight is within 20% of the ideal body weight. However, younger children may require less. Of this amount, 50% to 65% is given to meet the child's basal needs and 30% to 50% is given as bolus doses. Basal needs usually involve the administration of insulin glargine or NPH; bolus needs are usually met with lispro, aspart, or regular insulin. Other adjustments may be necessary during the honeymoon phase, puberty, and if the child develops diabetic ketoacidosis (DKA). (See *Adjustments in insulin requirements*, page 208.)

In DKA, additional factors must be considered. Children with DKA can present with an acute abdomen. Tenderness on palpation, decreased bowel sounds, muscle guarding, or a boardlike abdomen can all lead to a misdiagnosis that would require surgery. Children also present with acute dehydration and may have lost up to one-third of their body weight due to ketosis in new-onset type 1 diabetes. Children are more likely to experience cerebral edema if blood glucose levels are decreased too rapidly. Whenever blood glucose levels reach 300 mg/dl, I.V. glucose should be added to the regimen at a rate of 3 to 5 mg/kg/minute. Dextrose in concentrations greater than 10% shouldn't be used.

ADJUSTMENTS IN INSULIN REQUIREMENTS

For the newly diagnosed child with type 1 diabetes, insulin adjustments are necessary during certain periods. This chart highlights these times and changes in insulin requirements.

TIME PERIOD	INSULIN REQUIREMENTS	CONSIDERATIONS
Honeymoon phase	0.2 to 0.6 units/kg	May last 2 weeks to 2 years Occurs in 70% of type 1 patients
Puberty	Up to 1.5 units/kg/day	May require insulin levels to be increased rapidly
Mild diabetic ketoacidosis (DKA) (can still drink and retain fluids orally)	Daily dose supplemented by 0.25 to 0.5 units/kg every 4 to 6 hours	If using rapid-acting analogs, supplement every 3 to 4 hours
Moderate (can't retain oral fluids) to severe DKA (altered mentation)	0.1 to 0.2 units/kg or regular insulin per hour as continuous infusion	Check glucose levels every hour; should drop 75 to 100 mg/dl per hour

Adapted from Silverstine, J. et al. "Care of Children and Adolescents with Type I Diabetes," *Diabetes Care* 28(1):186-212, January 2005, with permission of the publisher.

PREVENTING COMPLICATIONS OF DIABETES

Children with diabetes are susceptible to the same complications as are adults. This chart summarizes recommendations for screening and treatment for some major complications.

COMPLICATION	AGE OF INITIAL SCREENING AND FREQUENCY
Microalbuminuria	■ Yearly beginning at age 10 with a history of diabetes for 5 years
Hypertension	■ Every diabetes visit
Hyperlipidemia and cardiovascular disease	■ Children older than age 2 with family history of cardiovascular disease, hypercholesterolemia, or unknown family history ■ At puberty (>12 years), repeating every 5 years if normal, or annually if abnormal
Retinopathy	■ Initial examination at age 10 or older and having had diabetes for 3 to 5 years ■ Follow-up with annual screening
Foot problems	■ Annually beginning at puberty (> 12 years))

In children who have had diabetes for some time and then present with DKA, several factors may have precipitated the insulin deficiency, including:

● insulin omission due to fear of weight gain

● insulin omission due to fear of hypoglycemia

● insulin omission due to rebellion from authority

● emotional stress

● eating disorders

● neglect or mismanagement

● interruption in insulin pump delivery.

Frequent bouts of DKA require investigation. Parents should remain involved with adolescents on insulin therapy, at least in a management or supervisory position.

Screening for complications

Like adults with diabetes, children are susceptible to the same long-term complications. Therefore, they need to be screened for possible risk factors and long-term complications. (See *Preventing complications of diabetes.*)

Hypertension

Identification and management of hypertension in children may be delayed until adulthood. However, parental hypertension is a good indicator for increased risk of hypertension in children. Children are defined as having hypertension when the average systolic or diastolic blood pressure measured on three separate occasions is greater than that of the 95th percentile for age, sex, and height. If the child's average systolic or diastolic blood pressure is greater than or equal to that for the 90th

TYPE OF SCREENING	TREATMENTS
■ Albumin-to-creatinine ratio using a timed overnight, 24-hour, or random spot urine	■ Angiotensin-converting enzyme (ACE) inhibitor
■ Appropriate-size cuff with patient seated and relaxed	■ Lifestyle interventions ■ ACE inhibitor ■ Additional antihypertensives if needed
■ Fasting lipid profile	■ Statin therapy for low-density lipoprotein >160 mg/dl ■ Additive cholesterol inhibitor if goal not achieved
■ Ophthalmologic screening	■ ACE inhibitor ■ Laser photocoagulation as needed
■ 5.07 monofilament test; assessment of pulses, skin integrity, nail condition	■ As needed ■ Nail problems such as ingrown toenails

percentile but less than that for the 95th percentile for age, sex, and height on at least three separate occasions, the child is considered to have high normal blood pressure.

Treatment recommendations for high normal blood pressure include dietary changes, increased activity levels, and weight control. Pharmacologic therapy is initiated if blood pressure isn't within acceptable levels after 3 to 6 months of lifestyle modification.

Pharmacologic interventions should be initiated as soon as the diagnosis of hypertension is confirmed. The first-line drugs of choice are angiotensin-converting enzyme (ACE) inhibitors. These agents are titrated to achieve a systolic and diastolic blood pressure that falls below the 90th percentile. Additional therapy may be necessary if target blood pressure goals aren't attained.

✳ **ALERT** *Keep in mind that ACE inhibitors are contraindicated in pregnancy. Therefore, assess for the possibility of pregnancy in all females who are menstruating.*

Cardiovascular disease
The incidence of cardiovascular disease in adults with diabetes is well documented, and has been related to the amount of glycemic control as well as blood pressure values. While data are lacking in young children, it's reasonable to assume some of the same pathology will apply. Screening for dyslipidemia in children should be performed on those older than age 2 if there's a family history of cardiovascular disease, hypercholesterolemia, or if family history is unknown. All children older than age 12 should be screened initially and then every 5 years if the results are normal.

Treatment for high lipid levels should be based upon the low-density lipoprotein (LDL) level. Limited amounts of saturated fats, weight control, glycemic control, and increased exercise can prove beneficial for some children. In the event the LDL is greater than 160 mg/dl, statin therapy should be started in children older than age 10 with the addition of ezetimibe if the cholesterol goal isn't achieved.

Special settings
Because children may spend extended periods away from home in school or at a day care, the ADA wrote the "Diabetes Care in the School and Day Care Setting" that highlights many important concepts. Several federal laws exist to help protect children with diabetes. They include:
● section 504 of the Rehabilitation Act of 1973
● the Individuals with Disabilities Education Act of 1991
● the Americans with Disabilities Act.

Under these laws, children should be guaranteed safe, nondiscriminatory care. Diabetes care in the daytime setting for children is vital so that they can maintain good glycemic control and perform academically to their potential.

A key component of the child's plan requires coordination and communication among the child's parent or guardian, the child's diabetes health care team, and school or day care personnel. The plan needs to specifically define the responsibilities of all involved, including the child. (See *Sample diabetes management plan for the school setting*.)

Diabetes camps
Another environment for the child with diabetes where he might be away from parents or guardians for extended periods is at a diabetes camp. This type of camp provides an invaluable opportunity for the child to be with others who have the same condition that he does while still in a safe and enjoyable environment. At the same time, it's an ideal place to learn more about self-management skills. A diabetes camp also has written medical plans to guarantee safety for the camper and peace of mind for the parent or guardian. Dur-

SAMPLE DIABETES MANAGEMENT PLAN FOR THE SCHOOL SETTING

Children spend lots of time in school. To ensure good glycemic control and promote the child's optimal academic performance, a coordinated plan among all those involved must be identified. This chart provides a sample plan for managing diabetes in school.

PARENT OR GUARDIAN WILL SUPPLY	SCHOOL PERSONNEL WILL SUPPLY
1. All materials and equipment needed for diabetes care	1. Training to all who provide education or care to the student
2. Supplies to treat hypoglycemia	2. Immediate accessibility to the treatment of hypoglycemia by a knowledgeable adult
3. Information about diabetes and the performance of diabetes-related tasks	3. An adult and backup adult(s) trained in insulin administration if the Diabetes Medical Management plan indicates the need
4. Emergency phone numbers for parent or guardian and health care team	4. An adult and backup adult(s) trained to administer glucagon if the Diabetes Medical Management plan indicates the need
5. Information about the student's snack and mealtimes	5. A location in the school to provide privacy during testing and insulin administration if desired by the student
6. Signed confidentiality release allowing school personnel to communicate with the student's diabetes team	6. An adult and backup adult(s) responsible for the student who will know the schedule of the student's snack and mealtimes
	7. Permission for the student to see school medical personnel upon request
	8. Permission for the student to eat a snack anywhere, anytime if necessary to prevent hypoglycemia
	9. Permission to miss school without consequence for required medical appointments
	10. Permission for the student to use the restroom and have access to fluids as needed
	11. An appropriate location for insulin and glucagon storage if necessary

Adapted from American Diabetes Association. "Diabetes Care in the School and Day Care Setting," *Diabetes Care* 29(Suppl 1):S49-355, January 2006, with permission of the publisher.

ing camp, a written record is kept of all blood glucose levels, insulin dosages, and activities.

Hypoglycemia is the main issue when at camp due to increased levels of activity and decreased accessibility to food. As a result, initial insulin doses are commonly decreased by 10% to 20% upon arrival.

DIABETES IN ELDERLY PEOPLE

As people age, many symptoms of diabetes are mistakenly accepted as normal age-related changes. Increased urination may be attributed to bladder muscle relaxation, which can interfere with the person's ability to control urination, or the use of diuretics. Additionally, the decrease in visual acuity and increased levels of fatigue are thought to be normal alterations in physical abilities. As a result, the vague, nonspecific symptoms are dismissed as nonsignificant, thus delaying the diagnosis of type 2 diabetes. It's only when the older adult sees a health care practitioner for a complication of hyperglycemia that the diagnosis of diabetes is made.

Factors affecting the elderly patient

As type 1 diabetes generally develops in people younger than age 30, newly diagnosed diabetes in older adults is predominantly type 2. As people age and gain weight, the risk of type 2 diabetes increases, with at least 20% of people older than age 65 having diabetes.

Weight and activity

As a person ages, weight gain increases, especially around the abdomen, thereby increasing the distribution of fat to muscle and leading to central obesity. Visceral fat has been identified as a more reliable indicator for the risk of diabetes than subcutaneous fat. Women with higher levels of visceral fat have a threefold increased risk of diabetes, while men have a 30% increased risk.

Additional muscle changes, such as muscle wasting, decreased muscle mass, and changes in muscle fibers also contribute to increased insulin resistance. Impaired insulin resistance is further exacerbated by a decrease in physical activity. Arthritis, joint diseases, and de-

creased muscle mass and strength as well as changes in visual acuity can limit physical ability, thereby hindering activity levels experienced at a younger age. Although aerobic exercise is beneficial to anyone with diabetes, elderly patients may not be able to participate due to physical limitations. However, progressive resistance training can improve physiological and psychological function, change body composition, and improve glucose homeostasis, resulting in improved quality of life.

While many people may be hesitant to begin an exercise program or routine, stressing the social and personal aspects of such activities can provide additional motivation. Studies have shown that discussing the importance of making lifestyle changes has a positive effect on a person's decision to make those changes. Therefore, all health care practitioners need to be aware of the role they play in influencing positive lifestyle changes such as exercise. Moreover, studies reveal that small changes are seen as more acceptable and are more easily accomplished, leading to feelings of success rather than failure.

Changes in nutrition

Limited mobility not only affects insulin sensitivity, but it can impair the older adult's ability to get fresh foods, especially if he has transportation issues. These factors may lead to the use of frozen meals, canned foods high in sodium, and other ready-to-eat options. Commonly, the patient is aware of healthier food options but may not be able to access or afford them. Malnutrition may be further affected by depression, social isolation, alcohol use, or cognitive impairment. The death of a spouse, retirement, and other major changes can lead to loneliness, boredom, and depression, which in turn can impact nutritional habits. Various resources are available for the elderly person in relation to nutrition, including:

- food stamps
- Meals On Wheels

- social services
- community nutrition sites
- in-home aids
- adult day care centers.

In addition, changes in dentition can impact nutritional intake, both in food choices and the amount eaten. As teeth are lost or denture fit deteriorates, softer foods become easier to chew. In combination with a decreased ability to taste sweet, sour, salty, and bitter tastes, the older adult may experience an increased desire for higher concentrations of sugar and salt, which can further cause an elevation of blood sugar and blood pressure. Carbohydrates in particular are easy to chew, taste good, and can be inexpensive for someone on a fixed income. Coarse fiber and protein-containing foods may be avoided due to the increased need for mastication. Approximately 40% of people older than age 65 don't have the teeth necessary to chew foods. Health care practitioners should identify persons with rapid weight loss or weight gain or persons who are underweight, overweight, or who have had recent lifestyle changes and assess them for nutritional intake.

Sensory changes

In people older than age 65, 28% to 55% have some form of hearing impairment, particularly in relation to the ability to hear higher tones. If there's a question about the hearing ability of the patient, it's important to ask open-ended questions rather than yes-no questions to differentiate if the information was truly understood or if the person is too embarrassed to admit his inability to hear clearly. Speak slowly and clearly, but don't shout and avoid using higher pitches if possible. Facing the patient while speaking to him can help get his attention. It's important to remember that the patient with a hearing impairment doesn't necessarily have an impaired ability to understand the information given. Commonly the patient with low literacy level can retain large amounts of spoken information.

Neurologic changes

Neurologic changes can present the largest area of concern whenever working with older adults. As patients age, they experience slower learning and processing time, have slower reactions, and have an increased risk of organic brain diseases. Memory loss, especially of more recent events, can make teaching basic day-to-day living skills a challenge. Sensory overload from the array of new information can lead to a further inability to retain that information. This in turn can lead to frustration and irritation, causing the patient to feel inferior and unable to care for himself. In addition, hyperglycemia can lead to impaired learning and retention, deficits in concentration and attention span, and the use of verbal reasoning.

Information should be provided in short sessions, with clear, simple instructions. Literacy levels also decrease with time away from school, and it's been determined that the average person can be considered to be 3 to 5 grade levels below the grade they last completed. For example, if an older man attended school through the 8th grade, his reading level may actually be at the 3rd grade reading level. Avoid using medical language, and provide information in everyday language. Written information is important and should be easy to read and printed on colors that are easy to see despite age-related changes. Dark letters should be used on a light background to further assist the older person.

Glucose regulation to near-normal levels can help to maintain cognitive performance as well as improve learning and memory. Cognitive impairment can lead to poorer adherence to prescribed therapy, worsening glycemic control, and increasing the risk of hypoglycemia. An assessment of the cognitive and affective domains should be made on the initial visit and periodically thereafter. In adults with diabetes and its comorbidities, the prevalence of depression is double than those without diabetes.

Cultural considerations

The prevalence of diabetes in older Americans is higher among Blacks, Latinos, Pima Indians, Micronesians, Scandinavians, and male Japanese. Elderly Latinos have twice the rate of diabetes as non-Latino Whites. Blacks and Latinos tend to have poorer glucose control than do other groups.

In an attempt to identify racial differences, the Health, Aging, and Body Composition Study was done and involved a cross-sectional analysis of 468 patients with diabetes. Participants were nondisabled Blacks and Whites, ages 70 to 79. Results revealed that Blacks of all ages were two times more likely to have poor glycemic control compared to Whites. When attempting to identify the rationale for this, several factors were suggested. One was the increased likelihood of Blacks to be on insulin. (They couldn't identify if this was due to increased disease severity.) A second factor was related to quality of care delivered, and the third factor was the level of self-care for each group. A systematic review of diabetes self-care interventions for older Blacks or Latinos lacked information in this area. Only 12 studies were identified, thereby revealing the need for additional research.

Comorbidities

Comorbidities in the older population can also impede the diagnosis of diabetes or may contribute to an increased risk of long-term complications. Normal cardiovascular changes, including systolic hypertension, common in people older than age 50; decreased cardiac output; peripheral vascular disease; and conduction defects can all be exacerbated by chronic hyperglycemia. Older adults with metabolic syndrome have a 38% increased risk of a coronary or cerebrovascular event due to arterial wall stiffness and increased intima-media thickness. Hyperglycemia then leads to increased lipid levels and further atherosclerosis. The Diabetes Control and Complications Trial and the United Kingdom Prospective Diabetes Study have demonstrated the significant reduction in negative outcomes with improved glycemic control.

Adverse cardiovascular events are directly related to increasing levels of blood pressure, which is compounded by an age-related increase in systolic blood pressure. In adults with type 2 diabetes, approximately 30% to 50% have hypertension, and 20% to 40% of those with impaired glucose tolerance have hypertension. Studies show that people older than age 80 who are treated for hypertension experience a reduction of 34% in strokes, 22% in major cardiovascular events, and 39% in heart failure.

Complications

Elderly patients with diabetes can experience macrovascular and microvascular complications that can significantly impact quality of life.

Macrovascular

For people with diabetes, macrovascular complications account for more than 80% of deaths in this population. Coronary artery disease is two to four times higher, and peripheral vascular disease with diabetes leads to a 15 times greater risk of amputations. So it's important that such patients be educated about modifiable risk factors.

Microvascular

Microvascular complications account for many additional problems in older adults with diabetes. When diabetes is present for more than 20 years, there's a 90% prevalence of ophthalmic complications, including cataracts, macular degeneration, glaucoma, and retinopathy. What's more, renal complications are the most common single cause of end-stage renal disease in the United States and Europe, with 55% of all cases occurring in adults with diabetes older than age 60. Peripheral neuropathy, the most common complication among older patients, develops in approximately 60% to 70% of patients having diabetes for over 10 years.

Renal and urinary system changes associated with aging include a decreased glomerular filtration rate (GFR), altered ability to concentrate or dilute urine, decreased renin production, and decreased response to antidiuretic hormone, leading to increased nocturia, decreased bladder capacity, increased residual volume, and involuntary detrusor contraction. These complications can all lead to an exacerbation of preexisting hypertension, an inability to assess for urinary changes, and a decreased renal threshold. Adults age 55 who haven't been diagnosed with high blood pressure have a 90% lifetime risk for developing hypertension.

Neuropathy is usually caused by diabetes. However, cigarette smoking is also a significant risk factor. Treatment is palliative, supportive, and aimed at relieving symptoms.

Due to poor vision and reduced mobility, older patients may not be able to accurately perform a foot self-examination. Health care practitioners need to be increasingly vigilant in assessing and inspecting an elderly patient's feet. In a study of diabetes nurse educators, these areas were considered the most important to include in foot care education:
● foot and nail care, including daily washing, moisturizing, and routine inspection
● proper footwear (shoes), including cautions related to bare feet
● general health measures, including temperature control and ways to promote circulation
● prompt attention to problems and foot emergencies.

Hyperosmolar hyperglycemic nonketotic syndrome

Age-related changes also include incomplete vasoconstriction and vasodilation as well as an increased risk of heat loss. In hyperglycemia, dehydration is a common result; however, as typical symptoms of dehydration — common with hyperglycemia — aren't as readily identified, the risk of hyperosmolar hyperglycemic nonketotic syndrome (HHNS) increases. HHNS is overlooked at times, identified as other illnesses or conditions. In the elderly patient, especially in one who lives alone and doesn't check his glucose level on a regular basis, HHNS may go unrecognized for several weeks. In elderly patients, mortality rates are higher with HHNS than with DKA for several reasons, including delay in diagnosis, severe metabolic changes, and the complications of comorbidities.

HHNS is a life-threatening emergency that's characterized by four main clinical features — severe hyperglycemia with levels greater than 600 mg/dl, absence of significant ketosis, profound dehydration, and neurologic changes. At times, neurologic signs may present with hemisensory deficits, hemiparesis, aphasia, and seizures resembling an acute stroke. As the dehydration is treated and glucose level returns to normal, the symptoms revert to normal.

Dehydration is also more profound in HHNS because elderly patients experience a decreased thirst mechanism, have fewer GI symptoms than with DKA, and therefore delay seeking treatment.

Other precipitating factors for HHNS in elderly patients include:
● myocardial infarction
● severe burns
● severe diarrhea
● GI hemorrhage
● uremia
● arterial thrombosis
● hemodialysis or peritoneal dialysis
● infections
● hypertonic feedings (prolonged I.V. therapy with parenteral nutrition or high-protein or gastric tube feedings)
● alcohol abuse
● medications (steroids, diuretics, propranolol [Inderal], phenytoin [Dilantin])

- pancreatitis
- trauma.

Elderly patients and their families need to be educated on the possibility of HHS and the aggravating and precipitating factors to help prevent it.

Hypoglycemia

Just as high glucose level can be a medical emergency for the older adult, so too can hypoglycemia. Due to normal age-related changes, elderly patients have a slower glucagon response, may have slowed and erratic intestinal absorption, and a decreased response time. Older adults have more neuroglycopenic signs and symptoms (dizziness, weakness, delirium, confusion) associated with hypoglycemic reactions, which can be mistaken for a neurologic disease.

The decreased GI motility and absorption associated with aging can impact how a patient should treat hypoglycemia and may in fact contribute to episodes of hypoglycemia. If a person is using sulfonylurea or insulin therapy with set peak times and there's a delay in food digestion secondary to decreased motility, hypoglycemia can result. In addition, if the person has autonomic neuropathy manifested by gastroparesis, many of the symptoms of gastroparesis may be assumed to be normal age-related changes. These symptoms may include:

- heartburn
- reflux
- anorexia
- early satiety
- nausea
- abdominal bloating
- weight loss
- stomach spasms.

Similar to the manner in which hypoglycemia is treated with patients on alpha-glucosidase inhibitors, rapid-acting glucose, such as glucose tablets or milk, must be used to treat bouts of hypoglycemia and considered for the elderly patient with gastric motility.

The risk of falling is increased even with mild bouts of hypoglycemia. In persons with peripheral neuropathy, balance may already be an issue. When complicated by hypoglycemia, the ability to remain standing may not be possible. Falls are the leading cause of nonfatal injury in the older population, and persons with diabetes have an increased risk of fractures. This type of injury may lead to temporary placement outside of their usual environment for additional care, which in turn can exacerbate cognitive deficits.

Pharmacologic therapy

In the older patient with diabetes, renal changes impact pharmacologic therapy when medications are excreted primarily through the renal system. Insulin requirements are also affected by renal impairment, with less insulin required whenever the GFR is less than 50 ml/ minute. (See *Medication considerations for the elderly patient with diabetes*.)

Polypharmacy, the use of multiple medications, is common in older patients due to multiple conditions associated with diabetes. In addition, it can lead to adverse effects that further exacerbate comorbidities. When possible, combination drugs that can reduce the actual number of pills that a person has to take can help promote compliance.

Regular review of the patient's medications, including over-the-counter medications, is important. Question him directly about the use of herbal supplements, vitamins, minerals, and home remedies. When prescribing new medication, changing the dose of existing medication, or discontinuing a medication, provide the patient with written instructions as to how to take the medication in relation to food, time of day, and possible adverse effects to watch for or which medication should be stopped.

Also ask patients about adherence to the prescribed regimen, including if the medication is being taken as ordered. Commonly, when on a fixed income,

MEDICATION CONSIDERATIONS FOR THE ELDERLY PATIENT WITH DIABETES

This chart highlights some of the commonly used medications for elderly patients with diabetes and the precautions that are necessary when they're prescribed.

MEDICATION	ADVANTAGE	PRECAUTION
Sulfonylurea	■ ↑ Glycemic control Usually well tolerated	■ Hypoglycemia ■ Metabolized in liver, excreted by kidney
Non-sulfonylurea secretagogues: Nateglinide (Starlix)	■ Short half-life ■ Rapid onset, rapid absorption ■ Taken only if meal is eaten ■ Fewer GI adverse effects than with repaglinide	■ Use with caution with moderate to severe liver disease ■ Excreted primarily in urine ■ Hypoglycemia possible, less likely than with sulfonylureas
Repaglinide (Prandin)	■ Short half-life ■ Rapid onset, rapid absorption ■ Taken only if meal is eaten ■ Can be used with caution with impaired kidney or liver function	■ Excreted primarily via bile, metabolized by liver ■ Hypoglycemia possible, less likely than with sulfonylureas
Metformin (Glucophage)	■ ↓ Triglycerides and low-density lipoproteins ■ ↓ Hypoglycemia ■ ↓ Weight gain	■ Contraindicated in heart failure or renal insufficiency ■ ↑ Risk of lactic acidosis ■ ↑ GI adverse effects
Thiazolidinediones	■ ↓ Triglycerides ■ ↓ Risk of hypoglycemia ■ May be used with impaired renal function	■ Contraindicated in heart failure (class IV/V) ■ Discontinue if alanine aminotransferase > 2.5 times upper normal limits
Alpha-glucosidase inhibitors	■ ↓ Risk of hypoglycemia in monotherapy	■ GI-related adverse effects ■ Contraindicated in renal dysfunction, inflammatory bowel disease, colonic ulcerations, cirrhosis ■ Require treatment with glucose or dextrose if used in combination therapy
Insulin therapy	■ ↑ Glycemic control ■ ↑ Quality of life, if symptoms of hyperglycemia had been limiting ■ Variety of delivery devices available	■ Assess cognitive ability, manual dexterity, and visual acuity ■ ↑ Risk of hypoglycemia

elderly people will take their medication less often to help decrease costs. A cross-sectional national survey of adults with diabetes regarding problems paying out-of-pocket medication costs showed that a total of 19% cut back on medication use in the previous year, 11% cut back on diabetes medications specifically, and 7% reported cutting back on their diabetes medications at least once a month. Another disturbing finding was that 28% of participants had gone without food or other essentials to pay their medication costs, resulting in 14% increasing their credit card debt and 10% borrowing money to pay for their medication. Of those with identified financial burdens, few reported having a health care practitioner give them information or other assistance to deal with medication cost pressures.

Clinicians need to actively identify patients with diabetes who are facing medication cost pressures and assist them by modifying their medication regimens, helping them understand the importance of each prescribed medication, providing information on sources of low-cost drugs, and linking patients with appropriate programs to cover therapy. Explaining the rationale behind the use of medications despite a lack of symptomatology as well as various lifestyle changes and the impact they may have on the reduced need for medications may assist patients in choosing to eat healthier, increase their activity levels, and take medications as prescribed.

Implications for treatment
As America ages, more patients will be diagnosed with type 2 diabetes. This complex, progressive, and multisystem disease requires vigilant health care practitioners to assist and enable these patients to lead better quality lives. A complete geriatric assessment should be made at the initial visit because it's been shown to reduce mortality, increase the chance of remaining independent and at home, reduce hospital admissions, and improve quality of life. Open communication needs to remain integral in all aspects of care because each person has a concept of what his last decades of life should be. Emphasis needs to be placed on diabetes, which may be considered of lesser importance than age-related problems. In 2004, the European Diabetes Working Party for Older People recommended that all

health care practitioners achieve these global standards:
- Treat patients with dignity and respect at all times.
- Inform patients about all services that may benefit them, acknowledging their rights to choice.
- Work in partnership with other health care practitioners and agencies to plan care and services.
- Plan diabetes care that's determined by a patient's physical, emotional, mental, and social needs.
- Ensure the availability of appropriate, reliable, and timely services, which are equally accessible to all patients with diabetes.

THE HOSPITALIZED PATIENT WITH DIABETES
The patient with diabetes who requires hospitalization poses significant challenges. Although the exact prevalence isn't known, diabetes was listed as a diagnosis on hospital discharges in approximately 12% of cases. The patient admitted to the hospital may have a medical history of diabetes that was previously diagnosed, undiagnosed diabetes, or hospital-related hyperglycemia. Hyperglycemia in the hospital may be the result of stress or problems with managing type 1 or type 2 diabetes. Additionally, it may be the result of iatrogenic causes due to the administration of certain pharmacologic therapies, such as corticosteroids or vasopressors.

Hypoglycemia also is common in the hospital setting. This may be due to a wide range of possible factors, such as altered nutrition, cardiac failure, renal or hepatic dysfunction, malignancy, infection, and sepsis. Other possible triggers may include:
- reduction in corticosteroid dose
- the patient's inability to report symptoms
- reduced oral intake or a change to nothing-by-mouth (NPO) status
- vomiting
- changes in the administration of I.V. glucose solutions

● interruption of enteral or parenteral nutrition
● altered level of consciousness due to anesthesia.

Regardless of the reason, goals of therapy focus on managing the underlying condition requiring hospitalization, avoiding hypoglycemia, and maintaining optimal glycemic control. A multidisciplinary approach is necessary.

Recommendations for pharmacologic therapy

For the patient with type 2 diabetes, oral antidiabetic agents are discontinued and replaced with insulin. If the patient is NPO, such as in preparation for a procedure, a regular insulin infusion or a reduced dose of long- or intermediate-acting insulin and short-acting insulin in conjunction with an I.V. infusion of dextrose 5% in water is given. If the patient can tolerate food, a subcutaneous injection of intermediate- and short-acting insulin may be given.

Patients with type 1 diabetes who are seriously ill or who are to receive general anesthesia and surgery should receive insulin administered as a continuous I.V. infusion or a subcutaneous injection of a reduced dose of long-acting insulin.

As with any medication, adjustments are highly individualized to meet the patient's needs. Evidence indicates that mortality, morbidity, and health care costs are improved when targeted glucose control is achieved in the hospital.

Nutrition

Nutritional therapy in the hospital must be addressed. Typically, a dietitian is a member of the multidisciplinary team. Nutritional therapy needs to reflect the patient's underlying condition and typical eating patterns and lifestyle habits. In addition, the patient's specific treatment goals, targeted glucose level, and medications must be considered.

Blood glucose testing

The patient with diabetes should have an order for blood glucose testing. The results should be readily available on his chart for all members of the multidisciplinary team. Due to the ease and ready access, bedside blood glucose monitoring is commonly done. If the patient is eating, blood glucose levels are obtained before meals and at bedtime. If the patient is NPO, then levels are tested every 4 to 6 hours. However, if the patient is receiving continuous I.V. insulin therapy, blood glucose levels are monitored every hour until they're stabilized. Then levels are checked every 2 hours.

Target goals for blood glucose levels differ depending on the patient's acuity. For the critically ill patient, targeted blood glucose levels should be as close to 110 mg/dl (6.1 mmol/L) as possible, with the uppermost range at less than 180 mg/dl (10 mmol/L). For the patient not considered critically ill, targeted goals are:
● 90 to 130 mg/dl (5 to 7.2 mmol/L) before meals
● less than 180 mg/dl (10 mmol/L) after meals.

In addition, if the patient with diabetes doesn't have an HbA_{1c} level available within the past 2 to 3 months, he should have an HbA_{1c} level obtained before discharge.

Education

As with any patient with diabetes, education is essential. It should include information about the disorder and treatment. The patient new to diabetes requires sufficient information to allow him to be safe at home. This type of education is termed "survival skills" education and is followed up in the home with additional care. If the patient is new to insulin or blood glucose testing, these areas also need to be addressed before discharge. Additionally, the patient hospitalized for an acute situation related to diabetes management or inadequate management at home also needs education. In most cases, a referral for home care follow-up is indicated. (See chapter 12, Daily care regimens, for information about daily care, and the appendix Patient-teaching aids.)

*Selected references*_____

Alberti, G., et al. "Type 2 Diabetes in the Young: The Evolving Epidemic," *Diabetes Care* 27(7):1798-811, July 2004.

American Association of Diabetes Educators. *A Core Curriculum for Diabetes Education: Diabetes and Complications,* 5th ed. Chicago: American Association of Diabetes Educators, 2003.

American Diabetes Association. "Gestational Diabetes Mellitus," *Diabetes Care* 27(Suppl 1):S88-90, January 2004.

American Diabetes Association. "Preconception Care of Women with Diabetes," *Diabetes Care* 27(Suppl 1):S76-78, January 2004.

American Diabetes Association. "Standards of Medical Care in Diabetes," *Diabetes Care* 28(Suppl 1):S4-36, January 2005.

Anderson, R.J., et al. "The Prevalence of Comorbid Depression in Adults With Diabetes: A Meta-analysis," *Diabetes Care* 24(6):1069-78, June 2001.

Barrs, V.A., and Blatman, R.N. "Obstetrical Management of Pregnancy Complicated by Diabetes Mellitus" [Online]. Available at: *www.utdol.com/ application/topic/print.asp?file= maternal/7964&type=A&selected.*

Bernstein, R.K. *Dr. Bernstein's Diabetes Solution.* Boston: Little, Brown, and Company, 2003.

Blazing, M.A., and O'Connor, C.M. "Coronary Heart Disease in the Elderly: Risk Factors, Presentation, and Evaluation" [Online]. Available at: *www.utdol.com/application/topic/print. asp?file=chd/13432.*

Blazing, M.A., and O'Connor, C.M. "Management of Angina Pectoris in the Elderly: [Online]. Available at: *www.utdol.com/application/topic/print. asp?file=chd/51332.*

Bloomgarden, Z.T. "Type 2 Diabetes in the Young: The Evolving Epidemic," *Diabetes Care* 27(4):998-1010, April 2004.

Briars, R. "Care of the Child with Diabetes in the Acute Care Setting." Presentation at the CDE networking dinner, Dyer, Ind., October 2005.

Buchanan, T.A., and Xiang, A.H. "Gestational Diabetes Mellitus," *The Journal of Clinical Investigation* 115(3):485-91, March 2005.

Castaneda, C., et al. "A Randomized Controlled Trial of Resistance Exercise Training to Improve Glycemic Control in Older Adults With Type 2 Diabetes," *Diabetes Care* 25(12):2335-41, December 2002.

Chin, M.H., et al. "Developing a Conceptual Framework for Understanding Illness and Attitudes in Older, Urban African Americans With Diabetes," *The Diabetes Educator* 26(3):439-49, May-June 2000.

Chobanian, et al. "The Seventh Report of the Joint National Committee on Prevention, Evaluation, and Treatment of High Blood Pressure: The JNC 7 Report," *JAMA* 289(19):2560-72, May 2003.

Clausen, T.D., et al. "Poor Pregnancy Outcomes in Women with Type 2 Diabetes," *Diabetes Care* 28(2):323-28, February 2005.

Dabelea, D., et al. "Increasing Prevalence of Gestational Diabetes Mellitus (GDM) Over Time and by Birth Cohort: Kaiser Permanente of Colorado GDM Screening Program," *Diabetes Care* 28(3):579-84, March 2005.

de Rekeneire, N., et al. "Racial Differences in Glycemic Control in a Well-functioning Older Diabetic Population: Findings from the Health, Aging and Body Composition Study," *Diabetes Care* 26(7):1986-92, July 2003.

Department of Reproductive Health and Research (RHR), World Health Organization. "Systematic Review on Maternal Mortality and Morbidity Monitoring and Evaluation" [Online]. Available at: *www.who.int/reproductive-health/global_monitoring/mortality. html.*

Dye, C. J., et al. "Insights from Older Adults with Type 2 Diabetes: Making Dietary and Exercise Changes," *The Diabetes Educator* 29(1):116-27, January-February 2003.

Halvorson, M., et al. "Unique Challenges for Pediatric Patients with Diabetes," *Diabetes Spectrum* 18(3):167-73, 2005.

Horvat, S.L. "Diabetes and Pregnancy." Lecture, Gary, Ind., September 2004.

Hypponen, E., et al. "Prenatal Growth, BMI, and Risk of Type 2 Diabetes by Early Midlife," *Diabetes Care* 26(9):2512-17, September 2003.

Jovanovic, L. "Medical Management of Type 1 and Type 2 Diabetes Mellitus During Pregnancy" [Online]. Available at: *www.utdol.com/application/topic/print.asp?file=maternal/6670.*

Jovanovic, L. "Prepregnancy Counseling in Women with Diabetes Mellitus" [Online]. Available at: *www.utdol.com/application/topic/print.asp?file=maternal/4940.*

Kanaya, et al. "Adipocytokines Attenuate the Association Between Visceral Adiposity and Diabetes in Older Adults," *Diabetes Care* 27(6):1375-80, June 2004.

Karch, A.M. 2007 *Lippincott's Nursing Drug Guide.* Philadelphia: Lippincott Williams & Wilkins, 2007.

Kaufman, F.R. *Diabesity: The Obesity-Diabetes Epidemic that Threatens America — and What We Must Do To Stop It.* New York: Bantam Books, 2005.

Kim, C., et al. "Gestational Diabetes and the Incidence of Type 2 Diabetes," *Diabetes Care* 25(10):1862-68. October 2002.

Langer, O., et al. "Overweight and Obese in Gestational Diabetes: The Impact on Pregnancy Outcome," *American Journal of Obstetrics and Gynecology* 192(6):1768-76, June 2005.

Manning, F.A. "The Fetal Biophysical Profile" [Online]. Available at: *www.utdol.com/application/topic/print.asp?file=antenatl/8316* [2005 November 23].

Martinez, N.C., and Tripp-Reimer, T. "Diabetes Nurse Educators' Prioritized Elder Foot Care Behaviors," *The Diabetes Educator* 31(6):858-68, November-December 2005.

McCulloch, D.K. "Definition and Classification of Diabetes Mellitus" [Online]. Available at: *www.utdol.com/application/topic/print.asp?file=-diabetes/9879&type=A&selected* [2005 November 23].

McCulloch, D.K. "Glycemic Control and Vascular Complications in Type 2 Diabetes Mellitus" [Online]. Available at: *www.utdol.com/application/topic/print.asp?file=chd/13432* [2005 November 23].

McCulloch, D.K., and Munshi, M. "Treatment of Diabetes Mellitus in the Elderly" [Online]. Available at: *www.utdol.com/application/topic/print.asp?file=diabetes/18477&type=A&selected* [2005 November 23].

Meece, J. (2003). *Type 2 diabetes and the older adult.* Retrieved November, 20, 2004 from Novo Nordisk Pharmaceuticals, Inc.

Ogunyemi, D. "Diabetes in Pregnancy. Lecture, Gary, Ind., January 2005.

Owen, K.R., et al. "Etiological Investigation of Diabetes in Young Adults Presenting with Apparent Type 2 Diabetes," *Diabetes Care* 26(7):2088-93, July 2003.

Pagana, K.D., and Pagana, T.J. *Diagnostic and Laboratory Test Reference,* 5th ed. St. Louis: Mosby–Year Book, Inc, 2001.

Palmer, J.P., and Hirsch, I.B. "What's in a Name: Latent Autoimmune Diabetes of Adults, Type 1.5, Adult-onset, and Type 1 Diabetes," *Diabetes Care* 26(2):536-38, February 2003.

Peveler, R.C., et al. "The Relationship of Disordered Eating Habits and Attitudes to Clinical Outcomes in Young Adult Females with Type 1 Diabetes," *Diabetes Care* 28(1):84-88, January 2005.

Piette, J.D., et al. "Problems Paying Out-of-pocket Medication Costs Among Older Adults With Diabetes," *Diabetes Care* 27(2):384-91, February 2004.

Riskin, A., and Haney, P.M. "Infant of a Diabetic Mother" [Online]. Available at: *www.utdol.com/application/topic/print.asp?file=neonatal/7268&type=P&selected* [2005 November 23].

Sarkisian, C.A., et al. "A Systematic Review of Diabetes Self-care Interventions for Older, African American, or Latino Adults," *The Diabetes Educator* 29(3):467-79, May-June 2003.

Saydah, S.H., et al. (2005). "Pregnancy Experience Among Women With and Without Gestational Diabetes in the U.S., 1995 National Survey of Family Growth," *Diabetes Care* 28(5):1035-40, May 2005.

Scuteri, A., et al. "The Metabolic Syndrome in Older Individuals: Prevalence and Prediction of Cardiovascular Events," *Diabetes Care* 28(4):882-87, April 2005.

Silverstein, J., et al. "Care of Children and Adolescents with Type 1 Diabetes," *Diabetes care* 28(1):186-212, January 2005.

Simon, E.R. "Gestational Diabetes Mellitus: Diagnosis, Treatment, and Beyond," *The Diabetes Educator* 27(1):69-74, January-February 2001.

Skelly, A.H., et al. "Self-monitoring of Blood Glucose in a Multiethnic Population of Rural Older Adults With Diabetes," *The Diabetes Educator* 31(1):84-90, January-February 2005.

Stanley, M., et al., eds. *Gerontological Nursing: Promoting Successful Aging with Older Adults.* Philadelphia: F.A. Davis Co., 2004.

Stuebe, A.M., et al. "Duration of Lactation and Incidence of Type 2 Diabetes," *JAMA* 294

Walker, J. "Health Literacy: An Overview." Lecture, Merrillville, Ind., September 2003.

Research

People with diabetes and those who care for them are eager for a cure. Since insulin's discovery in 1922, there's been considerable progress to understand and treat diabetes. The hope for a cure is realistic; however, considerable work remains.

PANCREAS-RELATED RESEARCH

Ideally, a replacement pancreas — one that senses the blood glucose level and responds with appropriate amounts of insulin and related hormones — is one goal of research. A replacement pancreas may remove symptoms of diabetes, hopefully for life. Research is investigating various methods of pancreas and islet beta-cell transplantation to help patients with diabetes.

Pancreas transplantation

Pancreas transplantation procedures began in the 1960s. However, it wasn't until the mid-1980s that the procedure was used more widely. This was in part due to the cost, with inadequate or no insurance coverage for reimbursement. Additionally, tremendous advancements have been made in organ preservation, surgical techniques, and immunosuppressive drugs. As a result, outcomes have improved dramatically.

Two methods of pancreas transplantation are available:
- whole-organ transplantation
- islet beta-cell transplantation.

Greater risk is involved with whole-organ transplantation, but it also offers the greatest benefit — the potential for insulin independence. Although about 6,000 potential cadaver donors are available each year, only 50% of those are suitable for transplantation.

Whole-organ pancreas transplantation

Typical candidates for pancreas transplantation are people without insulin secretion (people with type 1 and some with type 2 diabetes), who are non-obese, younger than age 50, and have difficulty controlling blood glucose. Because of the risk for severe hypoglycemia or diabetic coma in patients with type 1 diabetes, these candidates are preferred.

Contraindications for pancreatic transplantation include:
- uncontrolled heart disease
- active infection
- positive serology for human immunodeficiency virus or hepatitis B surface antigen
- malignancy within the past 3 years
- current or active substance abuse
- history of noncompliance or psychiatric illness
- active untreated peptic ulcer disease
- irreversible liver or lung dysfunction
- other systemic illness that would prevent or delay recovery.

Procedure

Whole-organ transplantation involves identifying a tissue-compatible donor (one that won't be rejected by the recipient's immune system) and surgically transplanting the organ.

The procedure can be done simultaneously with a kidney transplant, after a kidney transplant, or as a pancreas transplant alone. Another type of pancreas transplantation involves using only the distal portion of the pancreas supplied by a living donor. This type of transplantation is rare because of the controversy about using only a portion of the pancreas. In addition, the donor supplying the portion of the pancreas is at risk for developing problems with glucose tolerance.

Today, simultaneous transplantation of the pancreas and kidneys is the most common type of whole organ transplant being performed. Technical failures are lowest with simultaneous pancreas-kidney transplants. Results of studies demonstrating its effectiveness have shown that more than 75% of the patients receiving this type of transplantation have experienced normal glucose levels for approximately 1 year after the transplantation, with about 50% of the recipients continuing this level 5 years after the transplantation. Additionally, this type of transplantation is most advantageous because it provides the greatest life expectancy.

Two approaches may be used to transplant a whole pancreas depending on where the pancreatic drainage is directed: enteric drainage technique and bladder drainage technique.

Enteric drainage technique. The enteric drainage technique is preferred because it's associated with a decreased incidence of complications, compared to the bladder drainage technique, including acidosis, dehydration, and infection.

With the enteric drainage technique, the superior mesenteric and splenic arteries of the donor are connected to the patient's iliac artery. The donor's portal vein is attached to the patient's iliac vein. The segment of duodenum at the head of the donor pancreas is then anastomosed to a portion of the patient's small bowel, usually the jejunum. In this way, pancreatic secretions drain directly into the GI tract for reabsorption, allowing carbohydrates and lipids to be metabolized normally. (See *Enteric drainage technique for SPK transplantation.*)

Bladder drainage technique. The bladder drainage technique employs the same arterial and venous anastomoses as the enteric drainage technique. However, the donor pancreas and duodenum are anastomosed to the patient's bladder (duodenocystostomy) to allow drainage of the pancreatic secretions and enzymes.

Typically, regardless of the technique used, the venous drainage empties into the systemic circulation. In some cases, the venous drainage may be directed into the superior mesenteric vein, which allows drainage directly into the portal vein. Physiologically, this is more natural; however, performing this type of drainage is more technically difficult.

Risks and benefits

Controversy exists as to how beneficial the procedure truly is. Typically, patients report an improved quality of life because they no longer need to rely on insulin injections. They also report feelings of freedom related to not worrying about hypoglycemia or restricting their food intake. However, these subjective findings are difficult to measure quantitatively.

Numerous risks are associated with the surgery. Mortality and morbidity are high. In addition, patients typically require long bouts of hospitalization and are commonly readmitted for complications, such as intra-abdominal infection (including pancreatitis and intrahepatic abscess) and graft thrombosis. The procedure is expensive, even with more in-

ENTERIC DRAINAGE TECHNIQUE
FOR SPK TRANSPLANTATION

This illustration shows simultaneous pancreas-kidney (SPK) transplantation using the enteric drainage technique to anastomose the donor pancreas and small portion of the duodenum to the patient's intestine.

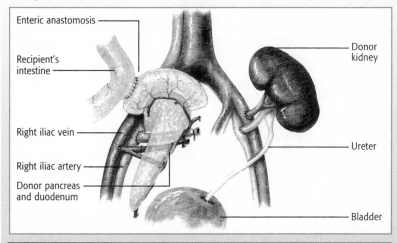

Adapted with permission from Kahn, C.R., et al. *Joslin's Diabetes Mellitus*, 14th ed. Philadelphia: Lippincott Williams & Wilkins, 2004.

surance providers now covering costs. Moreover, there's always the risk of acute or chronic rejection. (See *Key considerations after pancreas transplantation,* page 226.)

Immunosuppressive drugs are needed to prevent the recipient's body from rejecting the newly transplanted pancreas. Immunosuppression causes mouth ulcers, diarrhea, and other problems associated with immune system and bone-marrow suppression such as anemia.

Another risk is that the person may still develop posttransplant diabetes. Posttransplant diabetes has become more common as patients with transplantations experience increased survival rates. Pancreas transplantation also is accompanied by a high risk of death. The pathophysiology is complex, but is believed to be related to drugs used to induce immunosuppression. Posttransplant diabetes is higher among patients treated with the drug tacrolimus (Prograf) than those treated with cyclosporine (Sandimmune). Some have suggested that steroids used posttransplant should be cautiously reduced.

Islet cell transplantation

Islet cell transplantation began in the 1970s, but hasn't had the success of whole-organ transplantation. Technical problems have been numerous, such as extracting insulin-producing cells from the pancreas, which also makes protein-dissolving enzymes. Success is greatest using standardized collagenase, an enzyme that dissolves connecting tissue, and two to four donors' pancreatic cells in the transplantation.

KEY CONSIDERATIONS AFTER PANCREAS TRANSPLANTATION

The patient who has had a pancreas transplantation requires close, frequent monitoring. These are key areas to consider:

■ Metabolic acidosis may occur in a patient who has undergone transplantation with the bladder drainage technique. Pancreatic secretions are highly alkaline and eliminated along with urine. Some patients have an increased respiratory rate to compensate for this imbalance. If metabolic acidosis occurs, sodium bicarbonate is administered I.V.

■ In the immediate postoperative period, laboratory test results must be monitored closely, especially blood urea nitrogen (BUN) and creatinine levels as well as serum and urine amylase levels. If the patient has a wound drain in place, amylase levels in the wound drainage also are monitored.

■ Serial blood glucose, glycosylated hemoglobin, and C-peptide levels are used to evaluate graft function. In the immediate postoperative period, blood glucose level is monitored every 2 hours to evaluate the endocrine function of the pancreas, and insulin is administered if necessary. Typically, blood glucose level begins to decline in about 12 to 24 hours; the patient is euglycemic within several days of the transplantation.

■ An acute increase in pain with significant tenderness and swelling at the operative site and a marked rise in blood glucose and amylase levels suggest venous graft thrombosis, which is rarely reversible.

■ The patient's immune system has been suppressed by medication and, therefore, is at high risk for infection. Use of standard precautions and strict sterile technique is essential when changing dressings and peforming catheter care. The patient's white blood cell count is monitored closely.

■ Elevations in serum amylase and lipase may suggest rejection, but they may also suggest pancreatitis and thus aren't specific indicators for rejection. However, when the systemic bladder technique is used, urinary amylase levels may decrease. This decline typically occurs before hyperglycemia occurs and thus can be a useful marker for identifying acute rejection.

■ The only true way to confirm rejection is by pancreatic biopsy.

■ In patients having undergone pancreas-kidney transplantation, serum creatinine and BUN levels are monitored closely because rejection of the kidney and pancreas occur simultaneously and kidney function begins to deteriorate before pancreatic function does.

Procedure

Islet cell transplantation involves the injection of islet cells into the portal vein. The islet cells are obtained from the pancreas of a cadaver, which is subjected to an enzyme allowing recovery of the islet cells. A typical transplantation requires about 1 million islet cells. This usually involves the need for at least two cadaver pancreases.

After the islet cells are obtained, they're placed into the patient's liver by injection into the portal vein using a laparoscopic or transhepatic angiographic approach. The islet cells become wedged in the smaller portal vein tributaries. Here, they engraft, receiving their blood supply from the patient's vessels for growth. When implanted, the new islet cells begin to make and release insulin. (See *Understanding islet cell transplantation.*)

UNDERSTANDING ISLET CELL TRANSPLANTATION

This illustration shows the isolation of the islet cells from the donor pancreas that are then injected into the patient's portal vein for engrafting.

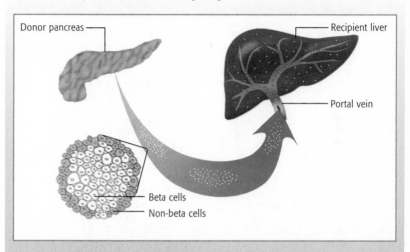

Donor pancreas

Recipient liver

Portal vein

Beta cells
Non-beta cells

Adapted with permission from Kahn, C.R., et al. *Joslin's Diabetes Mellitus,* 14th ed. Philadelphia: Lippincott Williams & Wilkins, 2004.

Risks and benefits

Islet cell transplantation, in comparison with whole organ-transplantation, is a much simpler procedure. The patient typically receives a local anesthetic, unless he can't tolerate it, in which case the surgeon may opt for general anesthesia. Usually, the procedure is less costly and considered by some to be less risky.

The development of independence from insulin is also less for islet cell transplantation when compared to whole-organ transplantation. Research has shown that the majority of patients receiving whole-organ transplantation achieved normal blood glucose levels almost immediately, whereas it took an average of 5 to 6 months for patients with islet cell transplantation to achieve this goal.

Unfortunately, the patient still requires immunosuppression to assist in keeping the islet cells functioning. Additionally, the supply of human islet cells from cadavers is limited. Thus, only a small number of patients can be treated. Moreover, not all cells transplanted engraft, with some of them being lost to local hypoxia, nonspecific inflammatory response, and localized clotting. Researchers are unclear as to why these events occur.

A University of Edmonton, Alberta, Canada group developed several refinements in islet cell transplantation. Known as the *Edmonton Protocol,* cells are transplanted immediately after extraction rather than frozen before transplantation. Patients receive at least 11,000 islets/kg of body weight. Immunosuppression is modified with the use of sirolimus (Rapamune) (low-dose tacrolimus) and corticosteroids, followed by steroid withdrawal after 3 months.

Although refinements improved survivability of the transfused cells, other problems related to immunosuppression still exist. These include the adverse effects these agents cause, such as oral ulcerations, diarrhea, edema, weight loss, hyperlipidemia, acne, menstrual irregularities, ovarian cysts, bone marrow suppression, and pneumonitis. In some cases, the complications are so severe that immunosuppression must be withdrawn. Procedural complications, such as peritoneal hemorrhage, partial portal vena cava thrombosis, and fatty liver also may occur.

Islet cell transplantation still has many problems to overcome. It's most beneficial to patients who already require immunosuppression such as those receiving kidney transplantations. Best results are obtained in centers well known for success with islet cell transplants, such as the Edmonton group.

Islet cells from other sources

The supply of available islet cells from humans for transplantation is limited. Therefore researchers are examining other sources for obtaining islet cells. These include cells from others species, such as pigs, cows, rabbits, rodents, and possibly fish.

Research has centered on the use of pig islet cells for several reasons:
● pig (pork) insulin has been used as a treatment for diabetes
● pigs have glucose levels similar to that of humans
● pigs are a component of the food chain.

However, working with pig tissue is difficult. In addition, new problems related to regulating the body's immune response to tissues from another species is cause for major concern. Moreover, a risk of retroviruses found in pig tissue may be a potential threat to humans.

Artificial pancreas

Whenever the function of glucose sensing is linked to a release of insulin, an "artificial pancreas" is created. Development of the artificial pancreas is highly anticipated. Two basic types are in development and include the closed-loop mechanical artificial pancreas and the polymeric artificial pancreas.

Closed-loop artificial pancreas

The closed-loop mechanical artificial pancreas is an electromechanical insulin pump that's controlled by a glucose sensor that's connected to a minicomputer. The minicomputer determines and controls the amount of insulin to be released into the patient's circulation.

Three types of closed-loop machines have been developed: the bedside, wearable, and implantable types. However, all of these machines have problems. The bedside type, known as the *Biostator*, was developed by Life Science Instruments. It has a double-lumen catheter: one provides continuous measurement of blood glucose and the other releases insulin. It's too large to be worn; hence, it's a bedside model.

A wearable machine was developed by Shichiri using an external glucose monitoring system based on dialysis sampling tubing. With this device, a dialysis hollow-fiber is implanted in the subcutaneous tissue, which is perfused with saline solution. Glucose concentrations are continuously measured with a needle-type extracorporeal glucose sensor. This model isn't fully developed, but will be small enough to be portable.

An implantable device, although possible, hasn't been satisfactorily developed due to the inability to create a device that's small enough with biocompatibility. Some implantable devices have resulted in the growth of "biofilms" (cellular blockage) into the release outlet, impeding insulin delivery. In other words, the autoimmune process of the host attacks the new insulin-secreting machine with immune antibodies against insulin.

Medtronic created an implantable insulin pump in the 1990s. Unfortunately, the device was 9 cm in diameter, and required surgical implantation with transcutaneous refilling of the insulin reservoir. It could be reprogrammed with a radio wave. Recharging the long-life lithium battery was problematic and sometimes requires a second surgery. Medtronic hopes to resolve problems with this pump and bring an implantable artificial pancreas to market by 2008.

Polymeric artificial pancreas
Several types of hybrid pancreatic tissue substitutes are in development. These include ethylene vinyl acetate copolymers impregnated with insulin that are sensitive to insulin levels, hydrogels that change from solid to gel based upon glucose concentration, hydrogels with phenylboronic acid, and pancreatic cells encapsulated in polymer materials for protection from the immune system. All of these pancreatic substitutes are still in development.

Islet cell replacement
Islet cell replacement research is currently being done to develop a means for producing islet cells that can be used to treat patients with type 1 diabetes. Currently, research is focusing on these areas:
- genetic engineering of nonpancreatic cells into cells that produce insulin and are sensitive to glucose
- changing stem cells or ductal cells of the pancreas into cells that produce insulin
- using nonhuman islet cells for transplantation to achieve normal glucose levels while preventing rejection.

The ultimate goal of this research is to develop procedures that would ultimately lead to restoring the body's ability to produce insulin for the patient with type 1 diabetes.

Islet cell replacement is an alternative because of the shortage of cadaver pancreases for whole-organ or islet cell transplantation. One researcher is attempting to develop human beta cells that could be transplanted. These cells would secrete insulin and function just like human beta cells. The ultimate goal is to develop this type of beta cell with the additional ability to reproduce so that there would be large numbers of cells available for transplantation. Research is also looking at the possibility of genetically manipulating these cells to reduce the risk of autoimmune attack. If successful, greater numbers of patients with type 1 diabetes would have the option of receiving an islet cell transplant to treat and potentially cure diabetes with a reduced risk of rejection.

OTHER EMERGING AREAS OF RESEARCH
The search for a cure for diabetes is ongoing. Research related to diabetes is wide ranging, including such topics as:
- earlier identification of type 2 diabetes
- improved methods for screening and identification
- reduction of risk factors for the development of diabetes
- measures to reduce the risk of complications
- types of drugs and alternative delivery systems
- noninvasive blood glucose sensing devices
- safety of fad diets for patients with diabetes.

The American Diabetes Association's Web site at *www.diabetes.org* provides a wealth of information related to current research on diabetes. In addition, the National Institutes of Health (*www.nih. gov*) and the National Institute of Diabetes and Digestive and Kidney Diseases (*www.niddk.nih.gov*) can provide additional sources for related research.

Insulin

Insulin administration can be problematic for patients. Research is ongoing to develop new, faster-acting insulins and alternative methods of delivery. Areas receiving attention include the development of transdermal, inhaled, and buccal forms of insulin. (See chapter 7, Insulin therapy, for more information.)

Diabetic complications

Complications cause numerous problems in patients with diabetes. A recent study suggested that the drug pioglitazone (Actos) significantly reduces the risk of myocardial infarction (MI) in patients with type 2 diabetes who have already suffered a previous MI. Another study is investigating the use of a class of antihyperlipidemic drugs, fibrates, to prevent diabetes-related complications, such as neuropathy and retinopathy. These drugs prevent or prolong the action of an enzyme, aldose reductase, which is responsible for changing glucose in the blood into sorbitol. Accumulation of sorbitol in the eye or nerve cells causes damage to these cells. Researchers believe that preventing or delaying this conversion can help prevent or delay the development of neuropathy and retinopathy.

Lower-extremity and foot ulcers are another area of morbidity and mortality for patients with diabetes. Although many treatments have been developed, the risk of infection and amputation is high. Studies involving the use of topical tretinoin (Retina-A) and human fibroblast-derived dermal substitute and silver dressings to treat foot ulcers show promise.

Obesity and nutrition

Studies are ongoing to determine the underlying mechanisms associated with obesity and insulin resistance. Obesity has been identified as a major contributing factor to the development of type 2 diabetes, including its development in children. In an effort to lose weight, many patients are turning to fad diets for help. This is true even for patients with diabetes. Researchers are investigating the safety of these diets, including the risk of hypoglycemia, the possibility of toxic effects due to overconsumption of vitamins and minerals, and the potential risks of nutrient deficiencies.

*Selected references*_____

Baldwin, E.J. "Fad Diets in Diabetes" *British Journal of Diabetes Vascular Disease* 4(5):333-37, 2004.

Bloomgarden, Z.T. "Transplantation and Islet Topics," *Diabetes Care* 28(1):213-19, January 2005.

Carson, S.N., et al. "Healing Chronic Infected Foot Wounds with Human Fibroblast-Derived Dermal Substitute and Sliver Dressing," *Wounds* 17(10): 282-82. Available at: *www.medscape. com/viewarticle/516861.*

Gaglia, J.L., et al. "Islet Transplantation: Progress and Challenge," *Archives of Medical Research* 36(3):273-80, May-June 2005.

Larsen, J.L. "Pancreas Transplantation: Indications and Consequences," *Endocrine Reviews* 25(6):919-46, December 2004.

Ryan, E.A. et al. "Beta-Score: An Assessment of Beta-cell Function After Islet Transplantation," *Diabetes Care* 28(2):343-47, February 2005.

Sutherland, D.E. et al. "Beta-cell Replacement Therapy (Pancreas and Islet Transplantation) for Treatment of Diabetes Mellitus: An Integrated Approach," *Transplantation Proceedings* 36(6):1697-699, July-August 2004.

Tom, W.L., et al. "The Effect of Short-contact Topical Tretinoin Therapy for Foot Ulcers in Patients With Diabetes," *Archives of Dermatology* 141(11):1373-377, November 2005.

Uchiyama, T., et al. "Implantable Polymeric Artificial Pancreas," *Journal of Biomaterials Science, Polymer Edition* 15(10):1237-262, 2004.

Weir, G. "Pancreas and Islet Transplantation," in Kahn, C.R., et al. *Joslin's Diabetes Mellitus,* 14th ed. Philadelphia: Lippincott Williams & Wilkins, 2005.

12

Daily care regimens

Patients with type 1 or type 2 diabetes require daily measures to achieve optimal blood glucose levels and prevent potential complications. These measures include self-monitoring of blood glucose (SMBG), checking urine for ketones, performing foot care, consuming an appropriate diet, engaging in physical activity, and administering prescribed medications. All of these measures are key components of patient education.

The American Diabetes Association (ADA), in collaboration with other organizations, federal agencies, and federally funded programs, has published 10 standards for Diabetes Self-Management Education. These standards were developed so that quality education concerning diabetes mellitus could be implemented in many settings with the goal of achieving successful diabetes self-management. (See *National Standards for Diabetes Self-Management Education*, pages 232 and 233.) These standards may be accessed at *www.care.diabetesjournals.org/cgi/ content/full/28/suppl_1/s72#SEC5.*

Daily care for the patient with diabetes involves a multidisciplinary approach involving various health care practitioners to develop a plan that's individualized to the patient's needs. This team includes the licensed nurse; dietitian; diabetes educator; physician, nurse practitioner, or physician assistant; social worker; and pharmacist. Some teams also include a podiatrist, behaviorist, and other health care practitioners, such as renal or neurologic specialists. Each team member provides different information and a slightly different approach, which typically results in achieving the maximum amount of education and patient and caregiver understanding. Clear, accurate communication among all team members is essential. As with any condition, assessment forms the foundation for designing effective care regimens.

ASSESSMENT

Providing care for the patient with type 1 or type 2 diabetes begins with a thorough assessment. This assessment must be comprehensive and include information about the patient's physical and psychosocial status, current level of self-care, and current knowledge level. Factors, such as stress, culture, spiritual beliefs, economic concerns, and impairments, also must be considered. Moreover, a key aspect of daily care involves the patient's ability to learn, which is directly affected by his readiness to learn and his literacy level.

Physical status considerations

Typically, the patient is instructed to check his vital signs at home. At each encounter with the patient, such as in the outpatient or hospital setting, evaluate his vital signs, including tempera-

NATIONAL STANDARDS FOR DIABETES SELF-MANAGEMENT EDUCATION

Self-management is a major aspect of diabetes care. To promote the best outcomes, standards have been developed to ensure that patients receive the most appropriate, relevant, accurate, scientifically based, and up-to-date information, regardless of the setting in which care is provided.

Standard 1
The Diabetes Self-Management Education (DSME) entity will have documentation of its organizational structure, mission statement, and goals, and will recognize and support quality DSME as an integral component of diabetes care.

Standard 2
The DSME entity will determine its target population, assess educational needs, and identify the resources necessary to meet the self-management educational needs of the target population.

Standard 3
An established system (committee, governing board, advisory body) involving professional staff and other stakeholders will participate annually in a planning and review process that includes data analysis and outcome measurements and addresses community concerns.

Standard 4
The DSME entity will designate a coordinator with an academic background or experience in program management and the care of patients with chronic disease. The coordinator will oversee the planning, implementation, and evaluation of the DSME entity.

Standard 5
DSME will involve the interaction of the patient with diabetes with a multifaceted education instructional team, which must always include a registered dietitian and registered nurse. Other team members may include a behaviorist, exercise physiologist, ophthalmologist, optometrist, pharmacist, physician, podiatrist, other health care practitioners, and paraprofessionals. DSME instructors are collectively qualified to teach the content areas.

Instructional staff must be Certified Diabetes Educators or have recent education or experience in diabetes education and management.

Standard 6
The DSME instructors will obtain regular continuing education in the areas of diabetes management, behavioral interventions, teaching and learning skills, and counseling skills.

Standard 7
A written curriculum, with criteria for successful learning outcomes, shall be available. Assessed needs of the patient will determine which of the following content areas are delivered:
- describing the diabetes disease process and treatment options
- incorporating appropriate nutritional management
- incorporating physical activity into lifestyle
- using medications (if applicable) for therapeutic effectiveness
- monitoring blood glucose and urine ketones (when appropriate) and using the results to improve control
- preventing, detecting, and treating acute complications

ture, heart rate, and respiratory rate. Obtain blood pressure readings while the patient is sitting, standing, and lying down. Compare these readings with the latest readings available from the health care practitioner as well as the patient's home recordings.

Assessment also should address the patient's and caregiver's knowledge about the rationale for checking blood pressure on a frequent basis — for example, once weekly — and his compliance with doing so and keeping a written log of readings. Ideally, the patient should have his own sphygmomanometer. However, if this isn't feasible, the patient may use a blood pressure device at a local pharmacy or hospital. Regardless of what's used to monitor blood pressure readings, it's important that the patient use the same sphygmomanometer or device each time to ensure accuracy. The patient or caregiver should bring

the written log along for review when visiting the health care practitioner at each appointment or whenever the patient goes to the hospital. The findings are then discussed.

The American Heart Association recommends that blood pressure in adults with diabetes mellitus should be maintained at 130/80 mm Hg or lower. Medication and lifestyle changes are key.

Also assess the patient's ability to take his temperature and his understanding of the rationale for doing so. The patient should take his temperature whenever he's isn't feeling well because slight elevations in temperature in a person with diabetes may signal the onset of significant illness.

Other key areas to assess related to the patient's physical status include evidence of slowed speech or responses, lack of ability to concentrate, or somatic complaints, such as sleep or eating.

Psychosocial considerations

Discuss feelings of guilt or loss of self-worth with the patient because these may suggest depression or anxiety. Depression and anxiety can occur in the patient with a chronic disease such as diabetes. Moreover, depression and anxiety may negatively effect learning ability, adherence to the care plan, and disease state.

Other important areas to address include the patient's living situation, degree of support from his family and friends, and possible stressors, such as financial concerns or the effect of changes on the patient's functional ability.

Self-care considerations

Various factors can affect a patient's ability to provide self-care. Some of these include mobility and functional status, vision, hearing, and coordination and dexterity.

Determine the patient's and caregiver's current level of self-care. Is the patient independent? Is he able to continue at this level of independence or is more care necessary at this time? Determine the extent and type of assistance that's provided by the caregiver. For example, does the caregiver provide transportation for activities such as to medical appointments and grocery shopping? Is the caregiver able and willing to continue, increase, or reduce the amount of care provided?

Assess the patient's current physical abilities. How well and safely does the patient ambulate? Is a wheelchair or other device necessary? Is the patient's vision affected and, if so, to what extent? Does this impair self-care and reduce safety?

Find out when the patient last had a retinal screening test and the results. Retinal screening tests are recommended on a yearly basis beginning with the diagnosis of diabetes mellitus. Determine if the patient complies with annual testing. If not, what's his reason for not doing so?

Also investigate if the patient has his vision tested annually as recommended. This annual testing helps to diagnose changes in vision caused by the disease. If not, what's his rationale?

If the patient wears glasses, assess the reason for the glasses and when the prescription was last changed. Observe the condition of the current glasses. For example, are the lenses clear without evidence of scratches? Do the frames fit and align properly? Does the patient notice changes in his vision? Has the patient's vision affected self-care abilities and safety? For example, can he read medication containers and medical instructions?

Assess the patient's hearing ability. Does the patient have hearing deficits and how well does he accommodate for these? When was the last time he had a hearing test?

Does the patient use a hearing aid? Is it in good working order, with a working battery? When did the patient begin using a hearing aid and what's the reason for its use? How often and under what circumstances does the patient use the hearing aid? For example, does he use it all the time or only for certain situations such as health care appointments? If the patient doesn't use the hearing aid as prescribed, determine the reason why. Not using the hearing aid correctly represents a safety issue that needs to be discussed with the patient and caregiver. In addition, does the patient understand that not using the hearing aid is a safety risk? Be sure to provide teaching about the need for proper use of the hearing aid.

Check the patient's eye–hand coordination and dexterity. Is this affecting self-care abilities and safety? For example, can he open medication containers, perform blood glucose checks, and administer medications?

Knowledge level considerations

To ensure adequate self-care, the patient and caregiver must have sufficient knowledge and the readiness and ability to learn. Assess the patient's and caregiver's general knowledge and understanding about the disease, rationale for treatment, and specific care plan and treatment goals overall and for this encounter. Also inquire about his daily management routine and practices, providing the necessary information.

To ensure adequate learning, consider the patient's literacy level and abilities. Can he read in the language used on his medication containers or teaching materials? Is larger print needed?

Also determine the patient's and caregiver's readiness and ability to learn. For example, anxiety, depression, or denial can affect the person's ability to learn, concentrate, and retain information. Would the patient's hearing or vision status affect teaching strategies?

When preparing teaching strategies, always consider patient location, room lighting, extraneous noise, room temperature, and overall patient condition. Make sure that the patient is comfortable and doesn't need to use the bathroom. Then adapt the teaching to the patient.

Daily care measures

The foundation of care for patients with diabetes mellitus remains self-care on a daily basis. Self-care should focus on SMBG, urine ketone monitoring, foot care, nutritional and dietary management, physical activity, and medication use.

Self-monitoring of blood glucose

The frequency and timing of SMBG is typically determined by the health care practitioner and individualized for each patient. It's suggested that the patient perform SMBG at a minimum of once per day, obtaining a fasting blood glucose level. This level should be set to the targeted glycemic level to achieve healthy outcomes. The target recommended by the ADA is 70 to 110 mg/dl (plasma glucose).

The ADA recommends that patients with type 1 diabetes perform SMBG at least three times per day. For pregnant women with gestational diabetes who are receiving insulin, the ADA recommends SMBG at least two times per day. For most patients with type 1 diabetes and pregnant women with diabetes who are using insulin, SMBG is recommended at least three times daily and possibly more frequently. A common routine for SMBG in patients with type 1 diabetes is testing before each meal, 2 hours after each meal, at bedtime, and during the night. Testing should be done more frequently when medication therapy changes or if the patient becomes ill, experiences unusual stress, or shows signs and symptoms of hypoglycemia.

Several glucose meters are available for SMBG. They vary in the amount of blood needed for testing, the speed to obtain results, size, ability to store results, and cost of the meter and testing strips. Newer meters are being produced with user-friendly functions, such as an increased memory for storing information, smaller size and ease of use, automatic timers, alarms, and safety features. In addition, some meters offer blood glucose level testing and insulin administration in one device.

Typically, blood for SMBG is obtained from the fingertip. However, new glucose meters allow blood specimen collection from alternative sites, such as the upper arm, forearm, base of thumb, and thigh. Although desirable, there may be some limitations with the use of alternative site testing. (See *Indications and contraindications for using alternative test sites*, page 236.)

⭐ **ALERT** *If the patient uses an alternative site, such as the forearm, teach him to rub his forearm before testing. Then advise him to choose an area that's free from hair and obvi-*

INDICATIONS AND CONTRAINDICATIONS FOR USING ALTERNATIVE TEST SITES

Although alternative site testing may cause less discomfort for the patient, be sure to warn him that these sites should *only* be used in certain circumstances, including:
■ before a meal
■ before an insulin dose
■ 2 hours after a meal, insulin dose, or exercise.
   Using alternative sites is contraindicated:
■ within 2 hours of a meal, insulin dose, or exercise
■ when blood glucose is changing rapidly
■ when blood glucose is falling
■ when there's a concern about possible hypoglycemia.
   In addition, urge the patient to use his fingertip for testing if an alternative site test result doesn't correlate with how he's feeling.

ous blood vessels. Also encourage the patient to keep the lancing device in place for approximately 5 seconds so that an adequate blood sample is obtained for testing.

Studies have shown that glucose changes in the blood are more rapidly demonstrated in the fingertips than in other parts of the body. Additionally, glucose levels in alternative sites appear to change more gradually than those at the fingertip after a meal, administration of insulin, and exercise. Alternative site testing also may require a certain type of glucose meter, such as One Touch Ultra and One Touch Ultra Smart, manufactured by LifeScan.

Patients commonly report discomfort and pain associated with the need for frequent sampling from the fingertips with multiple testing each day. This complaint can be a factor in adhering to the testing schedule. As a result, researchers have been exploring ways to obtain glucose measurements without the need for a fingerstick or ways that are minimally invasive. (See *Attempting to reduce fingerstick discomfort.*)

A major teaching aspect of SMBG is to make sure that the patient performs it

correctly. (See the appendix Patient-teaching aids.)

Reinforce the importance and rationale for maintaining tight glycemic control with the patient and caregiver.

ALERT *Keep in mind that targeted goals for glycemic control are less strict for children, especially in those ages 2 to 7. This population has a high risk of hypoglycemia due to the immaturity of counter-regulatory mechanisms and the lack of cognitive abilities in recognizing and responding to symptoms associated with hypoglycemia.*

Stress the need to document the results of each SMBG in a log or journal along with signs and symptoms that the patient is experiencing. Remind the patient to bring this log with him to office or clinic visits for review by his health care practitioner.

A key aspect of a daily care program is developing mutual outcomes or goals for care. Work with the patient and caregiver to develop appropriate goals for SMBG. These goals can help the patient view his progress in managing diabetes as well as help to promote

ATTEMPTING TO REDUCE
FINGERSTICK DISCOMFORT

The pain associated with fingersticks in self-monitoring of blood glucose (SMBG) can be a major stumbling block to patient adherence. As a result, researchers have been looking for ways to minimize this problem. The U.S. Food and Drug Administration has approved two devices — one that's minimally invasive and one that's noninvasive — for glucose testing. However, neither is intended to replace fingerstick monitoring.

The minimally invasive device uses a small catheter inserted just under the skin to collect a small amount of liquid. This liquid is then transported to a sensor in the device that measures the glucose level. The device records measurements over a 72-hour period. The results must be downloaded for review. This device is recommended for occasional use to discover patterns in glucose level during the day. The information may help the patient and health care practitioner determine the optimal times for performing SMBG.

The noninvasive device looks similar to a watch. It's worn on the patient's wrist and forearm area. Fluid is absorbed from the skin via a small sensor in a pad attached to the bottom of the device. The results can be viewed on the device. Blood glucose readings can be obtained every 10 minutes for up to 13 hours. This device is designed to track glucose level patterns and can be helpful in identifying episodes of hyperglycemia and hypoglycemia. However, the patient must check a fingerstick blood glucose level to confirm the results displayed on the device before taking action.

SETTING GOALS FOR SMBG

Encourage the patient to develop individualized goals for self-monitoring of blood glucose (SMBG). This list gives examples of appropriate goals.
- I will test my blood glucose ___ times per day and ___ times per week.
- I will record my blood glucose test results in my blood glucose log after each test.
- I will bring my blood glucose log to my health care practitioner at every visit or I'll download my blood glucose levels into my computer program every (week/month).
- My glycosylated hemoglobin will be __ % decreased in 3 months ___ (date).

compliance with the daily routine. (See *Setting goals for SMBG.*)

In addition to monitoring blood glucose levels via a glucose meter, the ADA recommends periodic testing of glycosylated hemoglobin (HbA_{1c}). This test provides an average estimate of blood glucose level and control over a 2- to 3-month period. Typically, the patient has this test performed at the health care practitioner's office or clinic setting. Testing kits are now available for home use. (See *Home HbA_{1c} testing*, page 238.)

Monitoring urine ketones

Another important aspect of daily care is urine ketone testing. The frequency and timing of testing for urine ketones is usually determined by the health care

HOME HbA₁c TESTING

Testing kits are now available for the patient to test his glycosylated hemoglobin (HbA₁c) level at home. With many of these home tests, the patient obtains a capillary blood sample (just as with daily glucose monitoring) and places the drop of blood on the test strip. Then the patient mails the test strip to the laboratory, and the results are mailed back to the patient. Some other kits allow the patient to test his blood and obtain the results at home, eliminating the need to mail in the test strip.

Although the tests have been found to be accurate, they don't replace daily self-monitoring of blood glucose. In addition, the patient needs to practice under the supervision of a health care practitioner to ensure proper technique, and thus, accuracy of results. The patient also must communicate with his health care practitioner by reporting the results to ensure that adequate glycemic control is being achieved.

practitioner. In general, testing for urine ketones is reserved for patients with type 1 diabetes who are experiencing blood glucose readings of greater than or equal to 240 mg/dl or as directed by the health care professional. The ADA recommends testing for urine ketones during times of illness and stress or when blood glucose is 300 mg/dl or more for all patients with diabetes, including pregnant women.

Tablets or strips are available for use. Some also test for glucose. Readings can be denoted by color changes and identified in various ways, such as negative, trace, small, moderate, and large or by 1+, 2+, and so on.

Make sure that the patient and caregiver understand how and when to test urine. Also make sure that the patient and caregiver can identify the color change appropriately. Remind the patient that certain medications and vitamins may cause false-positive results.

Testing for urine glucose is also available for home use, but isn't considered the gold standard; however, some patients and health care practitioners may want to use these tests as well as SMBG results.

Encourage the patient with diabetes who's testing for urine ketones to keep a written log or journal of the results, establish goals for testing, and share the results with his health care practitioner as instructed.

Foot care

Keeping blood glucose level within the target range reduces the amount of foot injuries in patients with diabetes. However, it's important that each patient with diabetes examine his footwear and feet at least twice daily — once before beginning daily activities and at the end of the day. This provides the patient with information concerning the condition of his feet so that appropriate actions may be taken rather than waiting for an actual problem to occur. If the patient can't see the plantar or lateral foot aspect, he should use a mirror or ask another person to inspect his feet. Tell the patient to look for red spots, blisters, swelling, dryness, hyperkeratosis (callus formation), corns, or cuts. (See *Causes of corns and calluses.*) If the patient notices cuts or breaks in the skin, ingrown toenails, or changes in skin or skin sensitivity, he should consult with his health care practitioner and seek appropriate care immediately.

Urge the patient to wash his feet at least once per day with mild, moisturizing soap, rinse thoroughly, and dry completely, including in between the toes. Moisturizing lotion should be applied to all foot surfaces except between toes. Advise the patient to keep his toenails smooth and trimmed straight. Tell him to trim his toenails after a bath or shower. Stress the importance of never trimming the skin around or at the end of the toenails as well as down to the corners of the nail. Warn the patient to check the temperature of the water being used to clean his feet and stress the need to avoid soaking them. If the patient desires to use foot powder after washing his feet, instruct him not to leave powder residue on his feet because this may cause excessive drying. The patient with diabetes should avoid hot water bottles, heating pads, and electric blankets to prevent burns. Tell him to avoid sunbathing his feet without sun block because this also may lead to skin damage.

Advise the patient to avoid over-the-counter foot remedies, such as ingrown toenail remover, wart remover, callus scrapers, and adhesive bandages, unless they are specifically prescribed by a health care practitioner.

If the patient's vision interferes with the ability to properly perform foot care, encourage the assistance of a caregiver or an appropriate health care practitioner to perform the care on a routine basis.

Furthermore, the patient with diabetes should elevate his feet while sitting, avoid crossing his legs, and perform ankle and toe exercises for 5 minutes two to three times per day to encourage blood flow and prevent possible circulatory problems.

As with any daily care regimen, the patient needs to develop mutual outcomes or goals for care. Work with the patient and caregiver to develop appropriate goals for foot care. These goals can help the patient view his progress in managing diabetes as well as help to promote compliance with the daily routine. (See *Setting goals for foot care*, page 240.)

Prevention and treatment of infection

Strongly encourage the patient to inform the health care practitioner of redness, swelling, drainage, corns, calluses, other skin damage, or ingrown toenails.

SETTING GOALS FOR FOOT CARE

Encourage each patient with diabetes to have goals relative to foot care. This list shows examples of appropriate goals.

■ I will inspect my feet ___ times per day and follow my health care practitioner's recommendations concerning treatment.

■ I will wear a different pair of shoes ___ times per day.

■ I will wear shoes that fit my feet and accommodate any deformities (bunions, hammertoes).

■ I won't self-treat foot problems without the express recommendation of _____, my health care practitioner.

■ I will make and keep appointments with _____, my foot care provider at least _____ times per year.

■ I will promptly inform my health care practitioner of any of these foot or leg symptoms that could suggest problems with peripheral neuropathy:
  – tingling or prickling
  – numbness or insensitivity to pain, heat, or cold
  – pain
  – burning
  – loss of balance or coordination
  – muscle weakness or changes in gait
  – increased sensitivity to light touch
  – sharp pains or cramps.

Prevention of ingrown toenails is important. Teach the patient that this condition can be caused by:

● wearing tight-fitting or high heeled shoes because they compress the toes together, causing toenails to grow abnormally

● trimming toenails so that the corners of the nail dig into the skin

● toenail infections, such as fungal infections, that cause thickening and widening of the toenail

● trauma to or near the nail

● genetics. (If a close family member has ingrown toenails, the patient is more likely to develop ingrown toenails.)

Instruct the patient about the signs and symptoms of a fungal infection, such as yellowing, peeling, or other discoloration of the nail. If any of these happen, warn the patient to consult

with his health care practitioner immediately. It's important for the patient with diabetes to understand that what may seem like a simple fungal infection may lead to a more serious bacterial infection.

If the patient develops toenail or foot fungus, such as athlete's foot, all shoes must be replaced as quickly as possible. The fungus remains in the footwear even though the patient with diabetes may be receiving treatment. For footwear that's impossible to replace, advise the patient to get an antifungal spray (refer to health care practitioner for recommendations) and to treat his footwear as indicated on the label. The footwear should also be left out in direct sunlight for a minimum of 8 hours after being treated to further destroy fungus. Hose or washable footwear should be washed in hot water with household bleach (1:10 bleach solution and hot water) and allowed to dry in direct sunlight for at least 8 hours.

The bathing facilities of the patient with diabetes who develops a fungal infection must be treated with a 1:10 bleach solution and hot water before and after each bath or shower. Additionally, bathing accessories, such as towels and facecloths, should be washed in the same bleach solution and dried either in direct sunlight or in a dryer set at the cotton drying temperature.

Footwear selection

The patient needs to be educated to wear closed-toe, closed heel, comfortable, well-fitting shoes with a broad toe box to prevent foot injuries such as blisters. Shoes should be checked before putting them on to evaluate for an intact lining, inappropriate wear, and foreign objects that might cause injury. Urge the patient to avoid going barefoot and to wear soft, cotton socks that wick moisture away from the feet.

If possible, encourage the patient to change footwear at least every 5 to 6 hours throughout the day and to have at least two pairs of shoes or footwear available at all times. For example, suggest that the patient wear one pair of shoes one day, and switch to the other pair the next day. In addition, when purchasing new footwear, the patient with diabetes should always have his feet measured because foot size changes with maturity and over time and not all footwear is manufactured to the same standard sizing. Remind the patient to be certain that the person measuring his feet is an experienced shoe fitter.

For an appropriate fit, footwear should fit the length and width of each foot, leaving room for all the toes. Shoes with pointed toes, high heels, or tight fitting around the toes should be avoided because they place too much pressure on various parts of the foot, which could lead to foot ulcers. Advise the patient to shop for new footwear at the end of the day because feet are commonly enlarged or swollen and fitting will be more accurate.

New footwear should be comfortable at the time of purchase, but should always be worn at home on carpeted floors for no more than 1 hour at a time to evaluate for rubbing or areas that could cause foot trauma. Initially the new footwear should be worn in this manner before wearing it for longer periods.

The patient with diabetes is more prone to shear and friction when walking, which may lead to forefoot calluses over time. To reduce the incidence of forefoot calluses, encourage the patient to avoid wearing shoes with a heel height greater than 1". Also suggest that the patient consider wearing cotton socks with a thick sole than those commonly available commercially. These socks may be referred to as "diabetic socks," but the consumer must know that such socks actually have thicker soles than standard socks or stockings.

There also are socks available that are impregnated with silver. However, there's no current evidence to indicate that such impregnation is more effective than plain cotton or wool socks. (See *Recommendations for shoes and socks,* page 242.)

The patient with diabetes also needs to consult with the health care practitioner before using over-the-counter foot orthotics, such as arch supports and heel protectors. Some of these may cause damage. It's important that he read the labels of foot, ankle, leg, and skin care products before using them.

Special shoes or devices may be necessary so that the patient can engage in necessary physical activity. Encourage the patient to discuss this with his health care practitioner and check with his insurance company about coverage for these items.

Diet

A good education tool for the patient or caregiver who desires a personalized diet is MyPyramid, according to the U.S.

RECOMMENDATIONS FOR SHOES AND SOCKS

Foot care for the patient with diabetes includes not just hygiene measures but also the use of properly fitting shoes and socks. Instruct him to:

- always wear socks or stockings with all footwear
- make sure that socks or stockings are ½" longer than his longest toe for proper fit
- avoid socks or stockings that are stretch or nylon or that have an elastic band or garter at the top because they restrict circulation
- avoid socks with inside seams because they'll cause pressure and may cause trauma
- never wear uncomfortable or tight shoes
- never wear shoes that rub, cut, or leave indentations or impressions on the feet
- always wear a minimum of one pair of clean socks and clean shoes every day
- change socks and shoes when they become wet because they may cause skin damage.

Department of Health and Human Services (HHS) available at: *www.MyPyramid. gov.* This site asks the patient to enter his age, current weight, and height and then produces a pyramid of what he should consume according to the most recent HHS findings. However, it's important that the patient with diabetes follow these general guidelines:

- consume many foods, selecting from the basic food groups while remaining within his body energy needs
- maintain daily physical activity
- manage his body weight through calorie intake management
- increase his daily intake of whole grains, nonfat or lowfat milk and milk products, and fruits and vegetables to meet minimum requirements and maintain good health
- carefully select carbohydrates
- select and prepare food with little or no salt
- safely prepare and store all food and beverages
- consume alcohol in moderation
- adhere to a balanced diet.

For patients with diabetes, regularity and timing of food is nearly as important as the amount of food consumed because this helps to stabilize the blood glucose level. (See chapter 5, Nutritional therapy, for a more in-depth discussion.) Foods that must be consumed in moderation are those with high levels of starch, such as biscuits, bread, cereal, pasta, rice, and certain vegetables. Low-fat cooking methods as well the removal of all visible fat from foods before cooking is strongly encouraged.

Encourage the patient with diabetes to avoid consuming foods and beverages high in sugar content, such as:

- white or brown sugar or syrup such as maple syrup
- sweet and sour sauces
- barbecue sauce
- desserts, such as cakes, pies, candy, pastries, pudding, donuts, cookies, fruit tarts, and sweet buns
- soft drinks, fruit drinks, tea, or coffee with sugar.

As with any daily care regimen, the patient with diabetes needs to develop mutual outcomes or goals for care. Work with the patient and caregiver to develop appropriate goals for diet. These goals can help the patient view his progress in managing diabetes as well as help to promote compliance with the daily routine. (See *Setting goals for diet.*)

Patient-teaching tip

SETTING GOALS FOR DIET

Encourage the patient with diabetes to set goals for diet and meal planning. This list gives examples.

■ I will eat three meals and _____ snacks on time every day. The times I will eat meals are _____, _____, and _____. The times I will eat snacks are _____.
■ I will follow my individualized Food Guide Pyramid to select healthy foods.
■ I will read the labels of all food to determine the contents and if it's a healthy choice.
■ I will control portion sizes and stop eating when I feel full.
■ I will keep a record of food and beverage intake along with my blood glucose log.
■ I will eat more low-fat foods and reduce added fat by _____ % within _____ days/weeks.

Physical activity

Physical activity is beneficial for anyone, but especially for the patient with diabetes. The ADA recommends at least 150 minutes per week of moderate intensity aerobic physical activity (at 50% to 70% of maximum heart rate) or at least 90 minutes per week of vigorous aerobic exercise (at greater than 70% of maximum heart rate). Activity should be done over at least 3 days per week with no more than two consecutive days without physical activity. The ADA also recommends resistance exercise three times per week for people with type 2 diabetes. For the patient with diabetes who can achieve this goal, results have shown:

● increased metabolism and muscle mass, which burns calories; increased glucose uptake; and lowered blood glucose levels
● improved body response to insulin
● reduced or eliminated need for diabetes medications in some patients
● maintenance of strong flexible muscles and joints
● reduced incidence of falls and fall-related injuries
● lower cholesterol levels and reduced blood pressure
● improved circulation
● reduced stress
● reduced risk of heart disease and stroke.

Encourage the patient who's sedentary to discuss the most appropriate fitness program with his health care practitioner and to select activities that are enjoyable, avoid injury, and complement his schedule and lifestyle. (See *Activities and calories expended,* page 244.)

Encourage the patient to keep track of his physical activity along with his blood glucose levels and share this information at every visit to his health care practitioner. Assist the patient with diabetes to become more active after a health check-up and with his health care practitioner's approval. Some of the ways to encourage the more sedentary patient to become more successful at adding exercise to daily life is to:

● assist him in choosing a physical activity that he wants to do
● suggest that he establish goals to include what clothing he'll wear or other items that will be needed — for example, tennis racket and balls
● assist him in selecting the days, times, and length of time for the activity and when he'll add to the activity
● assist him in determining a warm-up and cool-off plan for each activity
● encourage him to plan alternative activities if the weather doesn't permit the activity
● encourage him to seek out a partner (this is commonly the encouragement

ACTIVITIES AND CALORIES EXPENDED

When planning physical activity for a patient with diabetes, it's important to include activities that he can perform as well as enjoy. This helps to promote compliance with the routine. This chart highlights some common activities and an estimate of the amount of energy (calories) expended.

ACTIVITIES	CALORIES/HOUR*	ACTIVITIES	CALORIES/HOUR*
Sitting quietly	80	**Strenuous activity** Jogging (9-minute mile) Swimming	580
Standing quietly	95		
Light activity Office work Housework Playing golf	240	**Extremely strenuous activity** Running (7-minute mile) Racquetball Skiing	740
Moderate activity Walking briskly (3.5 mph) Gardening Cycling (5.5 mph) Dancing	370	*For example, in a healthy 140-lb (63.5-kg) female. If the patient weighs more than 140 lb, she'll probably burn more calories per hour. If the patient weighs less, she'll probably burn fewer calories per hour.	

that the patient needs to stick with an activity plan) and a method to measure his progress

● encourage him to determine how to reward himself for his accomplishments — for example, buying a new outfit in a smaller size, going out to a movie, or taking a trip to a museum or library.

As with any daily care regimen, the patient needs to develop mutual outcomes or goals for care. Work with the patient and caregiver to develop appropriate goals for physical activity. These goals can help the patient view his progress in managing diabetes as well as help to promote compliance with the daily routine. (See *Setting goals for physical activity.*)

SKIN CARE MEASURES

When blood glucose level is elevated in the patient with diabetes, the skin tends to be dry and more susceptible to bacte-

ria. Therefore, the first rule of skin care for the patient with diabetes is keeping his blood glucose level at target to prevent excessive dryness and infection. Patient goals related to skin and wound care typically include checking the skin for rashes, cuts, bruises, or other changes every day and attending to them immediately and keeping keep a skin and wound care kit readily available for use.

Bathing

Skin must be kept clean and as dry as possible at all times. Wherever skin touches skin, such as in the axillary, groin, or pannus areas, use of an after-bath or shower body powder is important to reduce friction, shear, and moisture accumulation.

Water temperature

When bathing, the patient should be warned to avoid hot water to prevent po-

SETTING GOALS FOR
PHYSICAL ACTIVITY

Encourage the patient with diabetes to set goals for physical activity. This list gives examples of appropriate goals.

- I will make and keep an appointment with _____, my health care practitioner, to discuss recommendations for increasing my physical activity by _____ (date).
- I will walk ____ steps per day for _____ months.
- I will obtain a pedometer to count my steps by _____ (date).
- I will park my car farther away whenever I'm driving.
- I will take the stairs rather than the elevator or escalator.

---

tential burns and excessively dry skin. It's important to keep home hot water heaters set at or below 110° F (43.3° C) to prevent potential burns.

The patient with diabetes needs to test all heated water before stepping or submerging into it to prevent skin damage. This is especially important when the patient is away from home and the temperature of the water is unknown.

Another reason for avoiding the use of hot water is that it tends to cause skin dryness, leading to further skin damage, such as cracks and tears. For this same reason, bubble baths also should be avoided.

Management and prevention of dry skin

The ADA recommends the use of moisturizing soaps, such as Dove or Basis, to reduce skin drying. After bathing, the use of an oil-in-water lotion or cream, such as Lubriderm or Alpha-Keri, is also recommended to further reduce skin drying. However, some experts prefer water-based lotions or creams. Urge the patient to discuss the use of moisturizers with his health care practitioner.

Instruct the patient to avoid applying the lotion or cream between his toes because this may encourage fungal growth. However, moisturizer should be applied to the top and bottom of the feet and allowed to absorb.

Furthermore, it's important to prevent dry skin. When the environment is cold, windy, or dry, moisturizing skin may need to be done more often than once or twice daily. During these times, bathing may need to be less frequent. In addition, the home environment should be kept more humid. Even in humid environments, patients with diabetes are more likely to have dry skin or dry skin in particular areas such as the feet. Scratching dry or itching skin should also be discouraged to prevent creating an open wound.

The patient with diabetes also should use skin moisturizers with adequate sunblock to prevent sunburn, another skin drying condition. The sunblock should be reapplied as indicated on the label. Wearing clothing that protects the skin from the sun is also recommended for all exposed areas. In addition, encourage him to wear dark-colored sunglasses whenever he's in the sun because this helps to reduce cataract development.

Female patients with diabetes are warned to avoid feminine hygiene spray. These are excessively drying and may alter the normal flora of the vaginal and perineal areas, possibly leading to yeast infections.

Mild shampoos are recommended to prevent excessive dryness of the scalp and hair. If skin, scalp, or hair problems don't completely resolve in a few days, urge the patient to contact the health care practitioner. The care of a dermatologist may be necessary.

Remind the patient that when he's taking prescribed antibiotics and his blood glucose levels aren't kept within target goal, fungal skin rashes may develop. Advise the patient that if he discovers such a rash with or without itching in skin folds or elsewhere, he should immediately consult with his health care practitioner or a dermatologist.

Treatment of problems

All cuts or wounds should be treated immediately. If the injury is minor, wash the area with tepid water and soap, rinse it thoroughly, and cover it with a sterile bandage. Cleaners, such as alcohol, hydrogen peroxide, iodine, or mercurochrome, should be avoided because they're too harsh and cause significant drying of the wound bed and edges. Antibiotic creams, ointments, or impregnated bandages should only be used on the advice of an appropriate health care practitioner. If an injury, burn, or infection is more than minor, a health care practitioner needs to be consulted immediately to prevent serious harm and complications, such as cellulitis or sepsis.

HEALTH PROMOTION SCREENING AND CARE MEASURES

Patients with diabetes are at risk for complications that can be life-threatening. Therefore, the patient needs to use measures to minimize the risk of developing complications. In addition, the patient should undergo screening as recommended to detect problems that may develop.

Oral health measures

Diabetes mellitus increases the risk of mouth infections and periodontal disease. These complications may result in tooth loss, bone or gum infections, and difficulty in keeping blood glucose lev-
els at target and under control. Patients with diabetes are also at greater risk for developing dry mouth syndrome, which may result in oral thrush. They may also have elevated levels of glucose in saliva, which may cause any of the above conditions. Therefore, it's important that patients with diabetes understand the need for dental care and health. (See *Oral care*.)

Additionally, suggest that the patient with diabetes contact the National Institute of Dental and Craniofacial Research for additional information and free booklets and wallet cards for oral health for diabetics. The site for this multilingual information is available at: *www.nidcr.nih.gov/*.

Vision and eye care measures

Diabetes mellitus is the leading cause of blindness in adults ages 16 to 74. Therefore, it's imperative that all patients with diabetes understand the symptoms, management, and prevention of vision and eye problems. The most common eye or vision problems experienced include glaucoma, retinopathy, cataracts, and blurred vision. The cause of the first three problems is thought to be elevated blood glucose levels. However, the cause for most of the complaints of blurred vision isn't definitive at this time. Some evidence suggests that blurred vision may actually be caused by a condition known as *dry eye*. If this is the case, it may be helpful to increase the consumption of foods high in omega-3 fatty acids, which are found in salmon, herring, tuna, and sardines.

The patient needs to be aware of the signs and symptoms of retinopathy. Advise him to notify his health care practitioner immediately if he experiences floating spots. This is commonly the first symptom. Other symptoms that should be immediately reported include:
- double or blurred vision
- rings, halos, or flashing spots

ORAL CARE

Keeping the mouth, teeth, and gums healthy is essential in preventing problems associated with diabetes. Make sure that the patient understands the need for good oral care. Include these topics in your teaching plan:

■ maintaining target blood glucose levels
■ informing the individual's dentist about the diagnosis, current medications or other treatments, and keeping the dentist updated
■ daily brushing and flossing of teeth; more often if recommended by the dentist
■ inspecting his mouth daily for evidence of a bad taste in the mouth; white patches; loose, sensitive, or painful teeth; or areas of soreness and reporting such symptoms promptly to the dentist
■ notifying the dentist promptly if:
  – gums are sore, red, or swollen
  – gums are bleeding
  – gums are pulling away from the teeth so that they appear longer than normal
  – his bite feels different.
■ notifying the dentist promptly of ill-fitting dentures and sores in the mouth (if a denture wearer)
■ keeping dentures and oral orthotics clean
■ getting regular dental check-ups
■ stopping smoking
■ adhering to the recommendations of his dentist about oral care.

● blank spots in visual field
● pain or pressure in or around one or both eyes
● vision loss in one eye
● difficulty seeing out of the corner of one or both eyes. (See chapter 9, Management of complications, for more information on diabetic retinopathy.)

Cataracts and glaucoma are other vision problems facing patients with diabetes. The major symptom of cataracts is loss of clarity or cloudy vision. Glaucoma causes a loss of vision from the sides of one or both eyes.

Additionally, changes in one or both eyes or changes in vision in a patient with diabetes should be immediately reported to an appropriate health care practitioner.

✷ **ALERT** *Advise pregnant women with diabetes to undergo appropriate prenatal care that includes vision testing within the first trimester.*

For patients and caregivers who want additional information about the potential effects of diabetes on eyes and vision, refer them to the National Eye Institute — 2020 Vision Place, Bethesda, MD 20892-3655, 301-496-5248. The Web site address is: *www.nei.nih.gov.*

Kidney health measures

Patients with diabetes need education about kidney function and how high blood glucose levels and high blood pressure may cause kidney damage, leading to kidney failure. The kidneys filter waste from the body and keep protein in. In the presence of high blood glucose levels or high blood pressure, the kidneys can't filter effectively, allowing protein to leak out of the kidneys and into urine. Called *proteinuria*, waste begins to back up into the body.

The best way to manage kidney damage is to prevent it. Educate the patient with diabetes to keep his blood glucose at target levels by following the care plan determined by his health care practitioner. It's also important for the patient to understand that maintaining target blood pressure will also help prevent diabetic nephropathy. This can be done by following the care plan determined by the health care practitioner and may include antihypertensive medication. It's vital that the patient continue taking prescribed blood pressure medication even if he feels fine.

In addition, the patient needs to inform the health care practitioner if he has signs and symptoms of a bladder or kidney infection, including:

● pain or burning with urination
● frequency of urination or the frequent urge to urinate
● cloudy or reddish urine color
● foul-smelling urine
● presence of pain in the back or side
● elevated temperature.

Urge the patient to complete all medical treatments prescribed for kidney or urinary bladder ailments — for example, finishing all antibiotics as ordered. Educate the patient with diabetes of the importance of adhering to the minimum of an annual visit with his health care practitioner that includes testing the urine for microalbuminuria.

MINOR ILLNESS MANAGEMENT

In the event of minor illnesses, it's important that the patient with diabetes mellitus has a sick day plan that's been developed before the need arises. (See *General sick day rules*.)

There are specific areas of self-management that must be included in this teaching plan that focus on medication and diet.

Medication

All medication for the patient with diabetes should be taken during times of illness, including insulin, regardless of the administration method. Oral medications should also be taken unless the patient is too nauseated or has vomiting and diarrhea for 6 hours and can't take the prescribed medications.

In this case, it's important to contact the health care practitioner for recommendations. The patient needs education about the use of over-the-counter medications. Advise him to always verify the sugar and alcohol content and use those that are sugar- and alcohol-free when possible. It's also important for the patient to be aware that some medications, such as decongestants, cold remedies, and corticosteroids, can raise the blood glucose level. Therefore, it's important for the patient to monitor his blood glucose level during illness.

In general, the patient with type 1 diabetes should test blood glucose and urine ketones every 4 hours during illness that alters his ability to eat, drink, or take prescribed medication according to the care plan. If the blood glucose level is at or above 240 mg/dl even though the patient has taken the extra insulin suggested in the sick day plan, the patient should notify the health care practitioner.

Blood glucose and urine ketones should be monitored at least four times per day for the patient with type 2 diabetes. If he takes oral medications and his blood glucose level is at or above 240 mg/dl before meals and remains at this level for 24 hours, he should notify the health care practitioner. If there are moderate amounts of urine ketones, the patient should also contact the health care practitioner. Maintaining blood glucose and urine ketone levels at target during illness requires the combined efforts of the patient and the health care practitioner.

Warn the patient to notify the health care practitioner when he experiences symptoms of ketoacidosis, dehydration, or other serious conditions, such as chest pain, difficulty breathing, fruity breath odor, or dry and cracked lips or tongue.

ALERT *Remind the patient that large amounts of aspirin or products containing aspirin may inter-*

GENERAL SICK DAY RULES

It's essential for the patient with diabetes to notify his health care practitioner when illness occurs. This list gives some general guidelines for managing sick days that can be included in the teaching plan.

- Notify the health care practitioner that you're ill.
- Monitor blood glucose level at least every 4 hours.
- Test urine for ketones, especially when your blood glucose level is greater than 240 mg/dl (13.8 mmol/L).
- Continue medications, such as insulin or oral antidiabetics.
- To prevent dehydration, drink plenty of sugar-free liquids every hour that you're awake.
- Continue to eat meals at regular times.
- If unable to tolerate solid food due to nausea, consume more easily tolerated foods or liquids equal to the carbohydrate content of a regular meal.
- Call the health care practitioner for any of these danger signals:
  - persistent nausea and vomiting
  - moderate or elevated ketones
  - blood glucose elevation after two supplemental doses of insulin
  - high (101.5° F [38.6°C]) temperature or increasing fever or fever for more than 24 hours.
- Treat symptoms (diarrhea, nausea, vomiting, and fever) as directed by your health care practitioner.
- Get plenty of rest.

act with other diabetes medications. This is specifically true with oral hypoglycemic agents. The patient taking these prescribed medications who ingests large quantities of aspirin may experience symptoms of hypoglycemia. Monitor the blood glucose level closely.

Diet

The patient with diabetes who's ill needs to consume his regular diet if possible. For the patient with type 1 diabetes, fluids are a vital component of a diet plan during illness. It's important for him to ingest at least 4 oz of clear liquids every hour and consume light foods, such as crackers or soup. If the patient can't tolerate solid food because of nausea, encourage him to eat more easily tolerated foods or liquids equal to the carbohydrates of the patient's regular meal.

For the patient with type 2 diabetes, continuing with the regular diet when

possible is also a key component of sick day management. If this isn't possible, he should replace carbohydrates with toast, crackers, or soup and replace fluids with no-calorie soda or ginger ale. The health care practitioner may recommend that the patient alternate no-calorie soda with sugar-added soda. Consuming crackers and easily digested soups helps to replace sodium and chloride, which can be lost during illness. If possible, the patient with diabetes should also ingest small amounts or orange juice or bananas to replace potassium that may be lost.

In both types of diabetes, the patient should eat and drink small amounts more frequently than when not ill even though he may have little or no appetite. To help ensure an adequate carbohydrate intake when ill, provide the patient with examples of foods and fluids that can be used. (See *Food and fluid options*, page 250.)

FOOD AND FLUID OPTIONS

To ensure adequate carbohydrate intake during illness, the patient may need some suggestions for appropriate food options. This list of foods and amounts are equivalent to 15 g of carbohydrates.

- ½ cup (4 oz) apple juice
- ½ cup (4 oz) orange juice
- ½ cup (4 oz) regular soda
- 1-stick Popsicle
- ½ cup (4 oz) Gatorade or similar sports drink
- 6 saltine crackers
- 1 cup skim milk
- ½ cup (4 oz) unsweetened applesauce
- ½ cup (4 oz) regular ice cream
- ¼ cup (2 oz) sherbet
- 1 cup (8 oz) plain or artificially sweetened yogurt (not frozen)
- ½ cup (4 oz) frozen yogurt
- ½ cup cooked cereal
- ½ cup (4 oz) regular Jell-O
- 1 piece of unbuttered toast

In the event of nausea, vomiting, or diarrhea, the patient should use small amounts of crushed ice or 1 to 2 oz of decarbonated regular soda or ginger ale. To accomplish decarbonation, stir or leave the beverage uncovered, allowing the carbonation to escape.

Make sure that the patient who lives alone has a contact person or persons available that he can call if he's ill. If the patient doesn't live alone, it's equally important to inform a competent person in the house of his illness. This plan is to enable someone to check on the patient with diabetes and respond appropriately if necessary.

Finally, it's important for the patient with diabetes to keep emergency contact numbers in an easily accessible location. This includes his health care practitioner and emergency health care telephone numbers and local emergency numbers such as paramedics.

Additionally, the patient should carry some type of medical alert identification with him at all times with pertinent information related to medical history, treatment, and health care practitioner for contact in case of an emergency.

MEDICATION REGIMENS

The type of diabetes, the length of time the patient has had the disease, how well he can maintain target blood glucose levels, cardiovascular risk factors, age, body weight, comorbid conditions, and physical activity all have a role in what medications are prescribed. Regardless of the medication prescribed, the patient must be able to:

- name each prescribed medication
- describe the rationale for the use of each prescribed medication
- explain unique or special storage requirements for each medication
- describe the action to take if a dose of medication is missed
- explain special or unique actions to be taken with each medication, such as self-monitoring of blood pressure if taking oral antihypertensives and watching for ease of bruising if taking aspirin or anticoagulants such as warfarin (Coumadin)
- describe the storage requirements of blood glucose monitoring meters and strips
- describe known drug allergies
- describe the symptoms of hypoglycemia and hyperglycemia, including actions to be taken and rescue medications to have available at all times.

Additional self-care measures for the patient taking insulin include demonstrating competency in preparing the insulin in the syringe, mixing insulins in one syringe, administering insulin correctly, and rotating injection sites. Insulin is described in greater detail in chapter 7; other drug therapy is discussed in chapter 6.

*Selected references*_____

American Diabetes Association. "Standards of Medical Care in Diabetes," *Diabetes Care* 28(suppl 1):S4-36, January 2005.

"Blood Glucose Meters and Data Management Systems" [Online]. *Diabetes Forecast Resource Guide*. Available at: *www.diabetes.org/uedocuments/rg06_meters.pdf.*

Kahn, C.R., et al. *Joslin's Diabetes Mellitus*, 14th ed. Philadelphia: Lippincott Williams & Wilkins. 2005.

Mensing, C., et al. "National Standards for Diabetes Self-Management Education," *Diabetes Care* 28(Suppl 1):S72-79, January 2005.

National Diabetes Information Clearinghouse (NDIC). "Preventing Diabetes Problems: Keep Your Eyes Healthy" [Online]. Available at: *www.diabetes.niddk.nih.gov/dm/pubs/complications_eyes/index.htm.*

National Diabetes Information Clearinghouse (NDIC). "Preventing Diabetes Problems: Keep Your Feet and Skin Healthy" [Online]. Available at: *www.diabetes.niddk.nih.gov/dm/pubs/complications_feet/index.htm.*

National Diabetes Information Clearinghouse (NDIC). "Preventing Diabetes Problems: Keep Your Teeth and Gums Healthy" [Online]. Available at: *www.diabetes.niddk.nih.gov/dm/pubs/complications_teeth/index.htm.*

United States Food and Drug Administration. "Glucose Meters and Diabetes Management" [Online]. Available at: *www.fda.gov/diabetes/glucose.html.*

"Urine Testing" [Online]. *Diabetes Forecast Resource Guide*. Available at: *www.diabetes.org/uedocuments/rg06_urine.pdf.*

Part

3

APPENDICES

TAKING CARE OF YOUR FEET

Dear Patient:

Because you have diabetes, your feet require meticulous daily care. Why? Diabetes can reduce the blood supply to your feet, so normally minor injuries, such as an ingrown toenail or a blister, can lead to a dangerous infection. Because diabetes also reduces sensation in your feet, you can burn or chill them without feeling it. To prevent foot problems, follow these instructions.

Routine care

- Wash your feet in warm, soapy water every day. To prevent burns, use a thermometer to check the water temperature before immersing your feet.
- Dry your feet thoroughly by blotting them with a towel. Be sure to dry between your toes.
- Apply oil or lotion to your feet immediately after drying to prevent evaporating water from drying your skin. Lotion will keep your skin soft. Don't put lotion between your toes.
- If your feet perspire heavily, use a mild foot powder. Sprinkle lightly between your toes and in your socks and shoes.
- File your nails even with the end of your toes. Don't cut them. Don't file the corners of your nails at a sharp angle or file them shorter than the ends of your toes. If your nails are too thick, tough, or misshapen to file, consult a podiatrist. Don't dig under toenails or around cuticles.
- Exercise your feet daily to improve circulation. Sitting on the edge of the bed, point your toes upward and then downward 10 times. Then make a circle with each foot 10 times.

Special precautions

- Make sure that your shoes fit properly. Buy only leather shoes (because they allow air in and out), and break in new shoes gradually, increasing wearing time by ½ hour each day. Check worn shoes frequently for rough spots in the lining.
- Wear clean cotton socks each day. Don't wear socks with holes or darns or those that have rough, irritating seams.
- Consult a podiatrist to treat corns and calluses. Self-treatment or application of caustic agents may be harmful.
- If your feet are cold, wear warm socks or slippers and use extra blankets in bed. Avoid using heating pads and hot water bottles. These devices may cause burns.
- Check the skin of your feet daily for cuts, cracks, blisters, or red, swollen areas.
- If you cut your foot, no matter how slightly, contact your health care professional. Wash the cut thoroughly and apply a mild antiseptic. Avoid harsh antiseptics, such as iodine, which can cause tissue damage.
- Don't wear tight-fitting garments or engage in activities that can decrease circulation. Especially avoid wearing elastic garters, sitting with your knees crossed, picking at sores or rough spots on your feet, walking barefoot, or applying adhesive tape or bandages to your feet.

PROTECTING YOUR SKIN

Dear Patient:

Exposure to the sun, or even to fluorescent lights, may make your condition worse. Excessive exposure, in fact, may cause rashes, fever, arthritis, and even damage to the organs inside your body.

However, you don't need to spend your waking hours in the dark to be safe. Just follow these precautions.

Prepare for going outdoors

Wear a wide-brimmed hat or visor to shield yourself from the sun's rays. Protect your eyes by wearing sunglasses. Put on a long-sleeved shirt and trousers to filter out harmful rays. In hot weather, choose clothing made of lightweight, loosely woven fabrics such as cotton.

Buy a sunscreen containing PABA (para-aminobenzoic acid) with a skin protection factor of 30 to 45. If you're allergic to PABA, choose a PABA-free product offering equivalent sun protection.

Before you go outside, rub the sunscreen on unprotected parts of your body, such as your face and hands. Read the label to determine how often to reapply it. Usually, you'll use more after swimming or perspiring.

Avoid strong sunlight

Try to stay indoors during the most intense hours of sunlight, from 10 a.m. to 3 p.m. The ideal time to garden, take a walk, play golf, or do other outdoor activity is just after sunrise or just before sunset.

Remove fluorescent light

At home, replace fluorescent fixtures or bulbs with incandescent ones. At work, however, avoiding fluorescent light may be difficult. Consider asking your supervisor about moving to a work area closer to a window so you can use natural light. If you have a fluorescent light above your

desk, turn it off and request a lamp that uses incandescent bulbs.

Be careful with soaps and drugs

Certain toiletries, including deodorant soaps, may increase your skin's sensitivity to light, so try switching to nondeodorant or hypoallergenic soaps. Certain drugs, including tetracyclines and phenothiazines, also make you more sensitive to light.

Always check with your health care professional or pharmacist before taking a new medication.

Recognize and report rashes

Stay alert for the key sign of a photosensitivity reaction—a red rash on your face or other exposed area. Report suspicious rashes or other reactions to light. Remember that prompt treatment can prevent damage to the tissues beneath your skin.

PREVENTING COMPLICATIONS
OF DIABETES

Dear Patient:
There's no way around it. Controlling your diabetes means checking your blood glucose level as directed by your health care professional and making these good health habits a way of life.

Care for your heart
Because diabetes raises the risk of heart disease, follow these American Heart Association guidelines:
- Maintain your normal weight.
- Exercise regularly, following your health care professional's recommendations.
- Help control your blood pressure and cholesterol levels by eating a low-fat, high-fiber diet.

Care for your eyes
Have your eyes examined by an ophthalmologist at least once per year. He may detect damage, which could cause blindness, before symptoms appear. Early treatment may prevent further damage.

Care for your teeth
Schedule regular dental checkups and follow good home care to minimize dental problems, such as gum disease and abscesses, which may occur with diabetes. Report bleeding, pain, or soreness in your gums or teeth to the dentist immediately. Brush your teeth after every meal and floss daily. If you wear dentures, clean them thoroughly every day and make sure that they fit properly.

Care for your skin
Breaks in your skin can increase the risk of infection, so check your skin daily for cuts and irritated areas. See your health care professional if necessary. Bathe daily with warm water and a mild soap, and apply a lanolin-based lotion afterward to prevent dryness. Pat your skin dry thoroughly, taking extra care between your toes and in other areas where skin surfaces touch. Always wear cotton underwear to allow moisture to evaporate and help prevent skin breakdown.

Care for your feet
Diabetes can reduce blood flow to your feet and dull their ability to feel heat, cold, or pain. Follow your health care professional's instructions on daily foot care and necessary precautions to prevent foot problems.

Check your urine
Because symptoms of kidney disease usually don't appear until the problem is advanced, your health care professional will check your urine routinely for protein, which can signal kidney disease. Don't delay telling your health care professional if you have symptoms of a urinary tract infection (burning, painful, or difficult urination or blood or pus in the urine).

Have regular checkups
Regular checkups help ensure the early detection and prompt treatment of complications.

PERSONALIZING YOUR
EXERCISE PROGRAM

Dear Patient:
Exercise is an important aspect of caring for your diabetes. You can make your exercise program suit your needs by determining your aerobic training level, adjusting your pace accordingly, and allowing adequate time to warm up and cool down.

Finding your pace
How do you determine the aerobic training level that's best for you? Your target heart rate range provides a guideline for achieving the greatest benefits during exercising while reducing risk. By monitoring your pulse and staying in this range, you'll achieve the greatest benefits from aerobic exercise. This chart from the American Heart Association provides target heart rate ranges according to age.

Heart rate range
Keep in mind, however, that these numbers provide a measure of what a healthy heart can do. Gradually slow down if you begin to experience pain. Ask your health care professional to help you determine an appropriate target heart rate. Some cardiac medications may not allow you to reach your target heart rate because of their specific action on the heart.

Warming up
Before starting a demanding physical activity, you want to perform warm-up exercises to stretch muscles and loosen joints. This lessens the risk of muscle strain or ligament damage and raises your heart rate slowly. A good warm-up offers psy-

TARGET HEART RATE RANGE		
AGE	TARGET HEART RATE RANGE (BEATS PER MINUTE) **50 TO 75%**	MAXIMUM HEART RATE (BEATS PER MINUTE) **100%**
20	100 to 150	200
25	98 to 146	195
30	95 to 142	190
35	93 to 138	185
40	90 to 135	180
45	88 to 131	175
50	85 to 127	170
55	83 to 123	165
60	80 to 120	160
65	78 to 116	155
70	75 to 113	150

Your maximun heart rate is about 220 minus your age. The figures above are averages, so use them as general guidelines.

(continued)

PERSONALIZING YOUR EXERCISE PROGRAM *(continued)*

chological benefits as well. Use this time to focus on the activities ahead and to get rid of tension. First, take your pulse, and then do 5 to 10 minutes of stretching exercises and light calisthenics.

Adjusting the pace

Gradually work toward your optimal aerobic training level. During your exercise period, take your pulse two or three times as directed. Adjust your pace according to your pulse rate and how you feel. If you exceed your target rate or if you have chest discomfort, breathlessness, or palpitations, slow down *gradually*. Don't stop suddenly unless signs or symptoms persist or worsen.

Cooling down

Never stop exercising abruptly. If you do, the amount of blood circulating back to the heart, which is still beating rapidly, won't be adequate to meet your body's needs. You need a cooldown period much as a horse needs to be walked after a race.

Gradually decrease the pace of your exercise for 5 to 10 minutes. This will lower your heart rate and blood pressure slowly. Then do 5 minutes of light calisthenics and simple stretching exercises. At this point, your pulse should be no more than 15 beats above your resting pulse. If you feel dizzy or faint after exercising, you may need a longer cooldown period.

Keeping records

Keep an exercise diary. List the date and time, the activity and its duration, your heart rate, and any symptoms you experience. Tracking your progress helps you to stay motivated, and the record gives your health care professional valuable information.

Patient-teaching aid

MIXING INSULINS IN A SYRINGE

Dear Patient:
Your health care professional has prescribed regular and either intermediate or long-acting insulin to control your diabetes. To avoid giving yourself separate injections, you can mix these two types of insulin in a syringe and administer them together.

Preparing the insulin

1. Wash your hands. Then prepare the mixture in a clean area. Make sure that you have alcohol swabs for both types of insulin and the proper syringe for your prescribed insulin concentration. Then mix the contents of the intermediate or long-acting insulin by rolling it gently between your palms.

2. Using an alcohol swab, clean the rubber stopper on the vial of intermediate or long-acting insulin. Then draw air into the syringe by pulling the plunger back to the prescribed number of insulin units. Insert the needle into the top of the vial, as shown below. Make sure that the point doesn't touch the insulin.

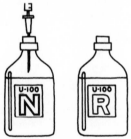

Inserting the needle

1. Push in the plunger, and remove the needle from the vial. Clean the rubber stopper on the regular insulin vial with an alcohol swab. Then pull back the plunger on the syringe to the prescribed number of insulin units. Insert the needle into the top of the vial, and inject air into the vial. With the needle still in the vial, turn the vial upside down. Withdraw the prescribed dose of regular insulin.

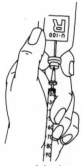

2. Clean the top of the intermediate or long-acting insulin vial. Then insert the needle into it without pushing the plunger down. Invert the vial and withdraw the prescribed number of units for the total dose. For example, if you have 10 units of regular insulin in the syringe and you need 20 units of intermediate or long-acting insulin, pull the plunger back to 30 units.

Additional points

- Never change the order in which you mix insulins.
- Always administer the insulin immediately to prevent loss of potency.

GIVING YOURSELF A
SUBCUTANEOUS INSULIN INJECTION

Dear Patient:
To transfer insulin from the medication vial to the syringe and then give yourself an insulin injection, follow these guidelines.

Getting ready

1. Wash your hands. Then assemble equipment in a clean area:
   - sterile syringe and needle
   - sharps container
   - insulin
   - alcohol swabs or wipes (or rubbing alcohol and cotton balls).

2. Check the labels on the syringe and bottle of insulin to make sure that they match. (If you're using U-100 insulin, you must use a U-100 syringe.) Also check that you have the correct type of insulin, such as NPH or Lente. (If your insulin is the cloudy-looking type, roll the bottle between your hands to mix it, as shown below.)

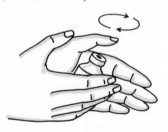

3. Mix gently to prevent large air bubbles from forming in the insulin.

4. Clean the top of the insulin bottle with an alcohol swab or wipe with a cotton ball and rubbing alcohol.

Cleaning the skin and preparing the syringe

1. Select an appropriate injection site.
2. Pull the skin taut. Using a circular motion, clean the skin with an alcohol swab or wipe with a cotton ball soaked in alcohol.

3. Remove the needle cover. To prevent possible infection, don't touch the needle; touch only the barrel and plunger of the syringe.

4. Pull back the plunger to the prescribed number of insulin units. This draws air into the syringe.

5. Insert the needle into the rubber stopper on the insulin bottle, and push in the plunger. This pushes air into the bottle and prevents a vacuum.

6. Hold the bottle and syringe together in one hand, and then turn them upside down so the bottle is on top. You can hold the bottle between your thumb and forefinger and the syringe between your ring finger and little finger, against your palm.

Injecting insulin

1. Pull back on the plunger until the top, black portion of the barrel corresponds to the line that indicates you have withdrawn your correct insulin dose.

2. Remove the needle from the bottle. If air bubbles appear in the syringe after you fill it with insulin, tap the syringe and push lightly on the plunger to remove them.

3. Draw up more insulin if necessary.

4. Using your thumb and forefinger, pinch the skin at the injection site. Quickly plunge the needle (up to its hub) into the subcutaneous tissue at a 90-degree angle.

GIVING YOURSELF A
SUBCUTANEOUS INSULIN INJECTION *(continued)*

Cleaning up

1. Place an alcohol swab or cotton ball over the injection site.
2. Press down on the swab or cotton ball lightly as you withdraw the needle. Don't rub the injection site when withdrawing the needle.
3. Dispose of the needle and syringe in a sharps container.

Additional points

- If you travel, keep a bottle of insulin and a syringe with you at all times.
- Keep insulin at room temperature. Don't refrigerate it or place it near heat (above 90° F [32.2° C]).

TESTING YOUR BLOOD GLUCOSE

Dear Patient:
In many cases, you'll be required to test your blood glucose level to determine how effective your diabetic regimen is. Regardless of how often or when you're to test your glucose level, follow these guidelines.

Getting ready

1. Be familiar with your glucose testing equipment. This typically includes a glucose meter, test strips, and a device to obtain the blood sample (called a *lancet*). Other supplies that you may need are cotton balls and alcohol wipes.
2. Read the manufacturer's instructions for using the meter and test strips.
3. Check to make sure that the test strips you have are designed to be used with the monitor that you have.
4. Periodically check to make sure that your meter is working properly. Follow the manufacturer's directions on how to do this and how often you need to check it.

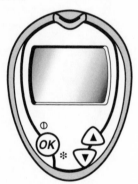

5. Always gather the necessary supplies before you begin. Have the meter turned on, the lancet ready, the test strip out of its wrapper or container, and several cotton balls ready to use. Identify the test site that you're plan-

ning to use, making sure that you using the same site each time.

Obtaining the blood sample

1. Wash your hands with soap and warm water and dry them completely. Or you can wipe the area you're planning to use with an alcohol wipe and then allow it to air-dry.
2. Hold the lancet device at a right angle (perpendicular) to the side of your finger and quickly prick your fingertip to create a drop of blood. If the manufacturer recommends, wipe away the first drop of blood with a clean cotton ball and milk your finger to create a new drop.

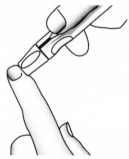

3. Position your hand with your finger facing down to help form an appropriate-size drop of blood. If necessary, milk your finger to get the blood to form a "hanging drop."

TESTING YOUR BLOOD GLUCOSE *(continued)*

4. Gently touch the drop of blood to pad on the test strip. Don"t smear the drop onto the pad or allow the skin of your fingertip to touch the pad. This might affect the accuracy of the results.

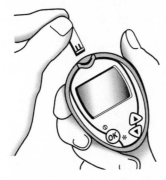

Obtaining the reading

1. Place the test strip into the meter as recommended by the manufacturer. Keep in mind that some meters require that you apply the drop of blood directly to a test strip that's already inserted in the meter.

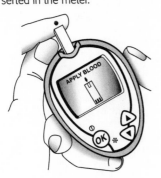

2. If required by the manufacturer, press a time button if appropriate.
3. Watch for the results to appear on the screen.
4. Use a cotton ball to apply pressure to the site where you obtained the blood sample.

Recording the results

1. Read the results on the meter and compare them with the levels recommended by your health care professional. Follow the appropriate actions based on the blood glucose level.
2. Record your results in your log or journal.
3. Discard the supplies and turn the meter off and store it and the supplies in a convenient but safe location.

Additional points

■ Be aware that some generic test strips are available for certain meters to help lower cost. Always check to make sure that the strip is compatible with your meter.
■ Always take your glucose testing supplies with you when your visit your health care professional.

USING INHALED INSULIN

Dear Patient:
If your health care professional prescribes insulin in the inhaled form, follow these guidelines.

Before you start
- Read the manufacturer's instructions carefully, making sure that you understand how to set up and use your inhaler. Know the parts of your inhaler.

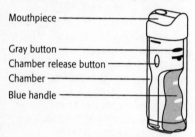

Mouthpiece

Gray button

Chamber release button

Chamber

Blue handle

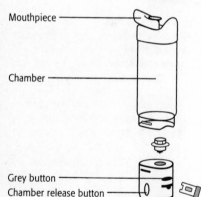

Mouthpiece

Chamber

Grey button

Chamber release button

Base

Blue handle

Black ring

- Use your insulin inhaler for the special insulin only and use the correct insulin pack; don't substitute an equal amount of a smaller pack for a larger single dose.

Using the inhaler
1. Set up the inhaler by holding it with the label name at the top and facing toward you; pull the ring at the bottom of the base down until the clear chamber is on top and you hear a clicking sound that indicates that the chamber is locked in place.

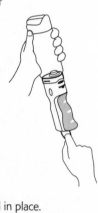

2. Insert the prescribed packet of insulin into the slot on the inhaler, making sure that the packet is facing printed side up and the notch faces the back of the inhaler.
3. Pull out the blue handle on the bottom half of the inhaler as far as possible, making sure that the mouthpiece at the top of the chamber is closed.
4. Squeeze the blue handle until you hear a snapping sound; this helps to create a pressure system inside the device.

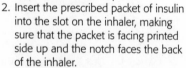

5. Prepare to administer the drug:
   - While sitting upright or standing, hold the inhaler so that the blue button is facing you.
   - Press the blue button and watch for a cloud of medication to fill the chamber.

USING INHALED INSULIN *(continued)*

– Exhale and open the mouthpiece (having it face you) and place your lips around it, forming a seal.

– Using one breath, slowly and completely inhale the cloud of medication from the chamber.

– Remove the mouthpiece, keep your mouth closed, and hold your breath for 5 seconds and then exhale normally.

6. Close the mouthpiece and press the gray button, which will release the used packet of medication.

7. Simultaneously squeeze the chamber release buttons on each side of the base and push the base into the chamber for storage.

Caring for the inhaler

■ Replace your inhaler annually.

■ Clean the inhaler weekly.

■ Take the inhaler apart: with the inhaler in the extended position (chamber fully extended on top of the base), simultaneously press the chamber release buttons and pull the base completely out of the chamber.

■ Clean the base by wiping it with a damp clean soft cloth, making sure that no water gets into the release unit; don't wipe the slot where the packet of medication is inserted.

■ Clean the mouthpiece and chamber with a damp soft clean cloth and mild liquid soap, wiping the inside and outside of the device; be sure to have the mouthpiece in the open position. Rinse the mouthpiece and chamber thoroughly and allow to air-dry. When dry, close the mouthpiece and reattach the chamber to the base.

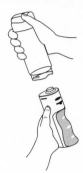

■ After the chamber and base are clean, reattach them by aligning the blue dot on the chamber with the blue button on the base and simultaneously squeezing the two chamber release buttons while pushing the base back into the chamber.

■ Replace the release unit every 2 weeks.

■ While the inhaler is apart, hold the base with the gray button facing you; turn the used release unit about one-quarter of the way counterclockwise, toward the unlock symbol.

■ Pull the unit up and out and discard it.

■ Obtain a new release unit and remove it from its packaging. While holding the unit with the top facing you, look for a blue line and then turn the top counterclockwise with your other hand as far as it will go.

■ Insert the unit into the base by lining up the blue line on the top of the unit with the unlock symbol on the base; the unit should drop into the base easily.

■ Turn the top of the unit until the blue line points to the lock symbol at the top of the base.

Additional points

■ Don't discard your insulin needles, syringes, or vials of medication. You may still need to give yourself insulin injections.

■ Continue to check your blood glucose level as directed by your health care professional.

SAMPLE MEAL PLAN: FOOD PYRAMID

This sample meal plan depicts an appropriate daily intake for the patient with diabetes using a food pyramid.

Breakfast	1 small banana 1 shredded wheat biscuit ½ cup nonfat milk Coffee or tea
Midmorning snack	2 graham crackers ½ cup nonfat milk
Lunch	2 slices turkey breast 2 slices light whole wheat bread 2 lettuce leaves 1 sliced tomato 1 small orange Sugar-free beverage
Midafternoon snack	½ cup plain yogurt
Dinner	3 oz flounder 1 mixed green salad 1 cup spinach 1 small dinner roll with 1 tsp low-fat margarine 1 small baked potato Sugar-free beverage
Evening snack	½ cup non-fat milk 3 ginger snap cookies
Total	6 bread, 3 vegetable, 2 fruit, 2 milk, 2 meat/egg, 1 fat

SAMPLE MEAL PLAN: CALORIE-BASED

This sample meal plan depicts the typical daily intake for the patient with diabetes who's allowed 1,200 calories, which may be used to promote weight loss.

Breakfast	½ cantaloupe 1 cup oatmeal ½ cup 1% milk Coffee or tea
Midmorning snack	1 hard-boiled egg
Lunch	3 oz tuna (in water) 1 cup iceberg lettuce 1 sliced tomato ¼ cup mushrooms 2 tbs low-calorie Italian dressing 1 light English muffin Sugar-free beverage
Midafternoon snack	1 cup strawberries
Dinner	3 oz hamburger 1 slice onion 1 cup mixed vegetables 1 small baked potato with 1 tbs sour cream 4 oz sugar-free gelatin with 1 tbs whipped topping Sugar-free beverage
Evening snack	1 cup fat-free popcorn
Total calories	1,200

SAMPLE MEAL PLAN: EXCHANGE LISTS

———•———

This sample meal plan highlights an acceptable daily intake for the patient using exchange lists as part of his nutritional therapy.

Breakfast	½ grapefruit 1 bagel with1 tbs cream cheese Coffee with 2 tbs half-and-half
Midmorning snack	¾ cup plain low-fat yogurt 3 graham crackers
Lunch	2 oz hamburger bun with 1 tsp mayonnaise 2 oz ground beef burger 1 large tomato 20 French fries 1 cup nonfat milk
Midafternoon snack	1¼ cups strawberries
Dinner	2 oz salmon 1 cup rice with 1 tsp low-fat margarine 1 cup salad greens ½ cup cauliflower 1 small apple Sugar-free beverage
Evening snack	1 cup nonfat milk 3 ginger snap cookies
Total exchanges	3 fruit, 10 starch, 3 milk, 7 fat, 2 lean meat, 2 medium-fat meat, 3 vegetable

SAMPLE MEAL PLAN: CARBOHYDRATE COUNTING

This sample meal plan depicts an appropriate daily intake for the patient who's allowed 130 g of carbohydrates daily.

Breakfast	½ cup orange juice 2 scrambled eggs 1 small bagel Coffee or tea
Midmorning snack	1 small peach
Lunch	3 oz canned salmon 2 slices light rye bread 1½ tbs mayonnaise 2 lettuce leaves Sugar-free beverage
Midafternoon snack	4 oz sugar-free gelatin with 1 tbs whipped topping
Dinner	2 slices turkey breast ½ cup rice 1 cup broccoli 1 mixed green salad 2 tbs blue cheese salad dressing Sugar-free beverage
Evening snack	2 chocolate chip cookies Coffee or tea
Total carbohydrates	130 g

Index

i refers to an illustration; t refers to a table.

---

i refers to an illustration; t refers to a table.

---

i refers to an illustration; t refers to a table.

---

i refers to an illustration; t refers to a table.

i refers to an illustration; t refers to a table.

---

i refers to an illustration; t refers to a table.

---

i refers to an illustration; t refers to a table.